IMMUNIZATION AND STATES

Globally, there has been a move away from national public sector vaccine development over the past 30 years. *Immunization and States: The Politics of Making Vaccines* explores vaccine geopolitics, analyzing why, and how this move happened, before looking at the ramifications in the context of Covid-19.

This unique book uses eight country studies – looking at Croatia, India, Iran, the Netherlands, Romania, Serbia, Spain, and Sweden – to explore the role of public sector vaccine institutes, past, and present. Raising questions about national sovereignty, the erosion of multilateralism, and geopolitics, it also contributes to debates around public interest and privatization in the health sector. An extended introduction sets the chapters in an international context, whilst the epilogue looks forward to the future of vaccine development and production.

This is an important book for students, scholars, and practitioners with an interest in vaccine development from a range of fields, including public health, medicine, science and technology studies, history of medicine, politics, international relations, and the sociology of health and illness.

Stuart Blume is Emeritus Professor in the Department of Anthropology, University of Amsterdam, the Netherlands.

Baptiste Baylac-Paouly is fixed-term Lecturer in History of Medicine at the Medical School Lyon-Est, France.

IMMUNIZATION AND STATES

The Politics of Making Vaccines

Edited by Stuart Blume and Baptiste Baylac-Paouly

Routledge
Taylor & Francis Group
LONDON AND NEW YORK

First published 2022
by Routledge
2 Park Square, Milton Park, Abingdon, Oxon OX14 4RN

and by Routledge
605 Third Avenue, New York, NY 10158

Routledge is an imprint of the Taylor & Francis Group, an informa business

British Library Cataloguing-in-Publication Data
A catalogue record for this book is available from the British Library

Library of Congress Cataloging-in-Publication Data
A catalog record has been requested for this book

ISBN: 978-0-367-67226-3 (hbk)
ISBN: 978-0-367-67227-0 (pbk)
ISBN: 978-1-003-13034-5 (ebk)

DOI: 10.4324/9781003130345

Typeset in Bembo
by KnowledgeWorks Global Ltd.

CONTENTS

List of figures *vii*
List of tables *viii*
List of contributors *ix*
Acknowledgements *xii*

Introduction 1
Stuart Blume and Baptiste Baylac-Paouly

1 The privatization of societal vaccinology in the Netherlands 20
Jan Hendriks

2 The rise and fall of state vaccine institutions in Spain (1871–1986) 44
María-José Báguena and María-Isabel Porras

3 Politics of vaccination in Sweden: the National Bacteriological Laboratory SBL (1909–1993) and current debates 65
Motzi Eklöf

4 The failed promises of a brighter future: the Institute of Immunology in Zagreb from a public asset to a privatized burden 89
Vedran Duančić, Snježana Ivčić, and Ana Vračar

5 Wilful neoliberal incapacitation of India's public sector vaccine institutions 110
Madhavi Yennapu

6 Start with the world and continue in isolation: the Pasteur and Razi Institutes' vaccine legacy in Iran 138
Payam Roshanfekr and Parisa Roshanfekr

7 Translating Pasteur's vision in Eastern Europe: the role of the Cantacuzino Institute in Romanian vaccination policies and vaccine production 155
Valentin-Veron Toma

8 Vaccine production in Serbia: political and socio-cultural determinants in historical perspective 176
Vesna Trifunović

Epilogue: states and vaccines in the age of Covid-19 199
Stuart Blume and Maurizia Mezza

Index *218*

FIGURES

1.1 FAIR founders (from left to right): Hans Cohen, Charles Mérieux, and Jonas Salk (1984) 24
1.2 Vaccinology training courses for international capacity building since the 1970s. 25
1.3 Relative contribution of vaccines produced by the public sector for diseases addressed by the Netherlands Immunization Programme (NIP) between 1950 and 2020. 32
5.1 BCGVL Chennai: Production, purchase order from the government, and supply of vaccines to the UIP 126
5.2 Central Research Institute (CRI) Kasauli: Production, purchase order from the government, and supply of DT vaccines to the UIP 126
5.3 Central Research Institute (CRI) Kasauli: Production, purchase order from the government, and supply of TT vaccines to the UIP 127
5.4 Central Research Institute (CRI) Kasauli: Production, purchase order from the government, and supply of DPT vaccines to the UIP 127
5.5 Pasteur Institute of India (PII) Coonoor: Production, purchase order from the government, and supply of DPT vaccines to the UIP 128
5.6 Pasteur Institute of India (PII) Coonoor: Production, purchase order from the government, and supply of DT vaccines to the UIP 128
5.7 Pasteur Institute of India (PII) Coonoor: Production, purchase order from the government, and supply of TT vaccines to the UIP 129

TABLES

1.1 Milestones in the deconstruction of Dutch vaccinology 37
5.1 Vaccine R&D and production in Public Sector Vaccine Institutions (PSVIs) established since 1800 112
5.2 The difference in vaccine prices between the public sector (PSVIs) and private companies per dose (0.5 ml) 120
5.3 Percentage share of vaccine production by private and public sector in India 125

CONTRIBUTORS

María-José Báguena passed away on 13 March 2021. She was at that time a full Professor of History of Science at the University of Valencia, as well as a member of the López Piñero Interuniversity Institute in Valencia. Her research was focused on the historical evolution of infectious diseases, the institutions and people who carried out microbiological research in Spain, and policies for the prevention and treatment of these diseases.

Baptiste Baylac-Paouly is a fixed-term lecturer at the Medical School of Lyon-Est, University Lyon 1. His research interest is the history of infectious diseases control strategies and policies. After working for 5 years on meningitis A in Africa and Brazil, he is now working on polio control strategies and policies in France in the second half of the twentieth century.

Stuart Blume is Emeritus Professor of Science & Technology Studies and a member of the Department of Anthropology at the University of Amsterdam. He has been an advisor on bioethics to the World Federation of the Deaf, a 'Professor 2' at the University of Oslo, and 'Prometeo' fellow at the University of Cuenca (Ecuador).

Vedran Duančić holds a PhD in history and civilization from the European University Institute in Florence (2016). He specializes in the modern intellectual history and the twentieth-century history of science. Between 2017 and 2021, he was a postdoctoral researcher at the Institute for the History and Philosophy of Science at the Croatian Academy of Sciences and Arts in Zagreb.

Motzi Eklöf is an associate professor in health and society. After 20 years in the academy, she is now working as independent researcher. Her research area is the social and cultural history of medicine and health, including ethical aspects.

Jan Hendriks is currently an independent researcher and consultant in vaccinology for non-profit organizations. Prior to his retirement in 2018, he had spent nearly 30 years in various international staff and management positions within the Dutch Vaccine Institute in Bilthoven.

Snježana Ivčić holds a PhD in public policy from the Faculty of Political Science in Zagreb. She has interests in the history of public health, the privatization of the healthcare system, the nurses' history, and the impact of the EU on the health policies of member states. She is a member of the Organization for Workers' Initiative and Democratization (OWID). From early 2013 until 2020, she was involved in a research project on The Continuity of Social Conflict in Croatia 1987–1991, conducted in cooperation with the Centre for Peace Studies (CMS) and the OWID. She currently works in Croatian Academy of Sciences and Arts.

Maurizia Mezza is a PhD candidate in medical anthropology at the University of Amsterdam. Her research focuses on pharmacovigilance systems for the monitoring of potential adverse reactions to vaccines, HPV vaccination in Colombia, and pharmacoepidemiology.

María-Isabel Porras is full Professor of History of Science at the University of Castilla-La Mancha, a member of the Regional Centre for Biomedical Research (CRIB) and Director of the Health, History and Society research group. She has been a guest professor at Emory University (USA), the EHESS, Geneva University, and the López Piñero Interuniversity Institute (Valencia).

Parisa Roshanfekr holds a PhD in International Law from the University of Tehran (Farabi Faculty). She wrote her thesis on 'Capacities of International Law to Combat Infectious Diseases as a Biosecurity Threat' and has also published articles in Farsi on 'Human Rights and Fighting Infectious Diseases: Challenges and Necessities'.

Payam Roshanfekr is an Assistant Professor of Social Determinants of Health (SDH) and a member of the Social Welfare Management Research Center at the University of Social Welfare and Rehabilitation Sciences (USWRs) in Tehran, Iran.

Valentin-Veron Toma is a senior researcher at the Institute of Anthropology 'Francisc I. Rainer' of the Romanian Academy, and Head of the Department of Social and Cultural Anthropology. His research interests include medical anthropology, cultural psychiatry, and medical history. In July 2020, he was an invited speaker at an online event 'No More Pandemics! Disease Prevention and Control Summit – America 2020' where he discussed the importance of local vaccine production in the context of the Covid-19 pandemic and the problems of inequitable access to vaccines in developing countries.

Vesna Trifunović is a Research Associate at the Institute of Ethnography, Serbian Academy of Sciences and Arts. Her field of research is anthropology of medicine and public health, with a special focus on the issues of vaccines and vaccination.

Ana Vračar is a cultural anthropologist and postgraduate student of public health at the School of Medicine, University of Zagreb. She works in the NGO Organization for Workers' Initiative and Democratization (OWID) and is currently the People's Health Movement's regional coordinator for Europe. Her primary interests include issues related to the health workforce, particularly the organization of health workers, and commercialization of health care.

Madhavi Yennapu is Senior Principal Scientist at the National Institute of Science, Technology and Development Studies (NISTADS, CSIR), New Delhi, India, as well as a professor and Coordinator of its Academy of Scientific and Innovation Research (AcSIR). She established vaccine policy research in India in the mid-1990s and served on committees of the Indian Council of Medical Research and acted as consultant to various NGOs.

ACKNOWLEDGEMENTS

The origins of this book lie in a two-day workshop held in Amsterdam in November 2019. The report of the workshop noted that public sector vaccine producers 'have been virtually written off as fossils of the past with little contemporary significance'. The last international discussion of their present and possible future roles had taken place at the WHO a full two decades earlier. There were six presentations at the Amsterdam workshop: three from Western Europe and three from post-socialist Europe. The similarities and differences, the comparative context, came as an eye-opener for everyone present. We were all familiar with discussions of the closure, or planned closure, of a national vaccine institute. But discussions had always related to the national context, to decisions taken by national politicians. Now we all saw that something larger was involved: influences that transcended national – that is to say local – politics.

Everyone present in November 2019 agreed that discussion of the significance of public sector vaccine institutions (henceforth simply PSVI), the implications of their closures and privatizations, was worth pursuing. Everyone present thought that we should consider expanding the discussion to include countries outside Europe that had or still have a national vaccine institute. We established a small group (consisting of Maria-José Báguena and Maria-Isabel Porras from Spain, Stuart Blume, Jan Hendriks, and Maurizia Mezza from the Netherlands, and Vesna Trifunović from Serbia) to explore possibilities for organizing a second larger workshop. Then came the pandemic, and all the restrictions it brought with it. We decided to move straight to the publication that would have been the major output of our second workshop. Almost everyone present in November immediately accepted an invitation to contribute to it. Only Anne Hagen Berg, who had given us a fascinating presentation of the Danish State Serum Institute, was unable to do so. We were however delighted to be able to interest the colleagues from India and Iran who have contributed chapters to this book.

Preparing this book has been a challenge. Its preparation has coincided precisely with the Covid-19 pandemic. Archives have been closed, and travel impossible. Many contributors have had to struggle, not only with the stresses of the pandemic but also with the tight deadlines we set for them. Remarkably however, everyone succeeded. In addition to the challenge it presented us all with, preparing this book has been an enriching experience.

One contributor and participant in the initial workshop who deserves a special mention at this point is Maria-José Báguena. Maria-José was actively involved in writing the chapter on Spain but has been unable to see the fruits of her work. Very sadly, Maria-José passed away on 13 March 2021.

We want to express our grateful thanks to the Health, Care, and the Body programme group of the Amsterdam Institute for Social Science Research (AISSR); to the Medical School of Lyon-Est and the University Lyon 1, as well as the Stichting Science Dynamics, for financial support; to Maurizia Mezza for helping organize the initial workshop and for preparing the Index; and to Zoe Goldstein for so skilfully editing some of the chapters. Finally, and on behalf of all contributors, we would like to thank Grace McInnes and Evie Lonsdale at Routledge for their encouragement and support from the very start of the writing process.

Stuart Blume and Baptiste Baylac-Paouly
Amsterdam and Lyon, May 2021

INTRODUCTION

Stuart Blume and Baptiste Baylac-Paouly

In the course of the twentieth century, vaccines became central to the control of infectious disease. They seemed to obviate the need for onerous and intrusive measures such as quarantine and enforced hygiene. The effectiveness of vaccination in controlling the spread of disease has been shown over and again. For years it has been seen as the most cost-effective tool that public health has at its disposal. The range of available vaccines continues to grow. Children born today in the industrialized world are likely to be given (or at least offered) twice as many antigens as their grandparents were when they were children. At the same time, vaccination has been extended to poor countries and even isolated communities in those countries. Serious cases of diseases such as polio and measles have declined dramatically. This narrative of progress forms the basis for most popular and historical accounts of vaccines and vaccination. That vaccines have become big business is less widely known. Lower estimates of the total amount of money spent on them in 2019 are between $25 and 30 billion (US), whilst some suggest as much as $48 billion. Even before the Covid-19 pandemic, business analysts forecast continued growth of the vaccines market.

Where do all these billions of doses of vaccine come from? Who produces them? Does that actually matter, so long as we have the ones we need? Two or three years ago most public health professionals would have shaken their heads: no, it makes no difference where they come from as long as we know they are safe and effective. Pressed further on who supplies the vaccines, most would probably have mentioned one or other multinational pharmaceutical company. How and for whom vaccines are developed and produced obviously did concern the upper echelons of the pharmaceutical industry. It also concerned experts tasked with purchasing vaccines, for example on behalf of international organizations such as the Pan-American Health Organization (PAHO) and the United Nations Children's Organization (UNICEF). For many years these have negotiated bulk

DOI: 10.4324/9781003130345-1

purchases on behalf of member countries. A few economists interested themselves in the vaccine industry,[1] though Muraskin was one of few historians or social scientists.[2]

At the end of 2020 the first vaccines against Covid-19 were approved, with many more in the development pipeline. Vaccine development seemed to reflect political rivalries reminiscent of the Cold War. For reasons both technical and economic, some of these first vaccines would be of limited utility in poor, tropical countries. It was immediately clear that, for months or longer, there would be insufficient vaccine to meet the world's needs. As the tragedy unfolded, as deaths globally climbed to a million, two million, a question which had scarcely been posed for decades was raised once more. If vaccines are so crucial to the preservation of human life, to the functioning of our societies, is reliance on profit-oriented corporations really wise? Ought states not to be involved in developing and producing, as well as delivering, the vaccines they need? In a number of countries the marginal existence, or complete disappearance, of a once prized national vaccine producer became a matter of public discussion. It is this new questioning, this widespread attention for an issue which had vanished from the global health agenda, which provides the rationale for this book. How has vaccine production figured in states' perceptions of their responsibilities for public health? What has changed – not only in the course of the Covid pandemic, but over a period of decades? What drove change? Where public sector institutions do, or did, develop and produce vaccines, do they follow a different logic, respond to different incentives, from private industry? Did they, and do they still, have a distinctive contribution to make to public health? These are among the key questions addressed in this book.

The early years

In the mid nineteenth century, as public health gradually became a field of state action, vaccines were of minor importance. Inoculation had emerged at the end of the eighteenth century. Edward Jenner, an English country doctor, set out to test what had become a popular belief among dairy farmers, that catching cowpox protected against smallpox. In 1796 Jenner showed that if fluid was taken from one person's cowpox lesion and rubbed into the scratched-open skin of another person's arm, the second person was also protected against smallpox. Jenner's results were tested by leading London doctors, and by 1800 vaccination was spreading worldwide. Not that everyone was convinced. Many physicians found the idea of deliberately introducing a potentially harmful substance into people's bodies ludicrous. Others thought it an ideal solution to a serious problem. The vaccination expedition that left Spain in 1803, bound for the Americas, would try to organize local smallpox vaccination at each port of call. Its success varied from place to place.[3] Not only was this new technique taken far afield, a number of governments made vaccination mandatory, with penalties for those who refused.

There were no other vaccines. Among the industrialized countries public health practices differed, with some tending to rely on sanitary measures, others on quarantine. Difficult to enforce, disruptive of commerce, these practices encountered powerful opposition.[4]

Cowpox and smallpox were known to be closely related conditions. If use of a mild infection to protect against a more serious one depended on the existence of such 'close relatives' it would have little further application. When Louis Pasteur demonstrated with his anthrax and rabies vaccines that weakened (or 'attenuated') pathogens could work just as well, he showed the way to vaccination as we know it today.

From the late nineteenth century to the first half of the twentieth century, two rival institutes – the Pasteur Institute in Paris and Koch's Institute for Infectious Diseases in Berlin – reigned over the new science of bacteriology. Pasteur's and Koch's ideas regarding the mechanism of disease causation, and in particular the influence of environmental factors, differed substantially. So too did the structures of the institutes that they directed, reflecting the different political and administrative traditions of the two countries (which had actually been at war with one another only a decade earlier). Investigations of the bacterial causes of diseases spread outwards from these two centres. Physicians travelled from far and wide to follow the training courses given there. In Paris a 3- or 4-month course began in 1889. Directed by Emile Roux, the course promoted Pasteurian principles internationally. Its many foreign students came especially from the Balkans, from Russia (prior to the Revolution), and from Ottoman Turkey. Few came from Britain or Germany, reflecting the political tensions and colonial rivalries of the time.[5] Pasteur had shown that vaccines against anthrax and rabies were effective, but these were not major sources of human disease and death. If bacteriology was to be really useful, the causative agent of each individual infectious disease would have to be identified and isolated. Two of the most serious were diphtheria and tuberculosis. In 1882 Robert Koch found the bacillus responsible for tuberculosis, and a few years later Albert Klebs in Zurich identified and isolated the one that caused diphtheria.

Diphtheria is an infection of the upper respiratory tract, with symptoms that include sore throat, coughing and difficulties in breathing and swallowing. In the nineteenth century it was a devastating disease especially of children. Common treatments at the time included scrubbing the throat, inhaling various vapours and, in the most serious cases, tracheotomy. Identification of the bacteria causing diphtheria made it possible to diagnose the disease by bacteriological analysis rather than by relying on symptoms alone. In 1890 Emil Behring and Shibasaburo Kitasato, working in Koch's laboratory, discovered an antidote. They found that when small amounts of the poison produced in culturing the bacilli were injected into healthy animals, a neutralizing serum was produced. This serum, or 'antitoxin', could then be used to kill diphtheria bacilli.

Since diphtheria was so dangerous for children there was great demand for the antitoxin. Its production became an important function of new public health laboratories in some places, and of private pharmaceutical companies in others.

The serum was used in hospitals to treat young patients, not to prevent infection. It was not until after World War I that prophylactic vaccination (other than against smallpox) began to gain credibility.[6]

Tuberculosis was another important focus of attention for the early bacteriologists. Because before the advent of bacteriological testing (and later chest X-ray) only the severest cases were found, it was impossible to tell how many people had milder infections. Though it was the single largest cause of death, tuberculosis (or 'consumption') was not commonly viewed as a 'public health' disease. Not only did it not appear to be epidemic, but many thought that it ran in families. Heredity gave the predisposition, but actual development of the disease was triggered by cold wind, bad air or injury to bronchi or lungs.

Although the microbial cause of tuberculosis (*tubercle bacillus*) had been isolated by Robert Koch in 1882, the disease remained a major cause of mortality. The overcrowding caused by housing shortages, and undernutrition suffered by many during World War I, facilitated its spread and exacerbated its effects. Despite years of research, the war was over before a vaccine with any protective benefits became available. The BCG (Bacillus Calmette–Guérin) vaccine was developed by scientists at the Pasteur Institute, which made it freely available in France, and later to physicians abroad. Calmette required only that countries should establish procedures for its production and distribution, and for monitoring the results. In Britain, where scientists questioned the vaccine's safety, as well as its efficacy, vaccination was not adopted. British scepticism toward the BCG vaccine also had a moralizing aspect.[7] People had to be taught to take responsibility for their own health, to learn the value of a healthy diet, and follow a healthy lifestyle! Using an argument later re-deployed in opposition to vaccination against sexually transmitted diseases, some claimed that BCG vaccination would give people a sense of false security and reduce their incentive to change their behaviour.

In 1883 Koch travelled to Alexandria and then to Calcutta. Applying the same method he had used with tuberculosis, he was able to isolate the organism responsible for cholera. The organism became known as the *Vibrio cholerae* or 'comma bacillus', because of its shape when viewed under a microscope. Attempts to develop a vaccine against this frightening disease soon followed. Waldemar Haffkine, a Russian emigre working in Emile Roux's laboratory, set about trying to develop a cholera vaccine. British colonial authorities permitted Haffkine to test his cholera vaccine in India. Travelling through the country, he faced numerous difficulties both technical and bureaucratic. Vaccinating thousands, Haffkine was trying to improve the conduct and reliability of his trials in order to assess the efficacy of anti-cholera vaccination. By mid- 1896 he had concluded that protection was possible, though it only lasted for 14 months. The work took its toll, however. Haffkine became sick from malaria and overwork and returned to Europe to recuperate. Because it was later found to provoke too strong a reaction Haffkine's vaccine was later abandoned.

For the colonial powers, transferring the new public health technologies to the colonies became integral to state policy. Though not a state institution, the

Pasteur Institute had a distinctly 'imperial' mission. Support from the French state was based on the hope that the institute would help restore the country's prestige, badly damaged by defeat in the Franco–Prussian war. From its very beginnings, the Pasteur Institute had planned to set up 'scientific colonies', or 'filiales', which would propagate the Pasteurian doctrine and initiate local research, especially in 'exposed tropical countries'. Scientists moved in both directions, through the Institute's worldwide network of bacteriological centres. Alexandre Yersin, for example, was sent to Hong Kong, where he identified the pathogen that causes bubonic plague. Returning to Paris, he prepared the first anti-bubonic plague serum, before leaving for French Indochina to establish a laboratory to produce it. This later became a branch of the Pasteur Institute. Other Pasteur institutes were established at the initiative of local governments – in Tunis, Senegal, Madagascar and elsewhere. Some initiatives failed, as a result of lack of political commitment or bureaucratic resistance. Historians have found a pattern in the diffusion of Pasteurian practices.[8] New institutes typically began by offering treatments for rabies, sometimes combined with a laboratory for producing vaccine and diphtheria serum. After the First World War, local initiatives had to submit their choice of director to Paris, and supply their own funding. As later chapters will show, ties with the Pasteur Institute played an important role in the beginnings of vaccine production in many countries. In Canada for example, Dr John G. FitzGerald, who had studied at the Pasteur Institute, set up a laboratory in Toronto in 1913. Fitzgerald wanted to provide his native country with the new tools of bacteriology at an affordable price. Within a few months, the University of Toronto had agreed to work with him, and what later became the Connaught Laboratory was established in the basement of the medical faculty building. The Connaught Laboratory produced diphtheria antitoxin, which it sold cheaply to Canadian public health authorities. As the value of the new sera and vaccines became more widely acknowledged, their production became accepted as a legitimate function of governmental and municipal laboratories. In some countries, that is. Elsewhere, as in Britain and Germany, commercial laboratories fulfilled this function, with the government's role limited to oversight and regulation.

In the 1930s the world entered yet another period of crisis. World War I had stimulated intensive efforts to develop vaccines against typhus and typhoid which would save the lives of soldiers fighting in insanitary trenches. Similarly, World War II led not only to new drugs (penicillin, streptomycin) but also to intensified vaccine research. This was to bear fruit shortly afterwards.

The Cold War era

Vaccine production

At the end of World War II, the pharmaceutical industry turned its attention to the new, powerful, and potentially very profitable, antibiotics. As resources were shifted to therapeutics, interest in vaccine development declined. For example, a pneumonia vaccine being developed in the 1940s attracted little attention. The new penicillin and sulfonamide drugs offered more attractive options. However, research was going on that was to change matters dramatically. At Harvard University John Enders and his colleagues were developing new and safer methods of culturing live viruses. This work would soon lead to the development of vaccines against viral diseases including polio, measles, and rubella. The prospects of breakthroughs in this area catalyzed renewed attention for developing and producing vaccines.

Polio was a particular focus of concern. It attacked children, in the most serious cases leaving them paralyzed, or only able to survive prostrate in an iron lung. In the United States, at the instigation of the National Foundation for Infantile Paralysis (NFIP) founded by Franklin D. Roosevelt – himself a polio victim and paralyzed in both legs – research on polio was a major priority. Development of a safe polio vaccine had been greatly hindered by the difficulty of safely growing the polio virus. Once Enders had shown how it could be done, a number of potential polio vaccines were soon under development. Jonas Salk's inactivated virus vaccine was first to be approved. Salk did not wish to patent his vaccine and was happy to share details of its production process with visitors from laboratories abroad. Not all virologists were convinced that an inactivated vaccine would be effective enough. Many, including Albert Sabin, continued trying to develop the attenuated viral vaccine which they thought was needed.[9]

Lack of patent protection, which would remain the norm in the vaccines field until the 1980s, was not viewed as a barrier to innovation. New scientific possibilities and active promotion of vaccination by the Federal government drew American pharmaceutical companies back into vaccine production. Industrial commitment, however, was to remain uncertain and unreliable. By the 1970s vaccines were becoming central to preventive health worldwide. Science was making gigantic strides forward. Nevertheless, vaccine development remained both commercially and technically challenging. It required:

> The cooperative team play of a wide variety of disciplines, including, at the very least, the fields of virology, cell biology, biochemistry, biophysics, pathology, clinical medicine, epidemiology and applied biology. The effort is doomed from the outset unless the cooperating scientists of these diverse disciplines can be brought to focus on the multifaceted problems which are involved and for whose solution the guidelines may be hazy or none-existent.[10]

Once more pharmaceutical companies began to turn their backs on vaccine production: something of particular concern in the United States. Like many countries the United States was almost completely dependent on private industry for its vaccines. And the private sector was losing interest. The Office of

Technology Assessment of the US Congress (OTA), investigating the matter, felt that:

> The apparently diminishing commitment – and possibly capacity – of the American pharmaceutical industry to research, develop, and produce vaccines … may be reaching levels of real concern.[11]

For 19 vaccines, including the polio vaccine, the United States was dependent on just one domestic supplier. What if that producer decided to exit the vaccine field? It had happened before. In the mid-1970s Eli Lilly was working on an experimental pneumococcal vaccine. Then the company decided to terminate almost all its vaccine R&D and production activities. Company executives told the OTA that this reflected the costs and difficulties of developing vaccines, market considerations, and carrying out the testing of each batch of vaccine as required by Federal regulations.[12] Vaccines were more difficult to develop, test and license than pharmaceutical products. They were also less profitable, and there were much greater risks of liability actions and huge damages if anything went wrong. After all, vaccines were typically administered to millions of healthy children. It was these concerns which would later lead to legislation protecting manufacturers against liability claims.

The international context

World War II left vast numbers of displaced, homeless, and malnourished people in its wake. Europe's devastated cities were breeding grounds for infectious disease. Alongside the huge reconstruction effort, facilitated by the Marshall Aid plan, came political realignments, the beginnings of independence movements across Asia and Africa, and the seeds of what would soon become the Cold War. Each of these developments impacted on public health. Tuberculosis was rampant, and as planning for what would soon become the WHO began it was clear that tuberculosis would be one of its first priorities.

Through the 1950s the world was becoming increasingly polarized. Eastern and Western bloc countries had different visions of how public health systems should be established and organized. This extended to health systems in areas of Africa, Asia, and Latin America where East and West competed for influence. Political leaders on both sides of the ideological divide were convinced that demonstrating success in controlling the spread of infectious diseases would reflect well on their respective political systems. For politicians vaccines had become symbols of ideological rivalry, their application loaded with political significance.[13] By contrast, vaccine researchers had little difficulty in co-operating across the ideological divide.

Objecting to what it saw as excessive US influence on the organization, the Soviet Union left the WHO soon after its foundation. In 1956 it re-joined. At the 1958 World Health Assembly (WHA), the Organization's 'parliament', the

Soviet delegation proposed that WHO commit itself to the eradication of smallpox. Despite the country's poor health infrastructure, the Soviet Union had succeeded in stopping the domestic transmission of smallpox. But because it was imported by visitors vaccination had to continue. Victor Zhdanov, a virologist and head of the Soviet delegation, argued that if 80% of the world's population were vaccinated costly vaccination could cease. At the 1965 WHA, the US delegation supported the Soviet proposal. US officials hoped that engagement in a humanitarian endeavour could mitigate the diplomatic damage caused by America's war in Indo-China. The WHO Director General was requested to draw up a plan for a smallpox eradication campaign, and a year later the plan was approved. Though by the 1960s smallpox had virtually disappeared from the United States and from Europe it was still rampant in parts of Latin America, in Africa, and above all in Asia. The USSR established facilities for producing freeze-dried smallpox vaccine on a large scale. Thanks to the leadership of D.H. Henderson, funding and skilled manpower from the United States, and vaccine supplied by the USSR, there was rapid progress. This was a programme in which the two superpowers could collaborate. It was neither visible nor strategically important enough to involve the top levels of political leadership. Though their reasons might have differed, each superpower saw eradication as in its interest.

In contrast to the Cold War rhetoric with which the United States and the Soviet Union positioned themselves in other realms of international relations, the two superpowers collaborated closely on smallpox eradication. Progressing toward the declaration of smallpox eradication in 1980, the programme successfully negotiated:

> Through some of the most violent postcolonial conflicts of the era, including the Nigerian civil war of 1967–70, the Indo-Pakistan war over the secession and independence of Bangladesh in 1971, and the conflicts in the Horn of Africa in the mid-1970s. Amid Cold War conflict, however, the [eradication programme] continued to rely on collaboration between the two superpowers.[14]

Did the smallpox campaign offer a model for other vaccination programmes? Infectious diseases were by far the most important public health problem in tropical countries. Mass vaccination of children would yield vast health gains. With this in mind, in May 1974, the WHA adopted a Resolution establishing what became known as the Expanded Programme of Immunization (EPI). The resolution recommended that WHO member states 'develop or maintain immunization and surveillance programmes against some or all of the following diseases: diphtheria, pertussis, tetanus, measles, poliomyelitis, tuberculosis, smallpox and others, where applicable, according to the epidemiological situation in their respective countries'.[15] The resolution also requested the WHO Director General to assist Member States obtain good quality vaccines at a reasonable price and 'to study the possibilities of providing from international sources and agencies an increased supply of vaccines, equipment and transport and developing local competence to produce vaccines at the national level'.

Some countries, including the USSR, Egypt, the Netherlands and Yugoslavia, had offered to supply vaccines. However, throughout the first years of the EPI development of regional or national vaccine production (or regional self-sufficiency) remained an element of the evolving strategy. Where no domestic vaccine production existed, funding by multinational or bilateral aid agencies should help countries establish it. At least, countries with large enough populations to make local production viable. Countries that already have production facilities could be helped upgrade these facilities.

The WHO expected national governments to take the lead in initiating vaccination programmes. No country would be pressed to introduce any particular antigen. Nor would WHO work proactively: its involvement would only be triggered by a request for assistance. A member state could approach WHO for help in determining whether, and if so how, it could adapt the arrangements put in place for smallpox eradication in order to boost vaccination against other diseases. The new proposals were discussed in the UNICEF-WHO Joint Committee on Health Policy, and by early 1975 UNICEF's participation had been agreed. A series of regional seminars was organized, designed to explain to national policy makers what an expanded immunization programme (beyond the existing smallpox and tuberculosis programmes) would entail. WHO offered national authorities help with planning, while UNICEF assisted with vaccine procurement. The United Nations Development Programme (UNDP) indicated it would be willing to fund some trial implementation programmes.

The global health era

Institutions

In the 1960s and 1970s relationships between public and (many) private vaccine producers were rooted in a common commitment to public health. Hans Cohen, who was for many years Director General of the Dutch Institute of Public Health responsible for supplying the country's vaccine needs, tells of his earlier relationships with industry, specifically with Pasteur Mérieux:

> They [Mérieux] got all our know-how, and we weren't always happy about that, but on the other hand we got a great deal of know-how back in return. For example, I got a rabies vaccine. We exchanged. It took three minutes. A matter of 'what do you want from me?' then the boss says 'I'll have some polio, and what do you want?' And I'd say 'Give me a measles strain, and some of that and some of that…' It was good. Really a free exchange.[16]

In the 1980s this changed. Knowledge was no longer freely available or freely exchanged. A 1983 survey of US vaccine manufacturers had revealed only two patents for 27 vaccine products. A decade later SmithKline Beecham (now GSK) had to assemble 14 patents to produce and market its recombinant hepatitis-B vaccine.[17] Vaccine development and production had become 'privatized'.

Increasingly profit-oriented, the private sector had become reluctant to share its knowledge. This was to generate new products, revenues and growth. Two knowledgeable insiders pointed to a growing disconnect between public health and decision making in the pharmaceutical industry:

> Public health objectives and advocacy…do not drive business decisions, and vaccine development often stalls when commercial firms calculate the relative advantage of investing in vaccines versus other products. Ultimately, industry executives, not public health officials, make the decisions about which products to develop.[18]

By the late 1980s the divergence of industry's priorities from those of public health had become glaringly obvious. It could be seen, for example, in the lack of industrial interest in developing vaccines against parasitic diseases such as malaria. Since their market would be almost exclusively in poor countries, developing vaccines against parasitic diseases would represent a poor investment. Resources could be more profitably deployed elsewhere. New mechanism and inducements were designed to bridge the growing gap between corporate interests and public health needs.

One of these mechanisms consisted of 'Partnerships' involving international agencies, donors, and industry. As well as introducing additional resources, they would bring industrial skills and expertise to bear on the health problems of the developing world. Numerous 'Global Public Private Partnerships' (GPPPs) emerged, many of them aimed at development and production of drugs and vaccines needed in the developing world.[19] Whereas previously public and private sectors had collaborated freely, now a formal mechanism had had to be devised in order to facilitate collaboration. The Children's Vaccine Initiative (CVI), established in 1990, pioneered the public-private partnership model in the vaccine field.[20] Linked with, but separate from WHO, the CVI was to stimulate the development of new and more effective vaccines, the ultimate goal being a universal vaccine containing all the antigens children require. It failed because unbridgeable disagreements emerged between the CVI's European and American donors. The Europeans felt that the organization was overly committed to technological solutions to public health problems. Despite shifting its focus from development of new vaccines to supporting vaccine introduction, the CVI was closed down in 1999.

Developments in science and technology also helped drive a wedge between public and private sector objectives. New techniques for manipulating genetic material pointed the way to new ways of producing vaccines. Unlike older methods of attenuation and inactivation, these new methods alleviated the need for bulk culturing of dangerous pathogens. In addition they could be precision-tailored to do a very specific job. Much of the research leading to new generations of vaccines was carried out in the United States. Legislation, the Bayh-Dole Act, required scientists whose research had been funded by the Federal government to commercialize it by making it available to industry. Many scientists who had been working on the manipulation of genetic material did this by moving out of their universities into small high tech 'spin off' firms. Producing nothing at the start, the sole resource of the new biotech firms was their expertise. This had to be carefully guarded through comprehensive patenting until a profitable product, or a take-over appeared. Unlike the traditional vaccine manufacturers, the new biotech firms had no established links with the world of public health.

Traditional vaccine manufacturers (private as well as public) had no expertise in these new techniques. In order to access them, established pharmaceutical companies had to collaborate with, or purchase, the small new companies with the skills, and the patents, they coveted. In some countries this happened more easily than in others. One of the few detailed studies of institutional responses to these changes is Louis Galambos' comprehensive history of vaccine development at Merck: one company that has maintained its commitment throughout. The study shows how Merck adapted as the focus in vaccine development shifted from bacteriology to virology, and then to recombinant DNA technology. Merck (and the companies it absorbed) modified their organizational structures and – crucially – their scientific capabilities and networks. Merck also had to adapt to changes in the vaccine market, and to government policies which affect it. Government policies, in the United States, had both negative and positive effects. On the negative side, Galambos refers to the growth of the public sector market, both nationally and internationally. Public sector agencies negotiate rock-bottom prices for their bulk vaccine purchases, and so drive down profits. In the United States the share of this public market was growing, to the extent that, according to Galambos, economic motives for remaining in the vaccine business were continuously eroding. On the positive side, Galambos refers to relaxation in antitrust laws in the 1980s and 1990s. These changes had made it possible for large companies like Merck to establish strategic alliances 'that broadened the front across which it innovates and enabled it to strengthen its position in global markets'.[21] This is what the company did. So did others, with greater or lesser success. A 1995 study found vaccine manufacturers engaged in a frenzy of acquisitions and alliance formations.[22] A diagram shows the links Merck established with other major manufacturers (including Pasteur-Mérieux in France), with a number of smaller biotech companies (including Biogen and MedImmune), and with public sector institutes, including the Dutch RIVM and CSL in Australia.

Writing in the late 1990s, Seung-il Shin, of the International Vaccine Institute (IVI), then recently established in Seoul (South Korea), characterized the changes which had taken place as follows:

> The most important thing driving the transformation of the vaccine enterprise (which encompasses the development, clinical testing, production, licensure and distribution of vaccine) is the increasingly complex

> scientific and technological base that is required [...] The second factor [...] is the changing nature of technology ownership [...] vaccine development has become primarily the purview of large industrial laboratories [...] In Pasteur's day, and even as recently as forty years ago when the polio vaccines were first developed, most of the new technologies needed to manufacture vaccines were owned by the public. The scientists and organizations that developed them often assisted and funded the technology transfer to institutions in developing countries [...]
>
> The third factor is the globalization of international commerce [...] The global vaccine industry in 1998 is thus dominated by a small number of large multinational companies, instead of the smaller, publicly owned and public-spirited national vaccine production centres that were until recently the norm. Consequently, some of the key decisions regarding which vaccines to develop and how to distribute (market) them are no longer made by scientists and public health officials but by business executives in boardrooms who must answer to their shareholders [...] Finally, the increasingly stringent international product safety standards required of vaccines.[23]

Reflecting these developments, the vaccine system was changing in shape and size, though in ways which varied from country to country. This was certainly the case for what Shin refers to as the 'publicly owned and public-spirited national vaccine production centres', once the mainstay of vaccine production in many countries. They suffered a variety of fates, privatization in particular, as discussed in later chapters of this book. There are others, not discussed here, which followed a similar trajectory. One is the Australian Commonwealth Serum Laboratory. Founded in 1916, in 1994 this was transformed into a private corporation, listed on the Australian Stock Exchange. It is now CSL Ltd. Among its acquisitions is Behringwerke, established by Emil von Behring in 1904. Connaught Laboratories, established in Toronto in 1913, has enjoyed a more complex recent history. In 1972 it was sold to the Canada Development Corporation (CDC), a state-owned organization established to develop and support Canadian-owned companies. In 1986, the CDC was dismantled and Connaught transferred to private ownership. In 1989 it was acquired by the Institut Mérieux, later became a component of Pasteur Mérieux Connaught, and is now part of the French multinational, Sanofi.

In the early 1990s, the bulk of the six EPI vaccines used globally was produced by public sector institutions in developing countries. And, in theory:

> Public sector vaccine developers, such as...RIVM in the Netherlands, or manufacturers in Brazil and Thailand, could play a major role in developing new vaccines with potentially great public health impacts, since they are not especially sensitive to considerations of market size. However, a recent analysis suggests that these institutions generally do not have sufficient resources to undertake major programs-by private sector standards-in these areas.[24]

Whatever the theory, the reality seemed to be that 'many vaccine manufacturers in the developing world cannot yet ensure consistent production of a high-quality product. Adherence to Good Manufacturing Practices is too often inadequate, and many countries lack national regulatory authorities that are truly independent of the vaccine producers'.[25]

Through the 1990s the view became widespread that public sector producers lacked the resources, the freedom from political interference, and the expertise, to produce good quality vaccines. Inquiries found this to be the dominant view among vaccine manufacturers in the industrialized world. With the growing influence of the private sector on national politics it was becoming the view of politicians too. It was a dogma which ignored the growing reluctance of private industry to collaborate with public sector producers. In 2005 two government scientists from the United Kingdom, which had had no public sector vaccine production for a century, argued the need for a strategic vaccine facility.[26] At the time their argument received no attention whatsoever.

The few institutions producing vaccines in the public sector which survived did so in the teeth of global capitalism. They include Russia's Gamaleya Institute, founded as a private laboratory in 1891 but now belonging to the state; Brazil's Fiocruz and Butantan Institute, both created in 1900; and Cuba's Finlay institute, established in 1991 and named after the Cuban pioneer in the investigation of yellow fever.

The political economy which became dominant in the 1980s led to what had once been 'knowledge' (specifically here the knowledge on which vaccine development would be based) being reconfigured as 'intellectual property'. In order to protect it, the newly established World Trade Organization (WTO) made membership conditional on modifications to national patent laws. In 1995, at the end of years of negotiation, the Agreement known as TRIPS, or Trade-Related Aspects of Intellectual Property Rights, came into force.[27] The restrictions it placed on the production of generic anti-retroviral medicines led to protests. A few years later the so-called Doha Declaration stated that it was permissible to circumvent TRIPS provisions in the event of a public health emergency. Multinational pharmaceutical companies felt that this revision damaged their interests. Their lobbying led a set of largely bilateral agreements between the governments of industrialized countries (notably the United States) and developing countries which contain additional and more stringent provisions. All of this has become known as 'TRIPS +'.[28]

The context: globalization

The transformation in the vaccine system that began in the 1980s was a consequence of two distinguishable, though interrelated, processes. One was the triumph of neoliberal economics, facilitated by the collapse of communist regimes, and which legitimized the privatization of knowledge (henceforth intellectual property). Second was the claim that vaccine producers were to be regarded as elements in a global system of supply. This in turn has to be understood in relation to emergence of the concept of 'global health'. Historians have suggested that the concept of global health was crafted partly in response to struggles for authority among international organizations.[29] The growing influence of the World Bank, combined with the diminishing prestige of the WHO, lies at the root of shift away from 'international' health, supposedly based on cooperation between independent nations.

In the early 1980s the WHO was losing resources and influence. Member States were losing confidence in the organization, to such an extent that in 1982 the World Health Assembly voted to freeze its budget. As the WHO shrank in size and influence the World Bank, which had far greater resources, moved into the space it left. The justification was that a healthy workforce was key to economic growth, and this of course was central to the Bank's mission. The Washington-based Bank was wholly committed to the new international political order, based on neoliberal approaches to economics, trade, and politics. The Geneva-based WHO was far less so. In tune with the new ideology, the Bank argued in favour of greater reliance on private-sector health care provision and the reduction of the public sector. The World Bank made its loans (which were becoming increasingly important in the health sector) conditional on privatization, decentralization and fee-for-service payments. No matter the effects of these measures on access to health care in much of the developing world. Countries were obliged to dismantle 'protectionist barriers' to the free flow of capital and goods. They were obliged to rewrite legislation that restricted the patenting of medicines. The question confronting the WHO was, how to arrest its decline? How to reposition itself at the heart of international/global health, given the influence of the Bank and an ideological climate anathema to many of its staff?

> In January 1992, the 31-member Executive Board of the World Health Assembly decided to appoint a 'working group' to recommend how WHO could be most effective in international health work in light of the 'global change' rapidly overtaking the world... The working group's final report of May 1993 recommended that WHO – if it was to maintain leadership of the health sector – must... above all increase the emphasis within WHO on global health issues and WHO'S coordinating role in that domain.[30]

Whereas the World Bank worked with and on individual countries, the WHO could claim global health as its domain. This was its answer.

Rather than examining the genesis of the concept, other scholars set about justifying a 'global' approach to world health. Basing his account on the SARS outbreak of 2003, and its containment, Fidler argues that the era of national approaches to public health problems (that he refers to as 'Westphalian public health') is now over.[31] Collaboration between nation states was no longer adequate in a world of vastly enhanced mobility. If this is assumed, then the need for global initiatives in the field of vaccine development is justified in a way they never could have been previously.

A new logic was being crafted which shows the significance of 'global health' with exceptional clarity. In the early 1990s, whilst working at the WHO, Batson and Evans developed a graphic representation, a Grid, on which countries were plotted according to their income and population size. This Grid played an important role in the work of the CVI Task Force on Situation Analysis (on the staff of which Batson and Evans served)[32] and, most important of all, it provided a guide to the optimal use of resources that donor organizations could use. Rich countries with large populations can be assumed to have the resources needed to produce vaccines for their own use, and populations large enough to make production viable. In other words, a large population implies a large enough market and so provides an economic justification for local production. Where the population is large but the country is poor, though the market potential for local production exists, technical assistance from outside is required for it to be realized. Such countries, for example Indonesia, should be helped to attain vaccine self-sufficiency. In poor small countries the assumption is that local production cannot be justified, so that donor support should be directed towards subsidizing procurement.[33] This graphic representational structure in which the proper place of each country and each organization, as well as the relationships between them, can be rationally characterized shows 'global health' at work.

Rooted in the same politico-economic changes, the idea underlying this representation – that vaccine producers, public and private, can be viewed in terms of their contribution to a single global system of supply – played a crucial role. The perspective was no longer to be national. The question was no longer to be 'what is the role of a national vaccine producer, given a country's health care needs and political aspirations?' Instead, the question had to be, 'what contribution can national producers make to the global system of vaccine supply?' The change of perspective entails a dramatic shift in the criteria for assessing the importance of national – often public sector – vaccine producers. It was from this new perspective that the CVI's 'Task Force on Situation Analysis' conducted its assessments of the 'viability' of individual national producers. Among the factors determining the 'viability' of national production, according to this analysis, are population size and wealth (measured as GNP/capita).

Only where resources and population are sufficient might a national producer be in a position to meet the challenges involved in vaccine production. These challenges they saw as costs and economies of scale in production; the need for increasingly rigorous quality control; and access to new knowledge. This new knowledge had of course been 'privatized'.

> To access research and development technology and scale up know-how, national producers will need to enter into agreements with commercial producers or wait until the knowledge enters the public domain. However, commercial producers will contemplate agreements only with national facilities who can assure quality and are economically viable.

As noted earlier, the CVI was closed down in 1999. It was replaced by a new public–private venture known as the Global Alliance on Vaccines and Immunization (now the GAVI Alliance) which was announced at the 2000 World Economic Forum held in Davos. GAVI's strategy, inspired by CVI, involved improving access to sustainable immunization services, expanding the use of all cost-effective vaccines, accelerating the introduction of new vaccines, speeding up efforts to create new vaccines, and making immunization a central part of assessing international development efforts. Its founding partners included WHO, UNICEF, the World Bank, The Bill and Melinda Gates Children's Vaccine Program, the Rockefeller Foundation, the International Federation of Pharmaceutical Manufacturers' Associations (IFPMA), and some national governments.

When the EPI began, national governments were offered technical help and support for public health priorities which they themselves identified: priorities that emerged from domestic politics. Moreover in the programme's early years, support for local vaccine production, and the establishment of local and regional vaccine markets, were taken to be important policy objectives. A decade or so later, in a very different ideological climate, discourse had shifted. These objectives had quietly been abandoned. Today, the GAVI Alliance offers funds principally to accelerate the introduction of new vaccines which it prioritizes. Strengthening local production is no part of its mission.

The vaccine system changed in shape and size through the last decades of the twentieth century, though the implications of these changes have varied from country to country. The 'publicly owned and public-spirited national vaccine production centres', once the mainstay of vaccine production in much of the world, have largely gone. It is their transformations and closures which form the substance of this book. It maybe, however, that views in the global health community are again shifting. Or that opinions are again becoming polarized, though in new ways. Thus, a report on vaccine technology transfer published by the WHO in 2011 concludes:

> Establishing local vaccine manufacturing is not necessarily cost effective; however vaccines should not be seen purely as commodities, and factors such as national health security need to be considered. The establishment of a vaccine policy by countries may assist countries in identifying how and when to consider local production.[34]

Structure of the book

Though some authors discuss the start of smallpox vaccination early in the nineteenth century, a later development represents a common point of origin. In all countries, and of course in many more not presented in detail here, laboratories for producing diphtheria serum were established just before or just after the start of the twentieth century. Some of them were, or soon became, public sector institutions. The subsequent histories of these institutions then diverged, from country to country. The challenges they faced, their fortunes, activities, and structures reflected the social, political, and economic transformations that many of the countries discussed underwent. Some have experienced revolutions and civil war; some became independent nations (e.g., India in 1947); some (such as Romania) were shaken by the violent overthrow of Communist regimes, whilst the collapse of Yugoslavia led to war and the formation of Croatia and Serbia as independent states. These events, and many others, whether of local or international importance, helped shape the fortunes of the institutes discussed in this book. The accounts given here differ not only because national histories differ so profoundly. They differ also because contributors come from different disciplines and different traditions within those disciplines. They bring different research conventions, experiences, and interests to bear. Some have made extensive use of interviews, others of archives, whilst yet others have drawn on personal experiences. We made no attempt to impose a common format on contributors. There is no standard way of writing the history of vaccine politics or of vaccine manufacture. As editors we are convinced that the contrast in styles adds to the richness of the book. Establishing an optimum sequence of chapters proved more problematic. Though there are no formal 'sections', because distinctions are blurred, the structure of the book is as follows. We begin with three cases in which, mainly or partly under the influence of neo-liberal ideology, public sector vaccine production has ended. In the Netherlands, Spain and Sweden, old institutes were privatized or sold. Then follow the cases of Croatia and in India, in which market and non-market ideologies appear to exist in an uneasy and fluctuating equilibrium. Finally, there follow three countries where, for different ideological reasons, vaccine production in the public sector has been retained, albeit sometimes marginally so: Iran, Romania and Serbia. This then is the structure we have given to the book. The final chapter is not a 'summary and conclusions'. Instead, in an Epilogue, the authors try to reflect on how the Covid-19 pandemic which began in early 2020 has impacted on the politics of making vaccines. It presages further changes still to come.

Notes

1 Daniele Archibugi and Kim Bizzarri, 'Committing to vaccine R&D: a global science policy priority', *Research Policy*, 2004, 33, 1657–1671; Ernst R. Berndt *et al.*, 'Advance market commitments for vaccines against neglected diseases: estimating costs and effectiveness', *Health Economics*, 2007, 16, 491–511.
2 William Muraskin, *The Politics of International Health: The Children's Vaccine Initiative and the Struggle to Develop Vaccines for the Third World* (New York: State University of New York Press, 1998).
3 Michael Bennett, *War against Smallpox: Edward Jenner and the Global Spread of Vaccination* (Cambridge: Cambridge University Press, 2020).
4 Peter Baldwin, *Contagion and the State in Europe, 1830-1930* (Cambridge: Cambridge University Press, 2005).

5 Anne-Marie Moulin, 'The International Network of the Pasteur Institute, Scientific innovations and French tropisms', in C. Charle, J. Schriewer and P. Wagner, eds, *The Emergence of Transnational Intellectual Networks and the Cultural Logic of Nations* (Chicago: The University of Chicago Press, 2004), 135–162.
6 Claire Hooker and Alison Bashford, 'Diphtheria and Australian public health: Bacteriology and its complex applications, *c.* 1890–1930', *Medical History*, 2002, 46, 41–64.
7 Linda Bryder, ''We shall not find salvation in inoculation': BCG vaccination in Scandinavia, Britain and the USA, 1921–1960', *Social Science & Medicine*, 1999, 49, 1157–1167.
8 Moulin, 'The International Network of the Pasteur Institute', 135–162.
9 Thomas Abraham, *Polio: The Odyssey of Eradication* (London: Hurst Publishers, 2018); Tony Gould, *A Summer Plague: Polio and its Survivors* (New Haven: Yale University Press, 1995); Thomas M. Daniel and Frederick C. Robbins, *Polio* (Rochester NY: University of Rochester Press, 1997).
10 Maurice Hilleman, 'Six decades of vaccine development: a personal history', *Nature Medicine*, 1998, 4, 507–514, 513.
11 Office of Technology Assessment (OTA), *Review of Federal Vaccine and Immunization Policies* (Washington DC: US Government Printing Office, 1979), 27.
12 *Ibid.*, 35.
13 Socrates Litsios, 'The long and difficult road to Alma-Ata: A personal reflection', *International Journal of Health Services*, 2002, 32, 709–732; Dora Vargha, 'Between East and West: polio vaccination across the Iron Curtain in Cold War Hungary', *Bulletin of the History of Medicine*, 2014, 88, 319–343.
14 Erez Manela, 'A pox on your narrative: Writing disease control into Cold War history', *Diplomatic History*, 2010, 34, 299–323.
15 WHO 1974, 27th World Health Assembly, Resolutions, Document WHA 27.57, Geneva, WHO.
16 Stuart Blume and Ingrid Geesink, 'Vaccinology: An industrial science?', *Science as Culture*, 2000, 9, 41–72, 60–61.
17 David C. Mowery and Violaine Mitchell, 'Improving the reliability of the U.S. vaccine supply: An evaluation of alternatives', *Journal of Health Politics, Policy and Law*, 1995, 20, 973–1000, 976.
18 P. Freeman and A. Robbin, 'The elusive promise of vaccines', *American Prospect*, 1991, 4, 80–90.
19 Benedicte Bull and Desmond McNeill, *Development Issues in Global Governance: Public-Private Partnerships and Market Multilateralism* (London: Routledge, 2007), chapter 4.
20 Muraskin, *The Politics of International Health.*
21 Louis Galambos with Jane Eliot Sewell, *Networks of Innovation: Vaccine Development at Merck, Sharp & Dohme, and Mulford, 1895–1995* (Cambridge: Cambridge University Press, 1995), 244.
22 Mowery and Mitchell, 'Improving the Reliability', 978.
23 Seung-il Shin, 'The global vaccine enterprise: a developing world perspective', *Nature Medicine vaccine supplement*, 1998, 4, 503–505.
24 William P. Hausdorff, 'Prospects for the use of new vaccines in developing countries: cost is not the only impediment', *Vaccine*, 1996, 14, 1179–1186, 1180.
25 *Ibid.*, 1184.
26 Jacqueline M. Duggan and Timothy J. G. Brooks, 'A strategic vaccine facility for the UK', *Vaccine*, 2005, 23, 2090–2094.
27 Julie Milstien and Miloud Kaddar, 'Managing the effect of TRIPS on availability of priority vaccines', *Bulletin of the World Health Organization*, 2006, 84, 360–365.
28 Jillian Clare Cohen-Kohler, Lisa Forman and Nathaniel Lipkus, 'Addressing legal and political barriers to global pharmaceutical access: Options for remedying the impact of the Agreement on Trade-Related Aspects of Intellectual Property Rights (TRIPS) and the imposition of TRIPS-plus standards', *Health Economics, Policy and Law*, 2008, 3, 229–256.

29 Theodore Brown, Marcos Cueto and Elizabeth Fee, 'The World Health Organization and the transition from "International" to "Global" public health', *American Journal of Public Health*, 2006, 96, 62–72.
30 *Ibid.*, 69.
31 David P. Fidler, *SARS, Governance and the Globalization of Disease* (Basingstoke: Palgrave MacMillan, 2004).
32 Violaine S. Mitchell, Nalini M. Philipose and Jay P. Sanford, *The Children's Vaccine Initiative: Achieving the Vision* (Washington D.C.: National Academies Press, 1993).
33 Amie Batson, Peter Evans and Julie B. Milstien, 'The crisis in vaccine supply: A framework for action', *Vaccine*, 1994, 12, 963–965; Julie Milstien, Amie Batson and William Meaney, 'A systematic method for evaluating the potential viability of local vaccine producers', *Vaccine*, 1997, 15, 1358–1363.
34 WHO, *Increasing Access to Vaccines through Technology Transfer and Local Production* (Geneva: World Health Organization, 2011), 24.

1

THE PRIVATIZATION OF SOCIETAL VACCINOLOGY IN THE NETHERLANDS

Jan Hendriks

Introduction

On 10 February 2009, health minister Ab Klink informed the Dutch parliament of his decision to end the production of vaccines by the National Institute of Public Health and the Environment (RIVM) in Bilthoven. This decision came 100 years after the establishment of the first national public health laboratory in Utrecht. In 2012, the vaccine production capability was acquired by the Serum Institute of India Ltd (SSIL),[1] marking the beginning of the end of a century of societal vaccinology[2] in the Netherlands.

Throughout the century, the mission of the Bilthoven Institute, in its different institutional constellations, remained 'purpose and not profit driven'. From the late 1950s onwards, tasks and activities were shaped predominantly, though not exclusively, by the requirements of the 'Rijksvaccinatieprogramma', the Dutch National Immunization Programme (NIP) for children. A polio epidemic in 1956/1957 had led to the NIP's creation, but its later successes can largely be attributed to the integrated national vaccinology knowledge and infrastructure that delivered the NIP's cornerstone component for decades to come: a home-made inactivated combination vaccine against diphtheria, tetanus, pertussis, and inactivated polio (DTPwP).[3]

This chapter describes the technological, policy, and institutional dynamics that characterize Dutch public vaccinology with a focus on the period of 1990–2020. Despite its achievements, in the early 2000s, the Institute failed to adapt its combination vaccine to new requirements, when the pertussis component had to be replaced by a safer version. How did that happen? Why did a national infrastructure that relied on locally made vaccines prove unsustainable? What were the circumstances, factors, and arguments that led the authorities gradually to privatize this national capability, and how did the Institute's top

DOI: 10.4324/9781003130345-2

management respond? I address these questions from the insider-perspective of an immunologist who worked in the institute from 1990 to 2018, largely in management of international projects and co-ordinating the Institute's training programme.

The first Dutch vaccinologist

Vaccinology in the Netherlands started with Geert Reinders, an uneducated but intelligent eighteenth-century farmer who developed a method of inoculating calves against rinderpest.[4] Inspired by the Enlightenment, he succeeded in elucidating several immunological principles, of which the underlying science would become clear only 150 years later. He was the first to observe that transfer of mother's milk from surviving (and therefore immune) cows to calves protects those calves from disease, even in close contact with sick calves or cows that subsequently died (*passive immunization*). He also showed that when calves in this protected period are infected with virulent rinderpest virus, they only get minor disease symptoms and that they are protected against later infections with virulent rinderpest virus (*active immunization*). He further discovered that vaccination should not be too early in the calf's life (to prevent negative interference of passive antibodies with live vaccine) and that a second vaccination (*booster*) is needed when calves were placed in the open air. For this early work into the concepts of immunology and vaccination, some Dutch authors call Geert Reinders the 'Founder of Immunology'. Today, smallpox and rinderpest remain the only diseases to have been declared eradicated globally. In both cases, a thermostable vaccine proved key to these successes.

Origins of the Bilthoven Institute

Production of cowpox vaccine on the skin of calves to protect against human smallpox was introduced relatively late, in 1868. So-called animal lymph was produced on a large scale in 13 'Parcs Vaccinogènes' until the death of the director of such a vaccination location in Amsterdam triggered a debate on how to improve the quality of the vaccine. Over the next decades, the number of Parcs fell from 13 to 3 and finally to one location in Utrecht. In 1954 this centralized smallpox vaccine production moved to Bilthoven, where it became part of new laboratory facilities of the national health institute that had its roots in the first decade of the twentieth century. In 1909, the 'Central Laboratory for the State Inspectorate', a laboratory for public health, had been established in Utrecht for research on cholera, diphtheria, tuberculosis, typhoid fever, and other serious diseases. This laboratory grew into an independent institution. Under the 1919 Health Act, the government decided that it would no longer leave the production of sera and vaccines in the hands of the private sector. The private 'Bacterio Therapeutic Institute' was purchased and converted into the 'State Serology Institute' that merged with the Central Laboratory in 1934 to form the National

Institute for Public Health (RIV).[5] The RIV (later to become RIVM) would become the Dutch national vaccine development and production centre. In the 1956 Public Health Act, the Health Council (*Gezondheidsraad*) was charged with providing the government with independent scientific advice on questions relating to vaccination. Since 2013 the Council's Vaccination Committee has followed a published methodology, involving seven criteria, when advising on the uptake of new vaccines in the NIP.[6]

Colonial aspects

The central smallpox vaccine laboratory in Bilthoven benefitted substantially from earlier research done in the Dutch East Indies, where several innovations had been first introduced. Variolation had spread through the Dutch Indies from the late 1770s/1780s, and from 1895 onwards local production with human lymph was centralized in 'Lands Koepokinrichting' on Java (which would later merge with the Pasteur Institute in Bandung). From 1928 onwards, new technologies developed in Java improved the vaccine. Dried lymph was ground to a fine powder and sealed in glass tubes, greatly improving thermostability. The entire Dutch Indies were supplied with this vacuo-dried vaccine and the Bandung facility became the world's largest production site for smallpox vaccines in the 1940s and 1950s. This 'colonial know how and experience' would greatly benefit the vaccine development competence of the RIV. Medical virologist Rijk Gispen, RIV's scientific director from 1951 to 1975, had previously spent more than 20 years researching smallpox and rabies in the Dutch Indies.

Vaccines for the National Immunization Programme

Vaccinology centralized

After World War II, thanks to financial support from Marshall Aid, the RIV was able to move to new buildings at its current location in Bilthoven. Funds had been provided to make the Netherlands independent of vaccine imports and, in case of a war with the Eastern Bloc, to make sufficient sera and vaccines for the military apparatus of NATO. New production facilities for smallpox vaccine[7] and bacterial vaccines were constructed. In the late 1940s RIV developed an improved diphtheria toxoid vaccine that was subsequently combined with a pertussis vaccine. From 1953 onwards a tetanus toxoid vaccine was added, resulting in a trivalent combination vaccine: diphtheria, pertussis, and tetanus (DTPw).[8] Soon afterwards, the RIV became the core supplier to the NIP.

Sole provider to the NIP and international recognition

Over time, the state-sponsored NIP had evolved from a simple package of a few classical vaccines in the 1950s to its current (2020) schedule, containing vaccines against 12 infectious diseases for children from birth to 12 years of age.[9] Although other vaccines are licensed and available on the Dutch market,[10] chief characteristics of NIP vaccines are that they are recommended by the Ministry of Health and provided free of charge, usually following guidance from the Health Council. A particular characteristic of the NIP is the policy to restrict the number of injections per contact moment to two, which puts limitations to the number of vaccines that can be applied in a single vaccination session.[3] This policy requirement would prove a powerful influence on the choice of combination vaccines.

A first (inactivated) combo vaccine is made locally

A serious polio epidemic in 1956 led the Health Council to recommend mass vaccination of all children up to 14 years of age with Salk's recently developed vaccine. Under the dynamic leadership of Hans Cohen, the NIPs 'founding father', head of RIVs vaccine production and later the Institute's director, a tetravalent polio-containing DTPw vaccine was developed by adding IPV to the DTPw vaccine (DTPwP). This reduced the number of injections to four instead of the previous seven or eight (four times DTPw plus three or four times IPV). In 1962, the locally made DTPwP vaccine replaced the separate DTPw and IPV vaccines in the NIP.[3]

Key to this success story was the development and introduction of innovative production technology by two RIV microbial process engineers Paul van Hemert and Anton van Wezel. Their innovations made industrial scale production of bacterial and viral vaccines technically and economically feasible. Van Hemert was the first world-wide to develop medium- to large-scale bacterial production and purification processes based on stainless steel fermenters (bioreactors) under standardized conditions and in closed systems, increasing product yield and quality. He called this the 'Bilthoven Unit System'.[11] This homogenous production system proved its value not only for DTPw but also appeared suitable for large-scale production of the tuberculosis vaccine BCG. Bioreactor-grown BCG later proved successful in the treatment of bladder carcinoma.[12,13] Van Wezel succeeded in producing large quantities of polio viruses (which need adherent cells) in these bioreactors by introducing small dextran beads ('micro carriers') on which cells, susceptible to polio viruses, had been grown. Initially this was done on primary monkey kidney cells, but later further efficiency and standardization was achieved by replacing these with continuously growing VERO cells, first developed in the Institut Mérieux in Lyon in the 1980s.[14] The use of micro-carriers increases the total surface on which cells are grown per given bioreactor volume, thereby dramatically increasing the yield of viral production and hence the vaccine potency. Van Wezel also improved the purification procedure. The resulting 'van Wezel process' was never patented and became a standard for inactivated virus vaccines. It is used today worldwide by most industrial manufacturers of inactivated polio and rabies vaccines.

A failed effort to reintroduce IPV into developing countries

During the 1960s, the Sabin live attenuated oral polio vaccine (OPV) replaced Salk's inactivated polio vaccine (IPV) almost everywhere. As it became apparent that, in a small number of cases, OPV could become virulent and itself cause polio, Salk campaigned for the reintroduction of his vaccine. He found allies in Charles Mérieux, former President of the Institut Mérieux, and Hans Cohen of the RIV. Together, they created the Forum for the Advancement of Immunization Research (FAIR) to develop the case for use of IPV in WHO's new Expanded Programme on Immunization (EPI).

IPV field trials FAIR carried out in Africa and other tropical countries suggested that a vaccination schedule covering all the recommended EPI diseases, including polio, and involving only two visits per year, would be effective. However, in the 1980s the WHO rejected this approach. Arguments, evidence, and strategies used on both sides in the light of the later recommendation to reintroduce IPV by WHO's global polio eradication campaign are described elsewhere (Figure 1.1).[15]

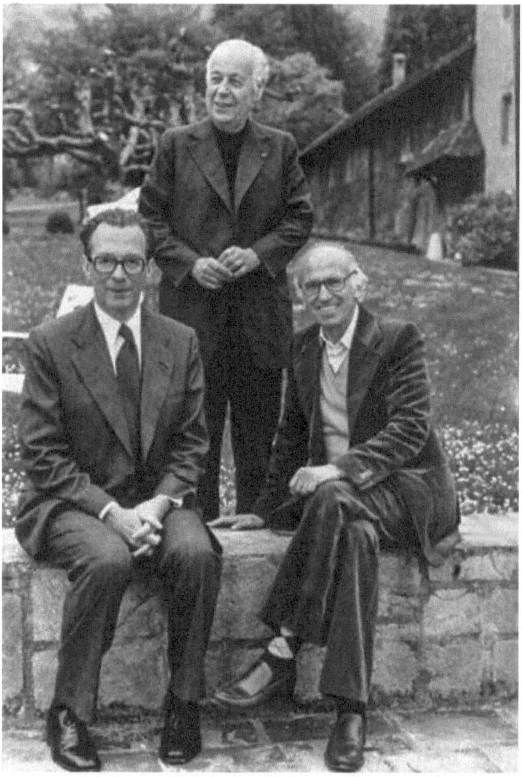

FIGURE 1.1 FAIR founders (from left to right): Hans Cohen, Charles Mérieux, and Jonas Salk (1984).

International recognition through knowledge sharing and technology transfer

The RIV innovations in vaccine production made large industrial scale vaccine production easier and offered economies of scale. The Institute's work attracted wide international interest from vaccine institutions in densely populated low- and middle-income countries (LMICs), particularly in Asia. For several decades, RIV (and its later successors) offered international vaccine courses partly based upon the 'Bilthoven Unit System' and the 'van Wezel process', both of which had not been patented (Figure 1.2).[16]

A second (live) combo vaccine follows, but can only be made under license

In a case study on vaccination against measles, mumps, and rubella (MMR), Blume and Tump analyzed the reasoning and complex negotiations that resulted in the eventual introduction of an MMR vaccine in the Netherlands in 1987.[17] By 1973, RIV had developed its own rubella vaccine from a HPV77 strain that had been obtained from the United States and had been further attenuated. By 1974 it was introduced in the NIP, initially for 11-year-old girls. A stand-alone vaccine against measles, purchased from MSD (Merck's European

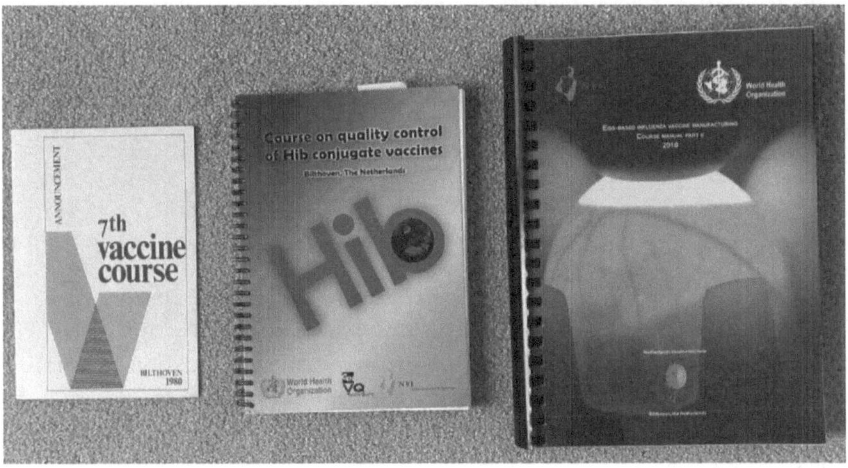

A B C

FIGURE 1.2 Vaccinology training courses for international capacity building since the 1970s.

Legend: **A**: Announcement seventh course on bacterial vaccine production (1980). **B**: Course book on quality control for cHib vaccines (2008). **C**: Course manual on egg-based influenza vaccine production (2011).

subsidiary) was introduced to the NIP in 1976. After an unsuccessful attempt at in-house development of an inactivated measles vaccine[18] that was to have been added to the existing DTPwP combination vaccine, RIV concluded a licensing agreement with Merck for making a live measles vaccine in Bilthoven with Merck's 'Moraten' strain. From 1981 onwards, RIV had started negotiations with commercial manufacturers to obtain a mumps vaccine strain, anticipating a recommendation of the Health Council that mumps vaccine should be added to the NIP. The initial idea was to combine an acquired mumps strain with the RIV rubella strain and a measles strain that was also being developed by RIV. However, MSD would not agree to licensing a single mumps component. Moreover, very costly Phase 3 field studies of the new combination vaccine would have had to be conducted. Joost Ruitenberg, from 1979 director of RIV's immunology and vaccine division (Cohen having become Director General), eventually negotiated a licensing agreement regarding MSD's combined MMR vaccine.[19] From 1987 onwards, RIV stopped making its own rubella and measles vaccines and supplied the NIP with MMR vaccine made under license from Merck.

The global health era

New technologies lead to more introductions in NIP but create supply challenges

In the late 1980s, genetic engineering and the conjugation of bacterial capsular polysaccharides to proteins emerged as two technological innovations that would lead to new categories of vaccines. With some delay, these would find their way into the Dutch NIP from the early 1990s onwards. However, none would be manufactured in Bilthoven, despite the substantial research and development conducted there.

Hepatitis B vaccine made by DNA recombinant technology

Hepatitis B vaccination was introduced relatively late in comparison with surrounding countries. For many years, the low prevalence of hepatitis B was the main reason that standard policy remained to restrict vaccination to certain risk groups, including children born to mothers who had tested positive in screening during pregnancy. Around 2000, as it became clear that about 25% of neonates did not receive the vaccine in time, discussion of mass vaccination by incorporating hepatitis B vaccine into the NIP re-emerged. The effectiveness, including the cost-effectiveness, of the 'target-group only' policy was re-evaluated around 2004. In 2007 the Health Council was still convinced that population-based immunization was necessary, but it changed its advice after applying a newly adopted assessment framework. On the basis of seven criteria, universal hepatitis B vaccination was introduced in the NIP in 2011 using hexavalent vaccine.[20]

Whether the non-availability of a locally manufactured hepatitis B vaccine played a role in this delayed introduction remains an unanswered question. RIV never initiated the development of such vaccine but had been somewhat involved in an initiative by the Central Laboratory of the Blood Transfusion Service (CLB) in Amsterdam. In the early 1980s, on its own initiative, the CLB had developed a safe and effective plasma-derived heat-inactivated hepatitis B vaccine, tested in over 3,000 individuals.[21] RIV contributed by transfer of quality control assays and in setting up potency studies in monkeys.[22] Although it compared favourably with other plasma-derived HepB vaccines at that time, the project came to an end in 1987 when the recombinant DNA HepB vaccine from MSD reached the market. While considerably cheaper, the disadvantages of making a safe and reliable vaccine from plasma obtained from donors were coming to seem too great. AIDS was on the rise.

Conjugate vaccine against Haemophilus influenzae *type b*

The first conjugate vaccine to be introduced in the NIP was a vaccine against *Haemophilus influenzae* type b (cHib) in 1993. It would also be the first NIP vaccine that had not been developed or produced within the Netherlands. In 1991, after cHib vaccination proved cost-effective, the Health Council advised the Ministry of Health that it should be introduced in the NIP.

Meanwhile, RIVM[23] had already prepared for the availability of a cHib vaccine by partnering with the small American pharmaceutical company Praxis Biologicals. They produced HbOC [Hib-oligosaccharides covalently coupled to the CRM197 protein, an atoxic variant of the diphtheria toxin]. The long-term goal was to develop a pentavalent vaccine, combining the Praxis Hib vaccine with RIVM's DTPwP combination vaccine. A Phase 1 trial in 1991 with several dozen children vaccinated with this 5-in-1 vaccine showed it was safe. This was one of the world's first pentavalent vaccines. Unfortunately, the collaboration between RIVM and Praxis Biologicals would end prematurely in 1992, and with it the further development of this vaccine. Jan Poolman, who had joined RIVM in 1986 to work on acellular pertussis and to develop vaccines against meningitis-causing bacteria, remembered in 2020:

> We had agreed to a licensing agreement in principle, where RIVM would get the production rights of HbOC for Europe against 10% royalty, but the Ministry and RIVM's management backed off with the argument that RIVM is not a commercial vaccine production organization. A similar unfortunate no-decision happened around acellular pertussis from Sclavo/Biocine. The two collaborations would have allowed RIVM to switch from the successful DTPwP of the 50-60's towards DTPaPcHibHepB in the 90-00's.[24]

Disappointed with this premature ending of an apparently promising collaboration, Poolman would continue seeking collaboration with industry. He laid out his overall strategy in RIVM's 1991 annual scientific report:

> During the next decade, three new bacterial vaccines are probably going to be registered for general use aiming at the prevention of diseases caused by Hib, *Neisseria meningitidis* (meningococci) and *Streptococcus pneumoniae* (pneumococci), together responsible for the bulk of the primary invasive bacterial diseases in man. In addition, a well-defined subunit vaccine is likely to replace the whole-cell pertussis vaccine. Developing four new bacterial vaccines goes beyond the capacities of the RIVM. This implies that cooperative projects with universities, institutes and industry would have to be started to realize this goal. For the Hib and the subunit pertussis vaccines licences from industry are being sought, while the vaccine development within RIVM will prioritize meningococcal and pneumococcal vaccines.

Disappointed by what he saw as missed opportunities, in 1996 Poolman moved to SKB/GSK where he played a key role in the development of their aP, Hib, MenC and Pneumo combination vaccines.

After the positive advice of the Health Council and the discontinuation of the partnership with Praxis, another vaccine was needed. By mid-1993, a cHib vaccine from Pasteur-Mérieux-Connaught (now Sanofi Pasteur) had been procured for inclusion in the NIP as an additional injection. The vaccine was given simultaneously with RIVM's DTPwP vaccine to all children born after 1 April 1993.

The institute had been unable rapidly to provide the NIP with a conjugate Hib vaccine. However, in 1998 Hans Kreeftenberg, who had returned from five years as head of Pasteur-Mérieux-Connaught's quality control division in Canada, convinced the Institute's management to start a cHib technology transfer project. This was in line with its International Vaccine Policy.[25] With outside funding, a robust Hib conjugate vaccine production process was developed and transferred to developing countries.[26] Perhaps RIVM's most important success in global health, this project eventually enabled several LMIC manufacturers such as Serum Institute India Ltd and Biological E Ltd to integrate cHib in their pentavalent DTPwHepB combination vaccine, obtain WHO pre-qualification, and subsequently supply global markets through UN procurement agencies and GAVI.[27] GSK had launched their pentavalent DTPwHepB combination vaccine in 2000 for use in LMICs and had for five years been a monopolistic supplier, refusing to lower its dose price of around $3.50. Only after the entry of LMICs manufacturers in 2008, GAVI/UNICEF prices dropped to around $2.20 per dose in 2012, enabling an increased and sustainable supply of affordable cHib-containing combination vaccines.[28]

Conjugate vaccines against Meningococci and Pneumococci

The conjugation technology would prove successful not only for Hib vaccines but also in the design of vaccines against other meningitis and pneumonia causing bacteria such as *Neisseria meningitides* and *Streptococcus pneumoniae.*

Meningococci

A second conjugate vaccine to be introduced into the NIP was a vaccine against meningococcal serogroup C (MenC) in 2002.

RIV had started studies in mice in the early 1980s by coupling MenC oligosaccharides to tetanus toxoid.[29] By the end of the 1980s, work on MenC was continued in a collaborative partnership with Praxis aimed at a conjugate meningococcal A/C vaccine. Such vaccine was also very much needed in Africa, where each year the MenA strain caused significant morbidity and mortality in the so-called 'meningitis belt'.[30] However, this collaboration with Praxis collapsed again for the same reasons as had happened earlier with cHib. When the Health Council advised the introduction of MenC vaccine in the NIP, it had to be procured from a commercial manufacturer.

More progress was made in the development of a vaccine against MenB, though not through conjugation to polysaccharides. For MenB, another approach had to be followed since MenB's polysaccharides show a structural similarity with sialic acid in glycoproteins from human neural tissue. Therefore, vaccines with this polysaccharide generate only a modest immune response, while at the same time increasing the likelihood of developing auto-antibodies. RIV developed a MenB vaccine candidate by making use of outer membrane vesicles (OMVs) containing outer membrane proteins of MenB. OMVs are spontaneously released during growth and present a range of surface antigens in a native conformation with natural properties like immunogenicity, self-adjuvation, and uptake by immune cells. This makes OMV's attractive for application in vaccines against pathogenic bacteria. Genetic engineering of OMV-producing bacteria can be used to improve and expand their usefulness as vaccines.[31]

RIVM genetically constructed a hexavalent MenB vaccine candidate based upon two OMVs each containing three different subtypes of pathogenic MenB strains. The construct showed promising results in Phase 1 and 2 clinical studies in infants, toddlers, and children in the United Kingdom and Rotterdam.[32] Uptake in the NIP appeared not far off. The rather abrupt departure of Poolman, who in 1996 became head of bacterial vaccine development with Smith Kline Biologicals (now GSK) in Belgium, slowed down RIVM's development work. Notwithstanding, this vaccine concept and production process would continuously be improved and optimized in subsequent years. Today, the OMV-based technology has been optimized by Intravacc[33] into a generic platform technology through combining MenB OMV vesicles with heterologous peptides or proteins from other pathogens, including SARS-CoV-2.

Pneumococci

A seven valent pneumococcal conjugate vaccine (PCV7) procured from Wyett-Lederle in the United States was introduced in the Dutch paediatric NIP in 2006, following advice from the Health Council and replaced in 2011 with a 10 valent vaccine (PCV10).

In none of these national introductions was RIVM involved as a vaccine provider, although substantial development work had been undertaken in the Institute. By the early 1990s a dual strategy for a pneumococcal vaccine had been initiated. A conjugation approach, coupling capsular polysaccharides from different serotypes to a carrier protein, was chosen for a vaccine intended for developing countries. Simultaneously, a protein-based approach was prioritized for the Dutch NIP using 'pneumolysin', a pneumococcal cytoplasmatic protein.

The conjugation strategy had been encouraged by an international initiative, the Task Force for Child Survival, and was implemented in a collaborative network with several Scandinavian Public Health Institutes working together towards a pneumococcal conjugate vaccine for developing countries: the Dutch Nordic Consortium project.[34]

For the protein-based strategy, a patent was acquired on pneumolysin. It promised to be an attractive protein as the basis for a new generation of pneumococcal vaccines because animal studies had shown that this highly conserved protein is immunogenic against all serotypes.

Around 1997, both approaches had made progress but the RIVM management realized it would not be in time since Wyeth Lederle's PCV7 vaccine would reach the Dutch market within two or three years. The Consortium's conjugate approach had by that time progressed to a tetravalent prototype vaccine ready for field testing. Several challenges brought this project to a near standstill. Despite successful small-scale Phase 1 studies in adults and toddlers in Finland, the intended field testing in Vietnam was not approved by the local authorities. Funds had meanwhile dried up, and the project was discontinued.[35]

For the common-protein approach, progress was even slower. Mutants (pneumolysoid) of pneumolysin were obtained by DNA-recombinant technology and investigated in animal models (mice and rats) for their immunogenicity and toxicity. Upscaling of the production of these proteins appeared difficult to implement, in part due to other internal projects competing for access to the process development laboratory. That laboratory was already heavily committed to delivering services to the China Vaccine Project, RIVM's largest vaccine technology transfer project, running from 1990 to 1997. So, choices had to be made.

Negotiations with Wyeth Lederle were considered to exchange RIVM's pneumolysoid patent and know-how for access to Wyeth Lederle's conjugate product. However, Wyeth Lederle had already started its Phase 3 trial and had chosen a different protein as the carrier. Indications pointed to a high efficacy, so there would be little interest in RIVM's pneumolysin. The development of this protein-based production process thereby came to an end.

Acellular pertussis replaces whole cell pertussis in the DPwTP combo vaccine

Ever since the first experimental whole cell pertussis vaccines were introduced, it had been recognized that this vaccine, far more than most others, gives rise to side effects.

Fears of encephalitis that had led to suspension of whole cell pertussis vaccination in Japan, Germany, and Sweden had in 1975 prompted the RIV to reduce the concentration of pertussis component in the DTPw-IPV combination vaccine, as a precautionary measure. The expected reduction in the number of serious complications did not materialize. In 1988 the Health Council advised that though it would be premature to introduce acellular vaccine at that time, in the longer term a switch would be advisable. By the end of the 90s, when a pertussis epidemic occurred in the Netherlands, questions arose about the apparently declining efficacy of RIVM's vaccine. In 1997 the Institute was instructed to work on the replacement of the whole cell pertussis component in its DPwT-IPV combination vaccine with an acellular component. This raised considerable technical and formulation challenges. When vaccine components are put together they influence each other, with possible safety or potency implications for each of the individual components. Since regulatory authorities consider the combination to be a new product, time-consuming and costly clinical trials are required. By 2004, the Health Council, noting that NVI had not succeeded in producing its own new vaccine in a reasonable time frame, recommended purchase of a commercially available combination vaccine. The Minister of Health followed this advice and from 2005 onwards a commercial DTPa-IPV vaccine was procured for the NIP.[35]

The reasoning of the Health Council and the choices made by the Ministry were highly influenced by public opinion and by the option to involve the domestic public manufacturing expertise, as discussed by Blume and Zanders.[36] The choice was either to purchase the whole combination vaccine from a commercial manufacturer, or to purchase the acellular component alone and mix it with the existing domestically produced diphtheria tetanus and polio vaccines. The latter course was chosen, but the desired vaccine could not be produced in time. The Minister soon found himself in a difficult position, as disagreement between the Health Council and the NVI became public. A little later, answering questions from Members of Parliament, the Minister stated that his decision had not been based on the substantive arguments of the Health Council, which he had not found sufficiently convincing, but on the need to reassure parents and to restore their faith in the vaccination programme as a whole.

The decision to procure the acellular pertussis-containing combination vaccine from industry implied that, as in 1987 with RIV's rubella and measles vaccines, the local production capacity for diphtheria, pertussis, tetanus, and polio had no further value in meeting the requirements of the NIP.

Gradual replacement by internationally procured vaccines

The hallmark of Dutch public sector vaccinology success is the innovative semi-industrial production processes in bioreactors developed in the 1960s and 1970s for bacterial and viral vaccines. Since none of these innovations were patented, they have since found global application by manufacturers both public and private. Nationally, the greatest value was the vaccine self-sufficiency of the NIP, which lasted for several decades. Development costs were not clearly known, and crucial technological competences were available in-house. Over time, as progressively more new vaccines were required, the capability to meet this national demand diminished. Finally, today, all vaccines and vaccine combinations used in the NIP are procured from international commercial manufacturers (Figure 1.3).

Institutional reforms following changes in government policy

The many take-overs in the international vaccine industry, ongoing since the late 1980s, were leading to its concentration in just a few multinational companies. In the late 1980s RIV management recognized that this would limit the options available to the government. It argued that maintaining a domestic source of vaccine supply would decrease dependence on the industry. Until that point, RIV had been a de facto monopolist in a commercially uninteresting market. However, commercially attractive new vaccines were appearing and by the early

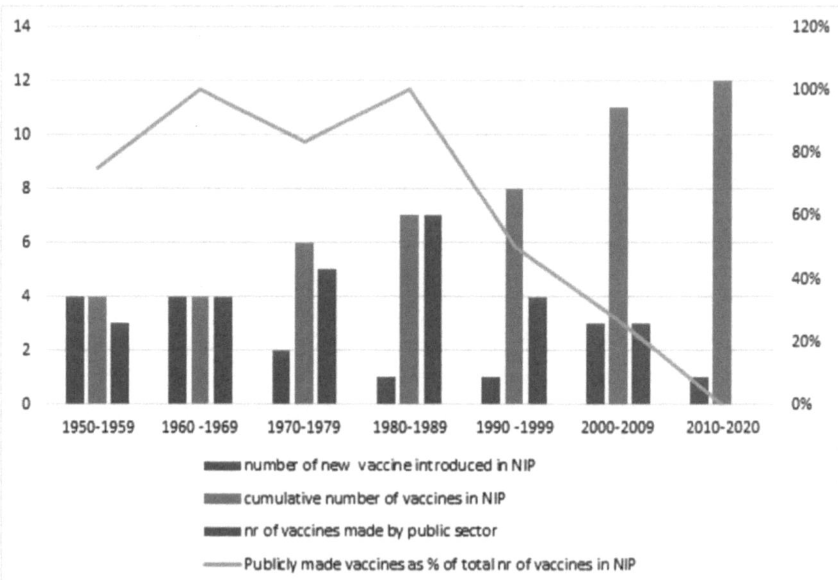

FIGURE 1.3 Relative contribution of vaccines produced by the public sector for diseases addressed by the Netherlands Immunization Programme (NIP) between 1950 and 2020.

1990s forthcoming EU regulations would make it difficult to keep competitors from the Dutch market. Yet as we have seen, the RIV was increasingly unable to meet the demands of the NIP. From the mid-1980s onwards, the Ministry of Health struggled with this dilemma and began to reconsider whether vaccine development and production should remain in the public domain and if so, how vaccine tasks and responsibilities could be best structured. The following three decades would see a succession of legal and institutional reforms, as government policies sought to adapt to new challenges.

A major reform had already taken place after the Council of Ministers decided in 1984 to cluster all the tasks in the field of public health and environmental hygiene. Three national institutions: The National Institute for Water Supply, the Institute for Waste Research, and the RIV were merged into 'The National Institute for Public Health and the Environment (RIVM)'. In the new structure, vaccine development and production were strategically defined as a component of infectious diseases control, and thereby a public task. Scandinavian governments had thought similarly, which is why RIVM reached out to those countries, leading to the Dutch Nordic Consortium initiative, agreed in 1990 during the celebration of the RIVM's eightieth anniversary. Meanwhile outside pressure continued, albeit not directly on the Ministry of Health. In the 1980s foreign manufacturers made several attempts to purchase the RIV vaccine business. These were directed not at the Ministry of Health but elsewhere, such as the Ministry of Economic Affairs, sensitive to the prospects of reducing costs through economies of scale. That stimulated the Institute's management to consider 'knowledge exploitation'. Being a small country in number of inhabitants, the Dutch vaccine market is too small to run an economically sustainable vaccine enterprise. By exporting knowledge and vaccines, cost-efficiencies could be reached. The Ministry of Health agreed in the mid-1980s that RIV could generate revenues through knowledge exploitation, up to a certain amount, without consequences for the annual lump-sum subsidy from the Ministry. Additional revenues were to be invested in vaccine research. Knowledge exploitation would later become the basis of the international vaccine policy, with technology transfer as its main instrument.

A foundation invented to meet austerity targets

When the austerity-oriented centre-right government tasked the new RIVM management with significantly reducing the number of public sector employees, a further step was taken to 'economize' vaccinology. Operational and technical production tasks were separated from vaccine research and development in a stepwise fashion through the creation in 1988 of a not-for-profit foundation, the 'Stichting voor Volksgezondheid en het Milieu' (Foundation for Health and Environment) or SVM.[37] The ultimate responsibility for SVM remained in the hands of RIVM's Director General, who chaired its Executive Board. The rationale was that, with the new foundation structure, the Institute's capacity could also be used for (private) customers. Previously, with the RIVM structure, this had not been possible. Nine years later, in 1997, the Council of Ministers confirmed that all operational production tasks were to be transferred to SVM, but that vaccine development and production for the NIP would remain the responsibility of the Ministry of Health. This was justified with several arguments: more options as regards the composition of the NIP; avoiding complete dependency on market forces; and as being potentially of great value in the event of a calamity, such as a suddenly emerging infection with endemic or pandemic potential.

Another reason for separating vaccine manufacturing from RIVM had to do with quality control. The national quality control laboratory, responsible for independently approving all vaccines released onto the Dutch market, was situated within RIVM's premises. This offered efficiency because resources, such as experimental animals and animal technicians, could be shared between the vaccine department of RIVM and the national quality control laboratory. By international standards however the interdependency of manufacture and quality control was seen as problematic: leading to a potential conflict of interest.

Development and production brought together again after September 11

Shortly after the 11 September 2001 attacks in the United States, the Dutch government decided that 'the possibility to develop and produce vaccines within the public domain needed to be preserved to ensure the timely availability of sufficient vaccines of assured quality'. The rationale was that maintaining a production capacity in the public domain would counterbalance the risk of market failure following any decrease in the number of commercial manufacturers. The perceived risk of a deliberately launched smallpox pandemic played a role in this decision. In mid-2001 the Ministry commissioned RIVM to establish a national smallpox vaccine stockpile.[38] The government's decision also led to the creation of the Netherlands Vaccine Institute (NVI), bringing together the SVM and the vaccine research and development department of the RIVM. All vaccine development and production-related facilities and staff were now merged into a distinct state agency separated from RIVM. NVI's mission was to guarantee (by procurement or production) the supply of vaccines necessary to protect the Dutch population against infectious diseases, both for use in the NIP and in crisis situations such as an epidemic or pandemic.

After September 11, the NVI embarked on an international strategy of seeking bilateral collaborations with industry for certain innovative vaccine concepts, such as the OMV-based MenB concept, while at the same time exploring, primarily within Europe, a public sector network approach to expedite vaccine development projects for emerging pathogens, based upon the network that had formed the earlier Dutch Nordic Consortium.[39]

The NVI did not have a long lifespan. In its seven years of existence, its performance came under increasing public and parliamentary scrutiny. Despite the advice from the Health Council in 2000 to switch to an acellular pertussis vaccine in the Dutch DTPwP vaccine, NVI's top management had remained sceptical about this. Instead, in 2004, it had proposed to prioritize development of a better whole cell pertussis vaccine rather than to develop a DTPaPcHib with an imported acellular pertussis, as the Ministry of Health had requested. When it became clear that NVI could not complete the development of this combination vaccine in time for its introduction by 1 January 2005, the Health Council recommended temporary purchase of a commercially available combination vaccine, until NVI was ready to supply its own DTPaPcHib vaccine. This 'policy disagreement' between Health Council and NVI reached the media and led to parliamentary questions about who is in fact in charge of setting vaccination policies. Since NVI was a vaccine manufacturer, which was also advising the government on new vaccine introductions, a perceived conflict of interest was suggested. NVI proved unable to produce the acellular pertussis component in the pentavalent combination vaccine, at an 'acceptable cost' and in time. Meanwhile other quality-issues further undermined the NVI's position. In 2005 the government's Health Inspectorate (IGZ) published a report highly critical of the overall quality of manufacturing (Good Manufacturing Practices).[40] This 'GMP-crisis' threatened NVI's vaccine manufacturing licence. After substantial investments, NVI managed to pass the follow-up IGZ inspection in 2006, but in 2008, the Medicines Evaluation Board rejected NVI's market authorization application for its DTPaPcHib combination vaccine.[41] To make matters worse, a batch of MMR was rejected by the national control laboratory, because its potency did not meet the required specification.

Combined, these quality and supply issues, in the context of the austerity-minded centre-right government, led to the 2009 decision to cease all vaccine manufacturing in the public domain. The main reason was economic. For years vaccine production had consistently been losing money.

Vaccinology deconstructed

NVI's vaccine manufacturing part was first turned into a state company, Bilthoven Biologicals (BBio Ltd) with the government as its only shareholder, before being sold to the Serum Institute of India Ltd for €32 million in 2012. At the same time, the Director-General Public Health of the Ministry and the Director-General RIVM together agreed to place NVI's vaccinology research and development capacity outside RIVM but directly under the Ministry of Health. From 1 January 2013 onwards a 'temporary working organization' continued as 'the Institute for Translational Vaccinology (Intravacc)', with as mission to 'bridge the translational gap between vaccine research in academia or small/medium enterprises including biotech and the vaccine industry'. In 2013, the Minister of Health announced her intention to privatize Intravacc as well. Nico Oudendijk, the Ministry's chief administrator managing privatization processes, commissioned Hans de Goeij, former Director-General of the Ministry of Health, to map the consequences of privatizing Intravacc. De Goeij concluded in his report that privatizing the vaccine research and development would be detrimental to the public interest. 'In the event of threats of virus outbreaks or calamities, the government wants to be able to continue to use a non-commercial organization', he wrote in 2015.

Nevertheless, the Minister decided to continue the privatization. In her view, Intravacc no longer had value for the public domain. Due to successive budget cuts, the organization lacked sufficient people and knowledge 'to be able to perform all the necessary tasks properly'. She announced her decision in a letter sent to parliament on 22 December 2016. While mentioning that public interests needed to be safeguarded after privatization,[42] she emphasized again the expected economic advantages for the government.

Unfinished business

Finding a buyer for Intravacc took more time than expected, but in late 2019, a prospective buyer who seemed prepared to guarantee the public and national interests to the Minister's satisfaction was found. Then in early 2020, the SARS-CoV-2 pandemic struck. The unfolding pandemic heightened concerns in media, public opinion, and parliament regarding the increasing dependency on foreign providers of essential medicines and vaccines. In October 2020, the Court of Auditors asked for assurances that Intravacc's know-how and intellectual property would remain responsive to the public interest after the sale. Despite these reservations, the Minister of Health informed parliament in December that the privatization process would be continued. As of 1 January 2021, Intravacc would be transformed into a public shareholding company with 'policy participation' from the Ministry of Health. In the Minister's opinion, this will give Intravacc the opportunity to further professionalize vaccine development and facilitate collaboration with private parties. All shares will remain in the hands of the State for up to two years. A definitive sales decision however was left to a new government, to be installed after the March 2021 general election (Table 1.1).

Conclusions and perspective

Vaccinology: what's in a name?

Vaccinology today is an industrial science characterized by the influence of the biotechnology revolution and the dominant role that private industry has come to play.[43] The dynamics of Dutch public sector vaccinology illustrate how these transformations have affected an affluent European country with a small population. For some three decades, a public health-driven vaccinology expertise centre with a semi-industrial infrastructure served national vaccine needs.

TABLE 1.1 Milestones in the deconstruction of Dutch vaccinology

1984	**RIVM** created as a merger of **RIV** with two environmental national institutes.
1988	**SVM** established as public foundation for austerity reasons. RIVM remains in control as chair of SVM's Board.
1996	Abrupt departure head of vaccine development Jan Poolman, who joins SKB/GSK.
1997	Council of Ministers confirms vaccine development and production to remain under ministerial responsibility. Development in RIVM and production in SVM.
2003	**NVI** is created, merging again RIVM's development and SVM's production.
2004	Pertussis controversy. NVI's and Health Council's diverging reports create dispute on pertussis vaccine choice in public domain.
2005	"GMP crisis". Inspectorate threatens to withdraw manufacturing license. Parliamentary questions on NVI's inability to timely supply DTPaP in 2006.
2006	NVI meets GMP standards again.
2008	NVI's MMR rejected by national control authority due to insufficient potency.
2009	Privatization starts. Health Minister decides to sell production and dismantle NVI.
2010	NVI's production capability turned into a state company: **BBio Ltd.** Development and other vaccine tasks reintegrated into RIVM.
2012	Serum Institute of India Ltd. acquires BBio Ltd. for €32 million.
2013	NVI's vaccine development capability turned into **Intravacc,** as "temporary work organization" under the Ministry, separate from RIVM.
2016	Health Minister decides to privatise Intravacc.
2020	COVID-19. Health Minister decides to turn Intravacc into a state company by January 2021 but leaves open its integration in a continuous public private partnership on pandemics.

Then, in the late 1980s technological, policy and economic challenges led to disagreements and struggle among the various governmental agencies. The eventual result was its dismantling and privatization. The government's dual relationship with the Institute in Bilthoven as both 'owner' and 'principal' for all vaccine tasks could no longer be reconciled. Tasks relating to advising the government on vaccination schedules and policies, monitoring vaccine coverage, and on procurement of vaccines, have remained public and are now re-integrated into the RIVM. Privatization of the Dutch vaccine production capacity (BBio Ltd) was completed in 2012, whilst at this time of writing privatization of the research and product development and technology transfer capacity (Intravacc) is pending.

The curse of combination vaccines and pressure to conform eroded national competence

The example of the Netherlands further shows that the politics of vaccine choice have changed, partly as the result of demands for public participation and personal choice. Because of its competence in vaccinology, in regard to polio the Netherlands was able to follow a course different from most countries. As vaccine politics changed, it became more difficult to diverge from majority opinion and practice. The existence of RIVM and NVI, closely allied to the Ministry of Health, rendered decision making more complex not only because of the institutional commitments entailed, but more fundamentally because—in theory at least—it also provided an alternative that is not available in most countries.

After successful introduction of two 'local' combination vaccines DPwTP and MMR in the NIP, the Institute was unable to license combination vaccines with procured components made by DNA recombinant and conjugation technologies. These new components were increasingly protected by patents, as discussed in the Introduction to this book. It was this failure that set the stage for the Institute's later decline. Whilst aware that DTPw-based combination vaccines including Hepatitis B and cHib were being promoted for use in developing countries, the Institute struggled to develop a clear strategy for the Netherlands. Moreover, the RIVM and later NVI did not recognize in time that an existing combination vaccine with a new component would be seen by regulatory authorities as an entirely new product, necessitating costly Phase 3 clinical trials in most cases.

Industry, on the other hand, in particular SKB in Belgium (later to become GSK), did respond. Supported by the Children's Vaccine Initiative (CVI), in 1988 SKB started development of a recombinant Hep-B–containing combination vaccine. Within just a few years, a whole array of these combination vaccines was licensed for use in the European Union.[44] The programmatic advantages and better safety profile of these commercial combination vaccines, together with the muscle and marketing power of a large multinational, strongly influenced Dutch policy makers.[45] This resembles a certain 'pressure to conform' also exerted by today's global agenda and institutions as has been described for developing countries. For example, a case study on Hepatitis B vaccination in India suggested in 2003 that policy is 'increasingly driven by supply push, generated by the industry and mediated by international organisations'.[46] Not only does the pressure to conform seem to overwhelm the capacities of developing countries, but it is also felt in a rich country like the Netherlands. The role of the specialized vaccinology expertise at the country's disposal, which had previously made autonomous choice possible, became controversial from the 1990s onwards, all the more because the institute's choices were sometimes at odds with recommendations from the government's main advisory body, the Health Council.

International networks and creation of global public goods could not turn the tide

At various times the Institute launched international collaborative initiatives that were mission-driven while at the same time intended to counteract increasing national pressures to conform and to meet austerity targets. The FAIR initiative in the 1970s and 1980s to 'globalize' RIV's inactivated polio vaccine-containing combination vaccine was met with scepticism and resistance from global policy makers, who preferred the cheaper (though less safe) oral polio vaccine. Only in the first decade of the new millennium would WHO re-convert to inactivated polio vaccine, finally recognizing that vaccine-derived polio cases have become the major obstacle to its now faltering Global Polio Eradication Initiative. As of December 2020, 23 countries were battling vaccine-derived polio outbreaks causing over 600 polio cases, five times more than in 2019.[47] The late 1980s and early 1990s were characterized by a collaboration strategy with national sister institutions in Europe in the Dutch Nordic Consortium and 'knowledge-exploitation' through capacity building and technology transfer to developing countries, contributing to the creation of Global Public Goods. RIVM's international network approach in the early 1990s was articulated in a widely distributed brochure and in a paper addressing the role of the public sector in 'shaping' the Children's Vaccine Initiative.[48]

The intangible yet significant contributions of Dutch vaccinology to global health since the 1960s has been described in several case studies.[49] The former colonial ties with Indonesia served as a basis to train staff and transfer large scale bacterial vaccine know-how and technology to the state company Perum Bio Farma Ltd. Today this is Indonesia's sole human vaccine manufacturer and one of the main suppliers of WHO prequalified vaccines to UNICEF and GAVI for global EPI vaccination programmes. RIVM's China Vaccine Project in the 1990s modernized large-scale vaccine production of EPI vaccines in three state vaccine institutes in China and successfully introduced the van Wezel microcarrier process technology for viral vaccines in at least one of those institutions. A final example is the initiating role RIVM played in 2000/2001 with WHO in founding the Developing Country Vaccine Manufacturers Network (DCVMN).[50] Today, DCVMN is globally recognized as a critical constituency providing vaccines for LMICs, including vaccines against Covid-19.[51]

When Europe became preoccupied with (re)-emerging health threats, post–September 11, RIVM (and later NVI) took the lead in a series of EU-funded collaborative projects between national vaccine institutions designed to increase national health security and pandemic preparedness.

Regrettably, the considerable value of these public health driven international activities, stretching over decades, was not sufficiently appreciated by the Dutch government itself. The Dutch Ministry of Health had no interest in seeking an alternative to privatization, either of production in 2009 or of research and development in 2016.[52] For the Ministry, focused on annual expenditures, the income and international prestige generated did not compensate for the extra costs and delays in supplying vaccines to the NIP.

Future: a Covid-19 inspired public-private vaccinology partnership?

The story does not end here though. The Covid-19 pandemic may lead to a new twist in this long privatization process. The letter that the Minister of Health sent to Parliament in December 2020 justified continuing with privatization. The Minister's argument was that the proposed legal structure (a state company with 'policy participation' from the Ministry of Health) will further professionalize vaccine development whilst also facilitating collaboration with private parties. At the same time, it wishes to safeguard the public interest, although it is unclear how. One day later, the government sent a report to Parliament entitled 'New Opportunities for Top Sector Life Sciences & Health'. The report had been commissioned by the Ministries of Health and of Economic Affairs to 'capitalise on the economic and social opportunities created by the arrival in 2019 of the European Medicines Agency in the Netherlands and to strengthen the Dutch Life Sciences and Health Sector'. Written by Clemènce Ross-van Dorp, a former State Secretary for Health, the report identifies infectious diseases control and vaccine development as a strength in the Dutch Life Science and Health ecosystem and refers to Intravacc as a biotechnological frontrunner for innovative vaccine technology. A '*continuous public private partnership*' around pandemic preparedness is proposed, which could include Intravacc in a national 'Vaccine Innovation Platform'.

As of January 2021, Intravacc is a public company with the state as its only shareholder. BBio Ltd and Intravacc are located today on one site in Bilthoven sharing a highly integrated infrastructure. In a 19 February press release, Intravacc announced the completion of a pilot plant for GMP production of vaccine candidates for clinical research. It also announced the formation of a consortium including BBio Ltd with the intention to design and build a new large-scale multipurpose vaccine production facility to be used immediately for national requirements in case of pandemics.[53] Perhaps the combined infrastructure and the expertise of BBio Ltd (a subsidiary of Serum Institute of India Ltd), and Intravacc Ltd, with its technology platforms and ties to a global network of low- and middle-income country vaccine manufacturers, lays the foundation for the proposed new public private partnership. In that way the legacy of Geert Reinders, Hans Cohen, Anton van Wezel, Paul van Hemert, and their successors would to some extent remain preserved.

Notes

1 https://www.reuters.com/article/poonawallas-serum-institute-buys-nvis-pr-idINDEE86304X20120704 (Accessed 18/05/2021).

2 For this paper, vaccinology is taken to include vaccine development and production with a strong connection to its application in societal immunization programmes.
3 M. van Wijhe *et al.*, 'Trends in Governmental Expenditure on Vaccination Programmes in the Netherlands, a Historical Analysis', *Vaccine*, 2019, 37, 5698–5707.
4 G. van Doornum, T. van Helvoort, and N. Sankaran, *Leeuwenhoek's Legatees and Beijerinck's Beneficiaries. A History of Medical Virology in the Netherlands* (Amsterdam: Amsterdam University Press, 2019).
5 https://www.rivm.nl/en/about-rivm/history/timeline-110-years-rivm (Accessed 18/05/2021).
6 M. Verweij and H. Houweling, 'What Is the Responsibility of National Government with Respect to Vaccination?', *Vaccine*, 2014, 32, 7163–7167.
7 RIV later played an important role in global eradication of smallpox by supplying vaccines to the WHO eradication campaign and by acting as a WHO smallpox quality control reference testing the safety and potency of smallpox vaccines from other suppliers to the programme.
8 Pw stands for whole cell pertussis vaccine, to be distinguished from the acellular vaccines (Pa) that would be developed much later.
9 The 2020 Dutch NIP contains vaccines against the following 12 diseases: diphtheria, tetanus, pertussis, polio, rubella, measles, mumps, *Haemophilus influenzae* type b infection, meningococcal disease, hepatitis B, pneumococcal disease, and human papilloma virus infection. A comprehensive timetable detailing the history of the NIP including target groups, vaccines and vaccination schemes, and modifications and year of introduction is provided by van Wijhe, 'Trends in Governmental Expenditure', 5698–5707.
10 There are other special national vaccination programs outside the children's NIP for special risk groups, such as annual influenza campaigns for the elderly.
11 Stuart Blume and Ingrid Geesink, 'A Brief History of Polio Vaccines', *Science,* 2000, 288, 1593–1594.
12 BCG production in bioreactors turned out to be a commercially attractive spinoff from van Hemerts' Unit System. RIV's BCG for bladder cancer is marketed today through the company MEDAC in Germany.
13 L. Schreinemachers *et al.*, 'Intravesical and Intradermal BCG-Application. A Phase I Study to the Toxicity of a Dutch BCG Preparation in Patients with Superficial Bladder Cancer', *European Urology*, 1988, 14, 15–25.
14 B. Montagnon, J. Vincent-Falquet, and B. Fanget, 'Thousand Litre Scale Microcarrier Culture of Vero Cells for Killed Polio Virus Vaccine. Promising Results', *Developments in Biological Standardisation*, 1983, 55, 37–42.
15 Baptiste Baylac-Paouly, Jan Hendriks, and Stuart Blume, 'Polio Vaccine Struggles FAIR and the Failed Reintroduction of Inactivated Polio Vaccine (IPV), 1975–1985', *forthcoming in Social History of Medicine.*
16 J.T. Hendriks, 'Technology Transfer in Human Vaccinology: A Retrospective Review on Public Sector Contributions in a Privatizing Science Field', *Vaccine*, 2012, 30, 6230–6240; J. Hendriks *et al.*, 'Vaccinology Capacity Building in Europe for Innovative Platforms Serving Emerging Markets', *Human Vaccines and Immunotherapeutics*, 2013, 9, 932–936.
17 Stuart Blume and Janneke Tump, 'Evidence and Policymaking: The Introduction of MMR Vaccine in the Netherlands', *Social Science & Medicine*, 2010, 71, 1049–1055.
18 Jan Hendriks and Stuart Blume, 'Measles Vaccination before the Measles-Mumps-Rubella Vaccine', *American Journal of Public Health*, 2013, 103, 1393–1401.
19 In 1989 Joost Ruitenberg left RIVM to become director at the Central Laboratory of the Netherlands Red Cross Blood Transfusion Service (CLB) in Amsterdam.
20 H. Houweling *et al.*, 'Preparing for the Next Public Debate: Universal Vaccination against Hepatitis B', *Vaccine*, 2011, 29, 8960–8964.
21 P. Lelie *et al.*, 'Immunogenicity and Safety of a Plasma-Derived Heat-Inactivated Hepatitis B Vaccine (CLB). Studies in Volunteers at a Low Risk of Infection with Hepatitis B Virus', *American Journal of Epidemiology,* 1984, 120, 694–702.

22 S. Blume, *Interview Joost Ruitenberg,* 1998.
23 The RIV would in 1984 be merged with two national environmental institutions and continue under the acronym RIVM (National Institute of Public Health and Environment).
24 Email of Jan Poolman to the author, 22 November 2020.
25 RIVM, International Vaccine Policy, *Brochure*, 1995, 1–18.
26 M. Beurret, A. Hamidi, and H. Kreeftenberg, 'Development and Technology Transfer of Haemophilus Influenzae Type B Conjugate Vaccines for Developing Countries', *Vaccine*, 2012, 30, 4897–4906.
27 Interestingly, SIIL's cHib vaccine was the second conjugate vaccine ever to be prequalified by WHO on 17 November 2008, only 7.5 months after Sanofi Pasteur's Act-Hib prequalification on 1 April 2008.
28 https://public.tableau.com/profile/supply.division#!/vizhome/UNICEFPricedata-overviewforvaccines/Fulldashboard (Accessed 18/05/2021).
29 E.C. Beuvery *et al.*, 'Vaccine Potential of Meningococcal Group C Polysaccharide-Tetanus Toxoid Conjugate', *Journal of Infection*, 1983, 6, 247–255.
30 B. Greenwood, 'Meningococcal Meningitis in Africa', *Transactions of the Royal Society of Tropical Medicine and Hygiene,* 1999, 93, 12.
31 L. van der Pol, M. Stork, and P. van der Ley, 'Outer Membrane Vesicles as Platform Vaccine Technology', *Biotechnology Journal*, 2015, 10, 1689–1706.
32 K. Cartwright *et al.*, 'Immunogenicity and Reactogenicity in UK Infants of a Novel Meningococcal Vesicle Vaccine Containing Multiple Class 1 (PorA) Outer Membrane Proteins', *Vaccine,* 1999, 17, 2612–2619.
33 The Institute of Translational Vaccinology (Intravacc) represents RIVM's former vaccine research and development unit, created in 2013 as a temporary agency after the government's decision in 2009 to privatize vaccine production.
34 Jan Hendriks and Stuart Blume, 'Why Might Regional Vaccinology Networks Fail? The Case of the Dutch-Nordic Consortium', *Global Health*, 2016, 12, 1–10.
35 Gezondheidsraad, *Vaccinatie Tegen Kinkhoest (summary in English),* The Hague, 2004, 1–117. https://www.gezondheidsraad.nl/documenten/adviezen/2004/04/07/vaccinatie-tegen-kinkhoest-inclusief-addendum (Accessed 18/05/2021).
36 Stuart Blume and Mariska Zanders, 'Vaccine Independence, Local Competences and Globalisation: Lessons from the History of Pertussis Vaccines', *Social Science & Medicine*, 2006, 63, 1825–1836.
37 This move was in fact not so much a real privatization, because the ultimate responsibility for SVM remained in the hands of RIVM's Director General, who formed the Executive Board. Thus, as a matter of governance, RIVM continued to have integral control in the field of vaccines.
38 RIVM (and later NVI) retained historical smallpox vaccine production competence and would after 27 months in 2003 deliver a stockpile of (first generation calf lymph) smallpox vaccines of sufficient potency, quality, and size to vaccinate the entire Dutch population in case of need.
39 Six EU projects against vaccine preventable re(emerging) diseases were realized between 2006 and 2014. They all were based on the principle of a consortium of collaborative public vaccine institutions. Their acronyms were SHERATON INITIATIVE, INSIGHT, FLUSECURE, BIOSAFE, IMECS, and FASTVAC.
40 The IGZ is the national authority under the Ministry of Health that inspects pharmaceutical manufacturers on GMP compliance.
41 The reason for withholding marketing authorization was an insufficient clinical safety data package. NVI had started the study in 2004 after discussing the proposal for a study in about 300 study subjects to the Medicines Evaluation Board. By the time of application in 2008, new EU guidelines for clinical studies had come into force, which required a sample size in the order of 2-3000 subjects, even for 'me-too' combination vaccines, of which the individual components had

already proven safe and effective for many years. Redoing the study would be too costly and very time consuming (*Carla Hoitink, personal communication, 25 November 2020*).

42 The Minister's letter specifies the following priority public interests to be safeguarded after Intravacc's privatization: (a) continued contributions to vaccine development and vaccine improvement, (b) access to critical facilities for vaccine development in case of calamities, (c) worldwide access to affordable vaccines of assured quality, and (d) reduction and replacement of animal experiments.

43 Stuart Blume and Ingrid Geesink, 'Vaccinology: An Industrial Science?', *Science as Culture,* 2000, 9, 41–72.

44 F.E. André, 'Development and Clinical Application of New Polyvalent Combined Paediatric Vaccines', *Vaccine,* 1999, 17, 1620–1627.

45 RIVM's head of vaccine development Jan Poolman became head of SKB/GSK's bacterial vaccine development in 1997 and was strongly involved in SKB/GSK's acellular pertussis containing hexavalent combination vaccine, and their conjugate vaccines MenACWY and PCV10 together now constituting most of the Dutch NIP.

46 Y. Madhavi, 'Manufacture of Consent? Hepatitis B Vaccination', *Economic and Political Weekly,* 2003, 38, 2417–2424.

47 L. Roberts, 'New Polio Vaccine Could Boost Faltering Eradication Drive Sabin's Oral Vaccine Has Itself Become a Source of Polio Outbreaks. A Modern, Stabler Version May Reduce the Risk', *Science,* 2020, 370, 751.

48 R.B. van Noort, 'The Children's Vaccine Initiative and Vaccine Supply: The Role of the Public Sector', *Vaccine,* 1992, 10, 909–910.

49 Jan Hendriks, *Societal Vaccinology: The Netherlands Public Sector Vaccine Development, Production and Technology Transfer in the Context of Global Health,* PhD Thesis (University of Amsterdam, 2017), 1–162.

50 T. Poeloengan *et al.*, 'Developing Country Vaccine Manufacturers Network (DCVMN), 26-27 April 2001, Bandung, Indonesia', *Vaccine,* 2001, 20, 285–287; S. Jadhav *et al.*, 'The Developing Countries Vaccine Manufacturers' Network (DCVMN) Is a Critical Constituency to Ensure Access to Vaccines in Developing Countries', *Vaccine,* 2008, 26, 1611–1615.

51 B. Hayman and S. Pagliusi, 'Emerging Vaccine Manufacturers Are Innovating for the Next Decade', *Vaccine X,* 2020, 5, 100066; S. Pagliusi *et al.*, 'Emerging Manufacturers Engagements in the COVID-19 Vaccine Research, Development and Supply', *Vaccine,* 2020, 38, 5418–5423.

52 An alternative solution was found in Denmark, a comparable country in Europe. While the vaccine production of Denmark's Staten Serum Institute was sold in 2016 to an Arabic investor (now AJ Vaccines), Denmark opted to keep vaccine research and development in the public domain.

53 https://www.intravacc.nl/news/press-release-press-release-intravacc-starts-concept-design-for-multifunctional-vaccine-plant-for-national-requirement/ (Accessed 18/05/2021).

2

THE RISE AND FALL OF STATE VACCINE INSTITUTIONS IN SPAIN (1871–1986)

María-José Báguena and María-Isabel Porras

Smallpox vaccination in Spain was carried out rapidly between 1799 and 1803, but declined through most of the following century. Many explanations have been put forward, including inadequate legislative and institutional frameworks and the generally underdeveloped state of healthcare, itself associated with slow industrialization and political instability.

This began to change in 1871, when, as elsewhere, the first National Vaccination Institute was created to promote vaccination against smallpox. This chapter focuses first on the period from 1871 to 1939, when the Spanish Civil War ended, and then from 1940 to 1986, when Spain's public health system was reorganized by a new General Health Law. The second period covers Franco's dictatorship, until Franco's death in 1975, the re-establishment of democracy and the reorganization of the country's public health system.

Conflicts among healthcare professionals, poor economic and human resources and political decisions all hindered the establishment of up-to-date vaccine producing institutions. We will show that Spain depended on help from international agencies, including the Rockefeller Foundation and the WHO, in establishing institutions in which bacteriology and virology could flourish and where vaccines could be produced. However, public in-house production of vaccines ceased in the 1980s, for the reasons discussed in the introduction to this book.

During the early period, several institutions were founded, some in response to scientific discoveries (e.g., the discovery of diphtheria serum in 1894 led to the National Institute of Hygiene and Bacteriology); or epidemics (the plague epidemic in Oporto in 1899 led to the Alfonso XIII Institute of Serum Therapy, Vaccination and Bacteriology); and some in response to political events (the loss of Spanish colonies in 1898 produced the Institute of Military Hygiene).

Smallpox vaccination and the application of diphtheria serum were the motive for the creation and improvement of Spanish scientific institutions. However,

DOI: 10.4324/9781003130345-3

their success was often compromised by the lack both of resources and political will, irrespective of regime change and economic situation.

The Alfonso XIII Institute was very successful prior to the Spanish Civil War, as were the municipal and provincial laboratories and the Institute of Military Hygiene (IHM), all of which were involved in vaccination policies. So also were the two private laboratories that produced serum and vaccines, created by a group of doctors from the Alfonso XIII Institute after the 1918–1919 flu pandemic. They continued after the Civil War, and a leading figure in the national institutions used one of them to try to produce a vaccine that he had failed to make in the state institution, rebuilt during Franco's dictatorship. The second period witnessed the maturing of Spain's vaccination policies but also the end of public vaccine production.

First State Vaccine Institutions

The National Vaccination Institute (INV) was created by Royal Order of 24 July 1871, at a point in Spanish history, the "six-year revolution" and the first years of the Restoration, when the social situation of the medical profession had improved and smallpox epidemics were common. The new Institute was established under the direction of the Ministry of Development and was also accountable to the Academy of Medicine, which had plans to establish its own Vaccination Centre. It was rarely active, being caught up in endless conflicts, both with the Academy and with the Valencian Medical Institute.[1]

The Valencian Medical Institute was a private scientific corporation promoted by a group of physicians and pharmacists. It gave free smallpox vaccination on its own premises and was a supplier of vaccine lymph to the Spanish King, the Military Health Department, and the General Directorate of Health and Charity. However, it was only in 1894, after fusion with the Medical Pharmaceutical Association (*Asociación Médico-Farmacéutica*), that it was officially recognized by the Ministry of Development. Two years later its vaccination activity ended.[2]

Another obstacle for the INV was the Royal Order of 14 December 1872, recognizing the free market for vaccine, thus giving physicians the right to establish private vaccination institutes without official permission. This decision was probably due to pressure from the medical profession, as well as the State's difficulty in ensuring sufficient production of good quality smallpox vaccine.[3] The first Spanish Republic also established the provincial statistical record of vaccinations, revaccinations, and smallpox cases, although not compulsory vaccination, as in many other countries.[4] However, this did not prevent people from rejecting vaccination, and some medical doctors still mistrusted the vaccine. This was still common in Spain in the early twentieth century: some doctors based their mistrust on German and French scientific literature, as well as on their personal experience.[5]

The last decade of the nineteenth century was crucial for several reasons. It started with the creation of the Central Vaccinological Institute of the Army in 1890, this time independent from the Royal Academy of Medicine.[6] This significant separation foretold other changes. A smallpox epidemic in 1890 led to the Royal Decree of 1891 aiming to overcome resistance to vaccination by involving medical practitioners. In exchange for actively involving themselves in extending smallpox vaccination and revaccination, they were offered considerable benefits.[7]

Also important was Emile Roux's 1894 presentation at the VIII Congress of Hygiene and Demography. Roux presented his results with anti-diphtheria serum, explaining how to produce it in large quantities. His presentation coincided with general acknowledgement of the severity of the diphtheria problem – 50% of infected children died.[8] The impact of Roux's presentation and the possibilities offered by the serum revolutionized the treatment of infectious diseases,[9] favoured hygienists as against clinicians, and encouraged new debates on the need for modernization in the context of the growth of Regenerationism.[10] Diphtheria was the first human disease to fully encompass the bacteriological medicine programme. After isolation of the bacteria, the serum is prepared as a specific treatment, followed by the vaccine as a prophylactic. It is easy to see why, after 1894, some Spanish doctors decided to go to Paris and Berlin to learn the new techniques. Among them was Vicente Llorente who set up the Llorente Institute, the first private laboratory to produce and apply the anti-diphtheria serum in Spain.[11]

The Spanish Government responded by sending a Commission of physicians from the Hospital of San Juan de Dios (Madrid) to Paris and Berlin and resolving to create a National Institute of Bacteriology and Hygiene (Royal Decree 23 October 1894). This was the first national centre of public health and would –as in other countries–be an important locus of bacteriological medicine.[12] The new institute was dedicated to "bacteriological and chemical studies and work applicable to healthcare services, to preventive inoculations against smallpox and other illnesses, to the use and application of all the therapeutic procedures arising from bacteriological knowledge (...)". However, it never really flourished, although the new treatment was authorized by the Royal Board of Health, and the production of anti-diphtheria serum was announced as being one of its responsibilities. In fact, the Bacteriological Laboratory of the San Juan de Dios Hospital was given provisional responsibility for production of the serum. This was due not only to the lack of resources and political support but also to bitter rivalry between ambitious hygienists and well-established clinical doctors. At the same time pharmacists and veterinarians competed with physicians for control of the Institute, unwilling to be mere dispensers of serum and vaccines. Seeing the newly acquired economic and social importance of these resources, they wished to be more actively involved.[13]

Financial concerns also blighted the new Institute. The intention was to use the budget of the INV, money allocated to a planned disinfection centre, plus part of the funds allocated to epidemics. There were concerns that lack of political commitment would lead to inadequate initial funding and that little attention would be paid to the Institute once created. In fact, the National Institute of Hygiene and Bacteriology never went into operation. However, the Government defended its creation as a way to modernize healthcare and to integrate bacteriological medicine into the fight against infectious diseases and thus into public healthcare, as had been done abroad.[14]

In other Western countries, new national health institutes relying mainly on clinical and laboratory technologies, experimental research, and bacteriology were becoming crucial to infectious disease control.[15] Their effectiveness depended on the State's active involvement in healthcare, but also on a willingness to allocate adequate resources. In Spain this proved insufficient for two initiatives taken at the end of the nineteenth century. One was the Institute of Military Hygiene (IHM), founded in 1898, when Spain lost its last overseas colonies. It was the result of the merger of the Central Vaccine Institute of the Army (1890) and the Anatomical-Pathological Institute of the Army (1888), under the Military Health Corps. The other was the Alfonso XIII Institute of Serum Therapy, Vaccination and Bacteriology, created in 1899, as a response to fears generated by the outbreak of the plague in Porto, as well as to pressure from France.[16] Despite initial limitations, this Institute became a key part of the renewal of civilian scientific healthcare in Spain before the Civil War, and of the public production of serum and vaccines, encouraging the development of virology before and after the war.[17] The IHM, meanwhile, was vital for the renewal of military healthcare and occasionally supplied vaccines to deal with civilian needs caused by epidemics. One of the key figures in the improvement of both institutions was the military doctor Manuel Martín Salazar who, after remarkable work in the IHM, moved to the civilian Health Service in 1909. He had considerable bacteriological training, expanded during visits to principal centres in Europe and the United States.

Municipal and provincial laboratories in the production and application of serum and vaccines

The production of serum and vaccines was also introduced into Spain by municipal and provincial hygiene laboratories, which prior to 1930 had their own production capacity. The most important of these were situated in Madrid (established in 1877), Barcelona (1886), and Valencia (1894). The latter two were created specifically for the production of vaccines and serum.

From the beginning the municipal laboratory of Madrid was run by pharmacists, and in 1896, it established an anti-diphtheria Serum Service so that doctors in the ten *casas de socorro*, or health centres, could give the serum (Roux or Behring) to poor patients of municipal charitable institutions. Initially, the serum came from the Pasteur Institute (Paris) and from Germany, and subsequently from the Madrid laboratory.[18] Later, the service was augmented by others, particularly from 1898, when the pharmacist César Chicote was appointed as director. Chicote, who was director until 1932, had previous experience as head of the municipal laboratory of San Sebastian, where he set up an anti-diphtheria service, and from his stay in Paris at the Pasteur Institute, where he learned about rabies vaccines and vaccination. He emphasized the competence of pharmacists to deal with serums and vaccines in his inaugural address to the Royal Academy of Medicine in Madrid.[19] As well as setting up the production and administration of the rabies vaccine, one of his first decisions, faced with the 1900 epidemic in Madrid, was the organization of a service to produce smallpox vaccine.[20]

A new building permitted increased production of various vaccines and serums for typhoid, streptococcus, pneumococcus, tuberculosis, brucellosis, etc.[21] This laboratory also played an important part in the flu pandemic of 1918–1919, by producing one of the vaccines used against the complications of flu.[22] Later new vaccines were added, including that against diphtheria. Changes following the establishment of the Second Republic in 1931, more sympathetic towards health-care matters, resulted in increased production, in turn justifying the foundation of a Vaccination Centre. Together with the Civil Registry a programme was established for the vaccination of new-born babies against smallpox.

The creation of the Barcelona municipal laboratory in 1886 led directly to the establishment of a rabies control service, following Pasteur's development of a rabies vaccine. Initially Jaime Ferrán, known for developing a cholera vaccine, was put in charge. Having developed a different rabies vaccine, he proposed the creation in Barcelona of an Institute similar to the Pasteur Institute in Paris.[23] The Barcelona City Council accepted his proposal and, in 1891, the Municipal Hygiene Institute was created.[24]

In addition to his rabies vaccine, Ferrán produced vaccines against typhus, diphtheria, and plague, but all had side effects, in some cases severe. When someone died after receiving the diphtheria vaccine Ferrán was replaced by the veterinarian Ramón Turró, director from 1905 to 1926.[25] The Institute played a leading role in production and in municipal vaccination policy. In 1917 it established a successful vaccination programme against smallpox for new-borns, and it played an important role during the 1918–1919 flu pandemic.[26] The quality of its work later declined, because the Franco regime marginalized the institute and some of its staff: it did not recover until the end of the regime.[27]

Valencia's Municipal Laboratory was established in 1894 to produce and apply serums and vaccines. Its director was Doctor José Pérez Fuster, who travelled to Paris to learn the techniques of production and application of Émile Roux's anti-diphtheria serum.[28] In 1898 the Republican Party, in control of the city council, set about modernizing Valencia's healthcare making use of the municipal laboratory, while reducing expenditure on disease control and dependence on laboratories elsewhere. Nevertheless, it was not until 1910, when the rabies vaccine was successfully prepared, that municipal services in charge of vaccine research and the various preventive resources were combined.[29] Although it initially required material and training support from the Alfonso XIII Institute and the Madrid Municipal Laboratory, its activity was consolidated in less than two years.[30] From that moment on, production of the rabies vaccine joined the other vaccines – smallpox, cholera, and typhoid – already being manufactured at the Valencian Institute of Hygiene.[31] The institution's activity was curtailed in 1912, when the Republicans lost control of the municipal government, and it was subsequently dissolved.[32] Its director, Pérez Fuster, again assumed the management of the municipal Bacteriological Laboratory, which continued with the immunizations already started and whose staff included Pablo Colvée, who later moved to the new Valencian Provincial Hygiene Institute.

Established in 1916, this new institute took over and extended the work of the old vaccination centre. Vaccines were produced and administered against smallpox, typhoid, rabies, brucellosis, etc.[33] The smallpox vaccine the institute prepared was a dermovaccine. They prepared the typhoid vaccine using the Vincent technique that Juan Peset Aleixandre had learnt in Paris in 1913.[34] The Provincial Hygiene Institute played a significant role during the 1918–1919 flu pandemic, during which it prepared a vaccine from the pneumococcus isolated in infected patients. The application of this vaccine, which was only useful against the complications of flu, was limited. It only became available when the second wave was ending.[35] The Institute's activity continued along similar lines until the arrival of the Second Republic in 1931, when its administrators changed, and its work intensified.[36]

The production and application of serum and vaccines in the Institute of Military Hygiene

The Institute of Military Hygiene (IHM) was established to reduce the mortality of Spanish soldiers from smallpox and typhoid fever. Although its production of serums and vaccines was intended for the military, it occasionally supplied the civilian health service in epidemic situations, such as the 1914 typhoid fever epidemic in Vigo.[37] Because of compulsory military service, it was the IHM that immunized most of the male population against smallpox, tetanus, diphtheria, and typhoid fever. Although the impact of this gendered immunization has not yet been quantified, it was probably significant in a country having no national childhood vaccination schedule until 1975, and with problems in organizing routine immunization lasting some years after that.[38]

Having overcome its initial lack of resources, the Institute grew during the first decade of the twentieth century, with new sections dealing with smallpox vaccination and diphtheria serum, as well as other serums and vaccines. Production of smallpox vaccine, which began in 1891 using a strain from the Military Vaccination Institute in London, continued until 1980 when the WHO declared the disease eradicated worldwide.[39]

Unlike in the civilian sphere, the manufacture of diphtheria serum was delayed until 1900, although it continued until 1964, when the IHM was asked to abandon production and start producing vaccine. This same request applied to anti-tetanus serum, whose manufacture had begun in 1915.[40] This was in response to Spain's introduction of the triple DTP vaccine in 1965, following WHO recommendations. The manufacture of tetanus vaccine ceased in 1990, when the request of the Head of the Vaccine Section to modify the type to be manufactured, in order to comply with WHO recommendations, was declined. This doctor also pointed out the advisability of travelling to national and foreign research centres to study new procedures before adopting them in the IHM. The Army Directorate of Health refused on grounds of expense.[41] In-house production of rabies vaccine in the IMH was also delayed until a Commission of military doctors had visited the Pasteur Institute in 1901 to study its efficacy and procedure. In 1923, it was decided to manufacture the modified Höyges vaccine, which was produced with minor changes until 1967, when it was decided that the Semple vaccine should be used and purchased by the National School of Health (ENS) or by Provincial Health Headquarters.[42]

Faced with the problem of typhoid fevers both in the military and civilian world, the IHM began manufacturing a vaccine in 1913. In 1920 it was replaced by Vincent's N° 2 anti-typhoid-paratyphoid vaccine (TAB), also manufactured at the Institute until 1988. This change required the adaptation of the facilities, with production ceasing a few years later due to inability to comply with national legislation.[43]

Lack of demand and the need to adapt to new types of vaccines and more stringent safety requirements eventually led to a substantial reduction in vaccine production by the IHM. However, attempts were made to prepare new vaccines and the Institute hoped to become an International Vaccination Centre recognized by the WHO, following an Agreement between the Ministries of Health and Defence.[44]

The Alfonso XIII Institute of Serum Therapy, Vaccination and Bacteriology

The Alfonso XIII Institute of Serum Therapy, Vaccination and Bacteriology, renamed the Alfonso XIII Hygiene Institute in 1911, succeeded partly because lessons were learned from the failure of previous civilian initiatives. Thus, the Commission of the Royal Health Council, which drafted the Basic Law providing for the creation of this Institute, consisted of doctors and pharmacists. The planned Institute would also involve participation from all three health professions –medical, pharmaceutical, and veterinary– and doctors from the IHM. Another crucial element in achieving scientific success and international credibility was the appointment of Santiago Ramón y Cajal as director.[45] Although he had not yet received the Nobel Prize, his scientific quality and prestige were beyond doubt, and he enjoyed the support of powerful sectors of the medical authorities in Spain, including that of the university and the College of Physicians.[46]

As a national institution, the Alfonso XIII Institute was justified by the value of bacteriology not only for medicine, but also for the national economy. It provided resources to treat and prevent infectious diseases in humans, but also in livestock and for agriculture. This was in line with other European countries, which saw these national health institutions as valuable instruments of state administration, both for their value in improving the health of the population, and also as source of public revenue.[47] Hence the insistence on the extent of state supervision, because "the cultivation of such highly valued products [could not] be completely abandoned to private initiative and left to the revitalising impulse of scientific interest",[48] referring to serum and vaccines. This was how the Alfonso XIII Institute began to operate. It played a key role at the start of what Rodríguez Ocaña called the "formative" stage of Spanish Public Health,[49] taking on the functions of research, teaching, healthcare, forensic, epidemiological studies, and the production of serum and vaccines, but also of quality control,[50] which was controversial from the beginning. The development of this ambitious programme was very difficult, due to lack of material and human resources, more marked at the beginning, but which continued throughout, given the usual lack of political will against that Cajal had to fight continuously.

In principle, the Institute was divided into three sections: bacteriological analysis and teaching, serum therapy and provision of serums and vaccines, and inoculations and vaccination.[51] In 1900, it officially began with this organizational structure, in a provisional building with inadequate conditions. Its work was only consolidated when its new building, planned in 1901 but without clear allocation of resources,[52] was finally completed in 1914. Fear of epidemics (cholera in Russia in 1907, in Barcelona in 1911, typhus epidemic in Gijón in 1911) encouraged the government to finance its construction. This, together with the national impact of the Nobel Prize awarded to Cajal, the support of the Inspector General of Health, Martín Salazar, the transformation in the medical business with the evolution of World War I and the increased value of serum and vaccines during the 1918–1919 flu pandemic, led to the consolidation and revitalization of the Alfonso XIII Institute. Changes included an increase in the number of Sections and Subsections and new internal regulations, though the Institute's controversial dual function as both producer and regulator of serums and vaccines remained.[53] It was not until 1925 that this was resolved with the creation of the "Technical Institute for the testing of serums and vaccines", later renamed "Institute of Pharmacobiology".[54]

Initially the Institute's main tasks were the production and application of smallpox and rabies vaccines, which became reference services. To manufacture the rabies vaccine, it used the Högyes method, giving better and cheaper results than that of the Pasteur Institute.[55] While anti-rabies immunization became less important for the Alfonso XIII Institute from the 1920s, as municipal laboratories took over the task, the opposite was the case of the smallpox vaccine, because in 1930, the Alfonso XIII Institute was designated as the sole supplier, so that other municipal and provincial laboratories and institutes could focus on smallpox immunization. Later, new vaccines were incorporated to tackle the most prevalent health problems: typhoid, cholera, dysentery, influenza, and tuberculosis.

Tuberculosis was added in 1927 and became more important during the Second Republic, when the government requested an official vaccination service that would allow the vaccine to be administered to all children.[56] Something similar happened with the production of serum, particularly after 1914, as the World War led to restricted access to pharmaceuticals, including serums and vaccines.[57]

Complementing its work in healthcare and as a producer of serums and vaccines, the Institute undertook epidemiological and bacteriological–virological research. It classified the pathogens causing the most important infectious diseases in Spain, including the agents responsible for the 1918–1919 flu and rabies. Research also focused on serums and vaccines, and developed further after the influenza pandemic of 1918–1919, when some of the doctors from the Alfonso XIII Institute created two new private laboratories: THIRF and IBYS,[58] aiming to offset the shortfall in the production of serums and vaccines. Lack of finance and difficulties in arranging imports meant that the Alfonso XIII Institute could not provide the quantities required during the World War I.[59] The two laboratories were merged in 1929 under the name IBYS, which also played a prominent role during the Franco regime, when Florencio Pérez Gallardo directed the Vaccine Section of IBYS at the same time as the Virus Service of the ENS.

In 1920, there was a change in the management of the Alfonso XIII Institute: Cajal was replaced by Jorge Francisco Tello. At that time, despite the shortage of full-time staff and funds to finance its activities, it had improved significantly, enabling Ramón y Cajal to affirm in 1923 that it was as good as the best foreign institutes.[60]

The quality of research had improved considerably, notably in developing new vaccines against smallpox and institutionalizing virology in Spain. The protagonists were Luis Rodríguez Illera, Eduardo Gallardo and Julián Sanz Ibáñez, who travelled widely for advanced training. With the help of fellowships from the Board for Further Studies[61] and the Rockefeller Foundation,[62] they went to the Pasteur Institute, the Robert Koch Institute and the Kaiser Wilhelm Institute in Berlin, the Neurologisches Institut in Vienna, and the Rockefeller Institute for Medical Research in New York. Rodríguez Illera prepared a dermovaccine against smallpox in 1922,[63] while in 1924, Gallardo prepared a neurovaccine that was faster and easier to make, purer than the dermovaccine, and not neurotropic, unlike that prepared by Levaditi.[64] Gallardo's innovation benefited from his having learnt the technique of culturing the smallpox virus in the allantoid membrane of chicken embryos during his stay at the Rockefeller Institute.[65] Gallardo's collaboration with Julián Sanz Ibáñez, who had specialized in tissue culture at the Kaiser Wilhelm Institute and the Neurologisches Institut, was also key to implementing Rivers' method of cultivating vaccinia virus *in vitro*, and that of Woodruff and Goodpasture of culturing it in the chorioallantoic membrane of a chicken embryo.[66] Sanz Ibáñez demonstrated that the latter was preferable to using rabbit serum.[67] This was a key element in the development of virology and the production of viral vaccines, with a great influence on research conducted after the Spanish Civil War.[68]

In short, after overcoming its initial difficulties, the Alfonso XIII Institute became Spain's most important public institution for bacteriological and virological research and for producing serums and vaccines. It also helped introduce new techniques for vaccine production into municipal and provincial laboratories, and it contributed to the relaunch of virological research and vaccine production at the ENS after the Civil War.[69]

Post-Civil War reconstruction and vaccine production in the Franco era

The Spanish Civil War, which began in 1936, curtailed progress in infectious disease control. The Alfonso XIII Institute building was destroyed by bombs, many scientists went into exile, and after the war the Institute was not rebuilt. Instead, institutional leadership was taken by the National School of Health (ENS), which had been founded in 1924 in Madrid, in collaboration with the Rockefeller Foundation. It offered scientific training in public health.[70] However, the work of the ENS suffered a significant decline after the Civil War because it too had lost many of its researchers.[71] Considering reconstruction and reorganization of the ENS to be necessary, in 1941 the regime appointed new personnel, with Gerardo Clavero del Campo as director. It redefined its functions in 1944, now including scientific research, epidemiological work, and the production of healthcare resources, including vaccines.

In the complicated post-war epidemiological situation, marked by the rebound in infectious diseases,[72] the National Health Law of 25 November, 1944 declared "mandatory vaccinations against smallpox and diphtheria" and "the enforceability of preventive vaccinations against typhoid and paratyphoid infections" when appropriate, due to frequent cases of these diseases or epidemics. Likewise, health authorities were told to recommend or impose existing vaccinations against other infections. To meet these demands, it was necessary to restore the production of vaccines, now in the ENS. Aware of public sector limitations, the regime decreed that "subject to prior compensation, the Ministry of the Interior may oblige producers to manufacture specific elements for health campaigns". During the entire Franco era (until 1975), there was no childhood vaccination schedule. Public administration of vaccines was limited to vaccination campaigns, functioning unevenly according to periods and geographical areas. At the same time, there was access to vaccines privately and at certain times through compulsory health insurance. This situation did not always guarantee access to vaccines for the majority of the population, making it difficult to control infectious diseases. Things improved in the mid-1960s, particularly after the first National Polio Vaccination campaign.

Little is known of how the ENS dealt with mandatory bacterial vaccines against typhoid fever, diphtheria, tetanus, and tuberculosis, also manufactured in official laboratories. There is evidence of limitations; and the existence of parallel channels for their administration meant greater expense and reduced effectiveness. This was because preventive and healthcare tasks were separated for political reasons, administration of prevention and public health being the responsibility of the General Directorate of Health of the Ministry of the Interior, while implementation came under the ENS. The latter was politically controlled by the Catholic Church and the military; while healthcare, administratively under the Ministry of Labour, thus in the hands of the Falangists,[73] was provided by Compulsory Health Insurance, which in the 1940s reached only a limited part of the population.

Against that background, in 1951 Spain joined the WHO. Clavero del Campo played a prominent role as a member of the Spanish delegation, as did Florencio Pérez Gallardo as advisor to the delegation.[74] Spain's relationship with the WHO would have to be negotiated: channels for scientific and technical cooperation were needed, and mechanisms regulating Spain's participation in WHO 'projects'.[75] This began with the signing of a Basic Agreement in 1952, initiating scientific and technical collaboration through 21 country programmes, carried out between 1952 and 1975 to tackle major health problems. It also provided access to WHO scholarship programmes, financing not only visits to Spain by WHO consultants to assess the situation and advise on improvements but also training visits for health professionals to leading research centres abroad. This was a key element in trying to correct, at least partially, the decline of science and healthcare after the Civil War.

Of the 21 Spanish collaborative programmes (Country Programmes), we will mention 'Spain 001', (1952–1958), aimed at controlling endemo-epidemic zoonoses, including rabies,[76] and 'Spain 025' (E25), from 1959 onwards, aimed at controlling respiratory diseases of viral origin. They all contributed to re-establishing virological research in Spain and the public production of viral vaccines in Madrid, although it took almost to the end of the Franco period to achieve it, given the lack of material resources, specialized personnel and again, above all, true political will. The leading figure in this renewal of scientific activity was Pérez Gallardo, who enjoyed the favour of the regime through support provided by Clavero del Campo. Pérez Gallardo replaced Eduardo Gallardo at the head of the Virus Service in this new stage of the ENS. It is worth emphasizing that the regime, as befits a centralist state, prioritized institutions located in Madrid over Barcelona when receiving help from collaborative programmes with the WHO, so the public production of viral vaccines took place only in the country's capital, first at the ENS and then at the National Centre of Health Virology and Ecology (Majadahonda, Madrid), also under the direction of Pérez Gallardo.[77]

In 1951, before Spain joined the WHO, the ENS Virus Laboratory, led by Pérez Gallardo, was declared by the WHO as an official national influenza centre. When an epidemic was declared, as in 1957–1958, it began manufacturing influenza vaccine. However, production and application on that occasion was limited. By the time of the 1968–1969 flu epidemic, when the Laboratory had moved into its new building in the centre of Majadahonda, production could be increased.[78] With the help of the rabies control plan, 'Spain E1.3', (1952–1958), and two WHO training grants, the Virus Service at the ENS succeeded in producing a rabies vaccine without adverse neurological side-effects and with more antibodies than other vaccines produced outside Spain.[79] However, as in the case of flu vaccine, quality and quantity of production only improved when, thanks to improvements provided by the E25 programme, the Pilot Centre at the National Centre of Health Virology and Ecology became operational in 1968.[80]

Although in the mid-1950s poliomyelitis became a serious social problem, the Franco regime would not acknowledge it. Unlike neighbouring European countries, Spain had not started immunizing with the Salk vaccine. Spain's medical science and economic conditions made it impractical. However, morbidity continued to rise and finally, on 28 December 1957, it was decided to introduce the Salk vaccine in Madrid through the National School of Childcare, albeit limited and not free.[81] In this context, the Spanish government asked the WHO to sign the E25 programme, although it did not mention that the reason was the need for major improvements to tackle poliomyelitis. The plan's objective was to carry out epidemiological studies on viral diseases of importance for public health, as well as the development of laboratory virological diagnostic services and the technical training of personnel. With these objectives, the E25 programme came at the right time for the country to prepare a polio vaccination campaign.[82] Pérez Gallardo wanted to produce his own polio vaccine like Pierre Lépine at the Pasteur Institute, with the help of the Juan March Foundation and funds from the General Directorate of health.[83] Between 1958 and 1960 he produced experimental polio vaccines, both inactivated and attenuated, at the ENS Virus Laboratory. The lack of suitable facilities and personnel prevented production being scaled up to an industrial level, since WHO quality guidelines could not be followed.[84] As a result, the first national campaign in 1963 to vaccinate children under seven with the Sabin oral vaccine had to be done with a vaccine provided by foreign and by private Spanish laboratories. Among the latter, a leading role was played by the Llorente Institute, which, as indicated earlier, had been the first to produce antidiphtheria serum in Spain at the end of the nineteenth century, and by IBYS laboratories, where Pérez Gallardo directed the vaccine section and was negotiating with Albert Sabin to produce his vaccine. However, Sabin felt that conditions in the laboratories were unsuitable to produce the vaccine, so it would just be bottled there.[85] The 1963 national polio vaccination campaign was very successful, but opting for this strategy, rather than establishing a childhood vaccination schedule, limited its effectiveness.[86] In fact, the first childhood vaccination schedule was only established in Spain in 1975 and the last case of polio occurred in 1988. However, the success of the 1963 campaign encouraged the health authorities to decide, in 1965, that vaccination campaigns against polio should be linked with diphtheria, already united with tetanus and pertussis in the combined DPT vaccine, following WHO recommendations.

In 1963 the Virus Service was expanded and became the National Virus Centre at the ENS. Its facilities were still very poor, as was the smallpox vaccine produced there, as Colin Kaplan, WHO consultant for vaccine production, noted during a visit in 1964. In his report he found that the premises where the Centre stabled the calves and obtained the vaccines were totally inadequate. The technique used was described as primitive.

Kaplan's report and the confirmation of the inadequacy of the facilities led in 1967 to the establishment of the National Centre of Health Virology and Ecology in a new building in Majadahonda. Also, under the direction of Pérez Gallardo, one of its functions was the production of smallpox vaccine. The vaccines produced from then on had to comply with standards the WHO had set in 1965. Products would have to be effective, sterile, and with a set expiry date.[87] Accordingly another building was erected within the National Centre of Health Virology and Ecology, the so-called "Pilot Centre", to produce and distribute vaccines, starting with smallpox and rabies. During the 1968–1969 influenza pandemic flu vaccine was also produced. Staff received grants from the WHO for training in virology techniques in foreign laboratories.

In the new centre vaccines were produced using animals, so three independent buildings were needed to handle them. The first housed quarantined animals. Adjacent were the facilities for the inoculation of animals with the virus, from which infected tissues were extracted after incubation. Separately, the facility also had rooms for the breeding of small laboratory animals.

Once the tissues with the virus were obtained, they were transferred to another building, the real "pilot", where the manufacturing and research processes were carried out on viral vaccines. Inspired by the facilities of the Karolinska Institute in Stockholm, it carried out the trituration of the tissue; inactivation of the viruses; and their purification, packaging, and labelling. Elsewhere, the potency of the vaccine was checked. This consisted of two areas, the first for smallpox vaccine and the second for rabies and other vaccines manufactured on a sporadic basis, such as that of influenza.[88]

In March 1968, Pérez Gallardo asked the Directorate General of Health to centralize the production of smallpox and rabies vaccines in the "Pilot Centre", given the quality of its facilities, which had now received the approval of Kaplan, and the training of its staff, which was carried out in Spain. Among other advantages, he observed that this would avoid the dispersion of credit given to the Provincial Headquarters of Health. He produced a comparative economic study of the production of smallpox and rabies vaccines in the Centre and in commercial laboratories, showing the economic benefits of production at the "Pilot Centre": here, the price per dose of smallpox vaccine was 0.27 pesetas, while in the Llorente Laboratory it was 1.38 pesetas. It was therefore suggested that orders be given that the two vaccines should no longer be manufactured in Provincial Health Headquarters. The Directorate General of Health approved this proposal in July 1968. After the official eradication of smallpox in 1980, obligatory vaccination against it ended in Spain. The Centre maintained vaccine production until its closure in 1982.

The National Virology Centre also conducted research on other viral diseases (rubella, measles, mumps) with the support of WHO through the E25 plan, but did not produce vaccines. These were purchased from private laboratories for the pilot rubella campaign in 1975, for the first national campaign for rubella vaccination (1977) aimed at 11-year-old girls, following WHO recommendations, and measles vaccinations after these were introduced in the vaccination calendar at nine months of age.[89] The WHO guideline was to administer the measles vaccine at 12 months, followed by mumps, and then by rubella, thus expanding the Expanded Programme on Immunization that had started in 1974.

In 1978, the Spanish press announced that the WHO recommended, for the first time, use of a trivalent vaccine for the subsequent season. In 1981, the combined triple viral vaccine (measles, mumps, and rubella) was included in the vaccination schedule to be administered at 15 months. It was imported from the United States for administration in primary care centres, after the transformation of the health-care model that had started in the period known as the Transition,[90] culminating in 1986 with the new General Health Law and the establishment of the National Health System, administered by the different Autonomous Communities that have made up Spain since the 1978 Constitution. 1981 was a pivotal point in the process of prevention of these three diseases. The list of notifiable diseases had been modified, incorporating diseases such as tetanus, pertussis, mumps, and rubella, given their epidemiological importance. In April a new vaccination calendar was announced including as a novelty the vaccine against mumps and rubella at 15 months, together with that of measles. In 1984, its sale in pharmacies was authorized for use in the private sector. Subsequently, a second dose with triple viral vaccine began to be administered to all 11-year-old boys and girls, but its introduction was uneven among the different Autonomous Communities, as a consequence of diversity in the transfer of responsibilities in Public Health between 1979 and 1985, Catalonia being the first to introduce it in 1978.

In Spain, vaccination is not mandatory. Currently, vaccines included in vaccination schedules, which have been expanding in recent years (14 vaccines were part of the lifelong Common Vaccination Calendar recommended in 2019) are 100% covered by public funds. For economic reasons there has been no vaccine production in public laboratories since the late 1980s. Autonomous Communities, responsible for public health since the 1980s, can obtain vaccines through agreements signed with the Government for the centralized purchase of vaccines.

Final remarks

In conclusion, the official production of vaccines in Spain encountered many difficulties from the start, some of which continued during practically the whole period studied. The initial creation of scientific institutions to incorporate bacteriology and with the capacity to produce vaccines was hindered by a lack of resources and a lack of political will, but also by conflicts of interests among medical professionals, and between them and the pharmacists and veterinarians. It was necessary to overcome the reticence of clinically oriented doctors to the introduction of the laboratory into the management of infectious diseases. Later, when the power of serums and vaccines against these pathologies became clear, the new field attracted the attention of pharmacists and veterinarians. Both – particularly the former – thought that they were better suited than physicians to oversee production. This called for negotiation and a division of labour among the three healthcare professions, as well as between civilian and military health authorities. Moreover, they had to overcome the opposition of the Royal National Academy of Medicine and of the directors of the leading medical journals, who lost power to the representatives of the fledgling Official Colleges of Physicians and the faculties of medicine.

Once all this had been achieved, state production of smallpox vaccine began, followed by other vaccines as they were developed and introduced to Spain. This was thanks to grants from international agencies, financing the specialist training of staff in foreign laboratories. The overall story, from the start of vaccination till the present day, is in some ways like that of other countries discussed in other chapters. However, Spain differs from other West European countries in that maintenance of the level of public production of vaccines was subject to the country's political vicissitudes. Ideology and administrative structures led to support being intermittent rather than sustained, leading to shortages of material resources and, even more frequently and seriously, of full-time well-trained personnel. These deficiencies prevented the optimal use of available facilities and equipment. Although the Spanish government understood that national production of serums and vaccines could be an important source of income, for most of the period prior to 1936, with the exception of its last 10 years, these deficiencies prevented the fulfilment of expectations. Spain remained dependent on the supply of resources from the main producing countries. Through the establishment of private laboratories by some of the health professionals from the Alfonso XIII Institute at the end of the World War I, it was hoped to increase the production of serums and vaccines to meet Spanish demand.

The Spanish case also shows the negative impact of the Civil War, not only in the destruction of material resources and the impoverishment of the country at the end of the war, but also in the serious scientific decline that came with the establishment of the Franco dictatorship. The resulting loss of the best scientists and health professionals, exiled or purged, seriously diminished Spain's ability to carry out public production of vaccines and serums. This was particularly the case for viral vaccines, given the greater complexity of their production. As before the Civil War, the support of international scientific and health organizations (this time the WHO) was again needed to overcome difficulties, and to adequately equip modern state vaccine institutions with material and personnel. Only in the late 1970s did production of vaccines reach international scientific standards. However, once again the lack of political will and of sustained adequate funding prevented the manufacture of all the viral vaccines necessary to attend to the public health problems present in Spain at the time. The support of private Spanish laboratories was once again necessary to complement the production of vaccines, but the country still depended on external supplies, now from foreign private pharmaceutical laboratories, to supply vaccines against polio, rubella, measles or mumps, of which Spain never had its own public production.

When, in the 1980s, under new political circumstances, Spain managed to modernize its health system, with capacity for producing (with certain limitations) and applying vaccines, the eradication of smallpox and the effect of world changes subsequent to the spread of neoliberal politics led to the end of state vaccine production in Spain. Subsequent mergers of pharmaceutical laboratories also led to the total disappearance of private vaccine production in the country. Under the impact of the avian flu of 1997 and the SARS epidemic in 2003 attempts were made in 2006 to modify the situation by establishing an agreement between the Ministry of Health and Berna Biotech Laboratories to install a factory to produce influenza vaccines in Madrid. This agreement came to nothing, as did the attempt with ROVI Laboratories to locate a flu vaccine factory in Granada at the time of the 2009–2010 flu pandemic. Both these failed attempts at public/private collaboration were cancelled for economic reasons.

The importance of vaccine production in the context of the current Covid-19 pandemic, with its tremendous impact on all levels of society, has rekindled the debate on the need for a properly endowed public health system and the importance of sufficient public funding, continued over time, to maintain quality scientific research, capable of responding more effectively to situations such as the current health crisis.

The interruptions to research into coronaviruses that some Spanish groups of recognized international prestige had begun years before, due to cuts in funding, could have been avoided. As in other countries, several of these groups are now developing vaccines against Covid-19, but the road they have to travel is longer and more complicated than it might have been. This final example succinctly sums up what happened throughout the period under review, and in the two distinct stages: first, from the beginning until the Spanish Civil War, and then from reconstruction until reaching maturity in the eighties, now in democracy.

Acknowledgements

This research has been produced within the context of the project "The standardization and application of serums and vaccines in Spain and Castilla-La Mancha and the role of international agencies (1918-2016)", financed by the Board of Community of Castilla-la Mancha–FEDER Funds (ref. SPBY/17/180501/000382).

Notes

1 Ricardo Campos-Marín, 'La vacunación antivariólica en Madrid en el último tercio del siglo XIX. Entre el especialismo médico y el mercantilismo', *Medicina e Historia*, 2001, 4, 1–15; Ricardo Campos-Marín, 'El difícil proceso de creación del Instituto de Vacunación del Estado (1871–1877)', *Asclepio*, 2004, 56, 79–109; María-Isabel

Porras-Gallo, 'Luchando contra una de las causas de invalidez: antecedentes, contexto sanitario, gestación y aplicación del Decreto de vacunación obligatoria contra la viruela de 1903', *Asclepio*, 2004, 56, 145–168.
2 María-José Báguena-Cervellera, 'El Instituto Médico Valenciano y la difusión de la vacuna', *Asclepio*, 2004, 56, 63–77.
3 Porras-Gallo, 'Luchando'.
4 Axel C. Hüntelmann, 'Smallpox vaccination in the German Empire. Vaccination between biopolitics and moral economy', *Asclepio*, 2020, 72, 292.
5 Arturo Balaguer-Mayo, *Vacunación de los recién nacidos* (Madrid: Imprenta J. Corrales, 1908).
6 Patrocinio Moratinos-Palomero, *Algunos datos para la Historia del Instituto de Medicina Preventiva «Capitán Médico Ramón y Cajal» (Instituto Anatomopatológico de Sanidad Militar)* (Madrid: Ed. Romagrof, 1988); Francisco Martín-Sierra, *Instituto de Medicina Preventiva de la Defensa "Capitán Médico Ramón y Cajal" 125 años de historia* (Madrid: Imprenta Ministerio de Defensa, 2010).
7 Porras-Gallo, 'Luchando'.
8 J. Guerra-Estapé, 'El Doctor Emilio Roux y la difteria', *Annals de l'Acadèmia de Medicina de Barcelona*, 1933, 367–390.
9 Esteban Rodríguez-Ocaña, 'El tratamiento de la difteria en la España de la segunda mitad del siglo Diecinueve', *Medicina e Historia*, 1994, 54, 21–28; Esteban Rodríguez-Ocaña, 'La producción social de la novedad: el suero antidiftérico, «nuncio de la nueva medicina»', *Dynamis*, 2007, 27, 33–44.
10 Regenerationism: an intellectual and political movement in late 19th and early 20th century Spain, seeking objective scientific explanations for Spain's decline as a nation, and possible remedies. María-Isabel Porras-Gallo, 'Antecedentes y creación del Instituto de Sueroterapia, Vacunación y Bacteriología de Alfonso XIII', *Dynamis*, 1998, 18, 81–105; María-Isabel Porras-Gallo, 'El Instituto Nacional de Higiene de Alfonso XIII: origen, creación y labor desempeñada', in Alfonso V. Carrascosa and María-José Báguena, eds, *El desarrollo de la Microbiología en España. Volumen I* (Madrid: Fundación Ramón Areces, 2019), 69–103.
11 Instituto Llorente, *70 años de trabajo en el campo de la inmunoterapia: 1894 suero antidiftérico, 1965 vacuna oral antipoliomielítica* (Madrid: Instituto Llorente, 1966).
12 Paul Weindling, 'Scientific elites and laboratory organisation in *fin de siècle* Paris and Berlin: The Pasteur Institute and Robert Koch's Institute for Infectious Diseases compared', in Andrew Cunningham and Perry Williams, eds, *The Laboratory Revolution in Medicine* (Cambridge: Cambridge University Press, 1992), 170–188.
13 Porras-Gallo, 'Antecedentes y creación'.
14 Porras-Gallo, 'Antecedentes y creación'.
15 José-Luis Barona, *Health Policies in Interwar Europe. A Transnational Perspective* (London: Routledge, 2019), 57.
16 Channelled by letter from Dr Brouardel, Head of the French Health Service and Dean of the Medical Faculty of Paris, to Dr Carlos María Cortezo, Directorate General of Health. Gaceta de Epidemias, *El Siglo Médico*, 1899, 2384, 573–575, 574.
17 María-Isabel Porras and María-José Báguena, 'The role played by the World Health Organisation country programmes in the development of virology in Spain (1951–1975)', *Historia, Ciencias, Saude – Manguinhos*, 2020, 27, 187–210.
18 J. Madrid-Moreno, *El Servicio del Suero Antidiftérico en el Ayuntamiento de Madrid* (Madrid: Imprenta Municipal, 1898).
19 César Chicote-Rego, *La vacuna anticolérica. Discurso de ingreso en la Real Academia de Medicina* (Madrid: Establecimiento Tipográfico Jaume Ratés Martín, 1911).
20 César Chicote-Rego, *Las vacunas y los sueros del Laboratorio Municipal* (Madrid: Imprenta Municipal, 1916).
21 *Ibid.*
22 María-Isabel Porras-Gallo, *La Gripe Española, 1918–1919* (Madrid: Libros de la Catarata, 2020).

23 Porras and Báguena, 'Role played by the WHO'.
24 Antoni Roca-Rosel, 'La higiene urbana com a objectiu: notes sobre la història de l'Institut Municipal de la Salut (1891–1936)', in Antoni Roca-Rosell, ed, *Cent Anys de Salut Pública a Barcelona* (Barcelona: Ajuntament de Barcelona, 1991), 75–103.
25 María-José Báguena, 'Jaume Ferrán' in José-María Camarasa and Antonio Roca, eds, *Ciència i Técnica als Països Catalans: una Aproximació Biogràfica* (Barcelona: Fundació per a la Recerca, 1995, vol.1), 652–679.
26 Esteban Rodríguez-Ocaña, 'La grip a Barcelona: un greu problema esporàdic de salut pública. Epidèmies de 1889–90 i 1918–19', in Antoni Roca-Rosell, ed, *Cent anys*, 131–156.
27 Porras and Báguena, 'Role played by the WHO'.
28 María-José Báguena-Cervellera, 'La microbiología', in José-María López Piñero *et al.*, eds, *Las Ciencias Médicas Básicas en la Valencia del siglo XIX* (Valencia: IVEI, 1988), 251–254; Gabriel Bernat-Condomina, 'El Ayuntamiento de Barcelona y la inoculación del suero antidiftérico en 1895', *Medicina e Historia,* 1991, 38, 6–28.
29 María-José Báguena-Cervellera, 'El Cuerpo Municipal de Sanidad de Valencia y la lucha contra las enfermedades infecciosas. El caso de la rabia', in Carmen Barona-Vilar *et al.*, eds, *Polítiques de Salut en l'àmbit Municipal València (1850–1936)* (Valencia: SEC, 2000), 71–109.
30 María-José Báguena-Cervellera, 'La prevención de la rabia y la sanidad municipal en Valencia (1894–1916)', *Cronos*, 1998, 1, 135–142.
31 *Ibid.*
32 *Ibid.*
33 Juan Peset-Aleixandre, 'El Instituto Provincial de Higiene de Valencia. Primer quinquenio de su funcionamiento (1916–1920)', *Anales de la Universidad de Valencia*, 1922–1923, 3, 453–475; Carmen Barona-Vilar, *Las Políticas de la Salud. La Sanidad Valenciana entre 1855 y 1936* (Valencia: Publicaciones de la Universidad de Valencia, 2006), 120–151.
34 Peset-Aleixandre, 'Instituto Provincial', 460–462.
35 María-Isabel Porras-Gallo, 'Sueros y vacunas en la lucha contra la pandemia de gripe de 1918–1919 en España', *Asclepio*, 2008, 60, 261–288.
36 Barona-Vilar, *Las políticas*, 143–151.
37 Manuel Martín-Salazar, *Críticas del estado actual de la vacunación antitífica* (Madrid: Imprenta y encuadernación Valentín Tordesillas, 1915).
38 María-Isabel Porras-Gallo *et al.*, *El Drama de la Polio. Un Problema Social y Familiar en la España Franquista* (Madrid: Libros de la Catarata, 2013).
39 Martín-Sierra, *Instituto de Medicina*, 84.
40 *Ibid.*, 85–94.
41 *Ibid.*, 94–95.
42 *Ibid.*, 89–90.
43 *Ibid.*, 86–90.
44 *Ibid.*, 13–14.
45 Gaceta de Epidemias, *El Siglo Médico*, 1899, 11.2284, 573–575, 574; Noticias, *El Imparcial*, 30 de agosto de 1899, 3.
46 Ramón y Cajal was close to Julián Calleja, Dean of the Faculty of Medicine of Madrid and President of the Madrid College of Physicians.
47 As Barona notes, these national institutions should be understood as the political response of liberal states when bacteriology had revealed its power to control infectious illnesses, and was opening the way to the international health movement. Barona, *Health policies*, 18–87.
48 Ministerio de la Gobernación. Dirección General de Sanidad, *Real Decreto de creación del Instituto de Sueroterapia, Vacunación y Bacteriología de Alfonso XIII y Reglamento para su aplicación* (Madrid: Imprenta Sucesora M. Minuesa de los Ríos, 1900), 7–11.

49 Esteban Rodríguez-Ocaña, 'La Salud Pública en la España de la primera mitad del siglo XIX', in Juan Atenza-Fernández and José Martínez-Pérez, eds, *El Centro Secundario de Higiene Rural de Talavera de la Reina y la Sanidad Española de su Tiempo* (Toledo: JCCM, 2001), 21–42.
50 Ministerio de la Gobernación, *Real Decreto de creación*, 7–11.
51 *Ibid.*, 7–11.
52 Grases, *Proyecto de un Instituto Nacional de Higiene* (Madrid: Establecimiento Tipográfico de E. Teodoro, 1901), 12.
53 This demand, particularly prominent during the influenza pandemic of 1918–1919, was supported using the example of Germany. Francisco Murillo, 'Necesidad de la intervención fiscalizadora del Estado en el comercio de los sueros medicinales', *Boletín del Instituto de Sueroterapia, Vacunación y Bacteriología de Alfonso XIII*, 1907, 11, 133–145, 140; Luis Siboni, 'Debate parlamentario sobre el Presupuesto de Sanidad', *La Farmacia Moderna*, 1920, 8, 97–100.
54 Javier Puerto, 'Instituto de Biología y Sueroterapia IBYS', in Antonio González-Bueno and Alfredo Baratas-Díaz, eds, *La Tutela Imperfecta. Biología y Farmacia en la España del Primer Franquismo* (Madrid: CSIC, 2013), 341–384.
55 Lucía Lebrero-Menéndez, *El Instituto Nacional de Higiene de Alfonso XIII* (Madrid: Facultad de Medicina, Universidad Complutense de Madrid, tesis doctoral inédita, 1984).
56 Lebrero-Menéndez, *Instituto Nacional de Higiene*, 84.
57 Porras-Gallo, 'Instituto Nacional de Higiene'.
58 Porras-Gallo, 'Sueros y vacunas'; Porras Gallo, *Gripe española.*
59 Puerto, 'Instituto de Biología'.
60 Santiago Ramón y Cajal, *Recuerdos de mi Vida: Historia de mi Labor Científica* (Madrid: Alianza Universidad, 1984), 211–212.
61 This was a Spanish institution created in 1907 to encourage the development of scientific research and education in Spain, headed by Cajal until his death in 1934.
62 María-José Báguena, María-Isabel Porras and María-Victoria Caballero, 'Innovación, producción y circulación de vacunas contra la viruela y la polio en España (1918–1963)', in Ricardo Campos *et al.*, eds, *Medicina y Poder Político* (Madrid: SEHM/Facultad de Medicina, 2014), 197–202; María-José Báguena-Cervellera, 'La producción y difusión de las vacunas en España: la vacuna antivariólica', in José Luis Barona and Ximo Guillem, eds, *Sanidad Internacional y Transferencia del Conocimiento. Europa, 1900–1975* (Valencia: PUV, 2015), 85–106; Esteban Rodríguez-Ocaña, 'Eduardo Gallardo Martínez y los inicios de la virología científica en España', in Ricardo Campos *et al.*, eds, *Medicina y poder político* (Madrid: SEHM/Facultad de Medicina, 2014), 467–472.
63 Luis Rodríguez Illera and Eduardo Gallardo, 'Del empleo del virus testicular de Noguchi como semilla para la vacunación de las terneras', *Archivos del Instituto Nacional de Higiene Alfonso XIII*, 1922, 1, 179–188.
64 Eduardo Gallardo, 'Valor práctico de la neurovacuna', *Archivos del Instituto Nacional de Higiene Alfonso XIII*, 1924, 3, 111–124.
65 Báguena-Cervellera, 'Producción y difusión', 94–97.
66 Eduardo Gallardo and Julián Sanz, 'Subcutaneous Smallpox vaccination with bacteria-free vaccine', *American Journal of Epidemiology*, 1937, 25, 354–361.
67 Báguena-Cervellera, 'Producción y difusión', 96.
68 Porras and Báguena, 'Role played by the WHO'.
69 The Alfonso XIII Institute of Hygiene also contributed to the introduction of virology into the Faculty of Medicine in Valencia after the Civil War. María-José Báguena-Cervellera, 'Estudios epidemiológicos y virológicos sobre la poliomielitis en Valencia (1959–1969)', *Asclepio*, 2009, 61, 39–54.
70 Josep-Lluis Barona, *The Rockefeller Foundation, Public Health and International Diplomacy, 1920–1945* (London: Routledge, 2015); Esteban Rodríguez-Ocaña, 'Por razón de ciencia. La Fundación Rockefeller en España, 1930–1941', in Ricardo Campos *et al.*, eds, *Medicina y Poder Político* (Madrid: SEHM/Facultad de Medicina, 2014), 473–477.

71 José-Luis Barona and Josep Bernabéu-Mestre, *La Fundación Rockefeller y la salud pública en España. En: La Salud y El Estado: el Movimiento Sanitario Internacional y la Administración Española (1851–1945)* (Valencia: PUV, 2008), 89–142.
72 María-José Báguena and María-Isabel Porras, 'La situación epidemiológica de las enfermedades víricas y los programas colaborativos de la OMS con España (1952–1986)', in María-Isabel Porras-Gallo, Lourdes Mariño-Gutiérrez and María-Victoria Caballero-Martínez, eds, *Salud, Enfermedad y Medicina en el Franquismo* (Madrid: Libros de la Catarata, 2019), 72–97.
73 The Falange Española was a fascist political party, and the only legal party under Franco.
74 Rosa Ballester, *España y la Organización Mundial de la Salud en el contexto de la historia de la salud pública internacional (1948–1975)* (Valencia: Real Academia de Medicina de la Comunidad Valenciana, 2016); Rosa Ballester, 'España y la Organización Mundial de la Salud. La cuestión española y la puesta en marcha de políticas y programas de salud pública (1948–1970)', in María-Isabel Porras *et al.*, eds, *Salud, Enfermedad y Medicina en el Franquismo* (Madrid: La Catarata, 2019), 43–56.
75 OMS, *Los Diez Primeros Años* (Ginebra: Organización Mundial de la Salud, 1958), 150.
76 María-José Báguena and Lourdes Mariño, 'Economía y salud: costes y beneficios de la erradicación de la viruela en España mediante la vacunación (1959–1982)', in María-Isabel Porras *et al.*, eds, *La Erradicación y el Control de las Enfermedades Infecciosas* (Madrid: Libros de la Catarata, 2016), 158–159.
77 Porras and Báguena, 'Role played by the WHO''.
78 Mercedes Ramírez and María-Isabel Porras, 'La vacunación contra la gripe y sus complicaciones en España (1918–2009)', in Ricardo Campos *et al.*, eds, *Medicina y Poder Político* (Madrid: SEHM/Facultad de Medicina, 2014), 191–195; María-Isabel Porras and Mercedes Ramírez, 'La lucha contra la gripe en España a través de las relaciones con la OMS (1951–1971)', in Alfonso Zarzoso and Jon Arrizabalaga, eds, *Al Servicio de la Salud Humana: la Historia de la Medicina ante los Retos del siglo XXI* (Sant Feliu de Guixols: SEHM, 2017), 109–115; María-Isabel Porras and Mercedes Ramírez, 'Los efectos de la pandemia de 1918–19 en la lucha contra la gripe en España: el papel de los cambios de percepción del riesgo y la posterior creación de la OMS', in Antero Ferreira, ed, *A Gripe Espanhola de 1918* (Guimaraes (Portugal): Casa Sarmento-Universidad do Minho, 2020), 13–34.
79 Rafael Nájera, 'Florencio Pérez Gallardo 1917–2006', *Revista Española de Salud Pública*, 2006, 80, 605–608.
80 Porras and Báguena, 'Role played by the WHO'.
81 María-Isabel Porras and María-José Báguena, 'La lucha contra la enfermedad mediante las campañas de vacunación en Madrid, Valencia y Castilla-La Mancha (1958–1975)', in María-Isabel Porras-Gallo *et al.*, eds, *El Drama de la Polio. Un Problema Social y Familiar en la España Franquista* (Madrid: Libros de la Catarata, 2013), 141–169.
82 This was one of the reasons given by the WHO consultant, Dekking, to justify the E25 programme. F. Dekking, 'Rapport sur une mission en Espagne (14 Octobre-15 Novembre 1959) par le Docteur...', EUR-Espagne-25. AT-292.54 (WHO Archive, Geneva, Switzerland, 1959).
83 'La ayuda "Ciencias médicas"', *ABC*, 1958, 2 April, 26.
84 Florencio Pérez Gallardo, *Estudios sobre la Epidemiología y la Profilaxis de la Poliomielitis en España. Informe Final de la Ayuda de Investigación: Grupo de Ciencias Médicas. Año 1958* (Madrid: Fundación Juan March, 1961).
85 María-Victoria Caballero-Martínez, *La Poliomielitis en España y Europa desde los inicios de la Vacunación hasta su Erradicación en la Región Europea (1955–2002)*, PhD thesis (Universidad de Castilla La Mancha, 2017).
86 María-Isabel Porras and María-José Báguena, 'El conocimiento sobre la realidad de las campañas de vacunación contra la polio, su cobertura y su seguimiento en las capitales y provincias españolas (1963–1975)', in Enrique Perdiguero-Gil, ed, *Política, Salud y Enfermedad en España: entre el Desarrollismo y la Transición Democrática* (Elche: Universidad Miguel Hernández, 2015), 170–215.

87 Báguena-Cervellera, 'Producción y difusión'.
88 Carlos J. Domingo Fernández and Gerardo Contreras Carrasco, 'Los tiempos del piloto', *Anales de la Real Academia Nacional de Medicina,* 2006, 123, 747–757.
89 María-Isabel Porras and María-José Báguena, 'El papel desempeñado por los médicos, el gobierno y la OMS en la implementación de las encuestas serológicas sobre polio, sarampión y rubeola en España (1958–1978)', *Asclepio,* 2020, 72, 294.
90 It started on 20 November 1975, when Franco died, and ended with the accession to power of the PSOE (Partido socialista obrero español) in 1982.

3

POLITICS OF VACCINATION IN SWEDEN

The National Bacteriological Laboratory SBL (1909–1993) and current debates

Motzi Eklöf

This chapter deals with Sweden's vaccine policy, specifically vaccine production in the National Bacteriological Laboratory, prior to its closure. Today neither Sweden nor any other Nordic country produces vaccine for national use – although this could change as a result of the Covid-19 pandemic.

Two state bacteriological laboratories were established in Sweden: one for human medicines in 1909 and one for veterinary medicine in 1911. Although the relationship with veterinary medicine is part of the history, the focus here is on the production of human vaccines in the period of 1909–1993. Soon after its foundation the name of the laboratory was changed to *Statens bakteriologiska laboratorium* (SBL). The laboratory was initially under the supervision of the country's highest medical authority, the Royal Medical Board (RMB) (with roots in the 1600s Collegium Medicum, in 1968 reorganized as the National Board of Health and Welfare). From 1954 SBL was an independent agency.

During the laboratory's first decades, the bacteriological preparations were handcrafted on a small scale, unlike the more industrial production in, for example, Germany and France. Early years saw a number of 'incidents' related to the production of diphtheria antitoxin (1916) and smallpox vaccine (1932). It was not until mid-century that the laboratory found real public success, with its own polio vaccine (IPV) developed as a competitor to the Salk vaccine. After the Swedish national childhood vaccination programme started in the 1940s and expanded rapidly thereafter, SBL met the country's entire need for vaccines, whether through manufacture or import.

In close collaboration with the nearby *Karolinska Institutet* (KI), SBL became a research node for the country's microbiologists, many of whom worked there. The laboratory's activities were broad, ranging from diagnostics, epidemiology, research, and production, through control, sales and to distribution. Whilst this breadth of coverage was seen as a strength by SBL, outsiders regularly questioned

DOI: 10.4324/9781003130345-4

it, and the laboratory was subjected to one investigation after another. Criticism of the laboratory's premises, animal husbandry, and production conditions has been recurrent. There have occasionally been tense relations between the parliament, the government, the RMB, independent experts, and SBL. And while the laboratory sought to expand, other actors highlighted the importance of other infectious disease control measures, including hygiene, contact tracing, isolation, and quarantine.

Eventually, the arguments for separating vaccine production from other disease control activities prevailed. In 1993, the laboratory was divided into a production company, SBL Vaccin AB, and a new Centers for Disease Prevention and Control. Some staff and much of the microbiological research were transferred to KI. Since then, further reorganization of infectious disease prevention and control has taken place, and vaccine production has ceased. In recent decades only marginal vaccine production has taken place at SBL vaccine, such as travel vaccine against cholera.

★

This chapter follows Swedish vaccine production from its beginnings until Sweden's response to the Covid-19 pandemic that began in 2020. The chapter is divided into three time periods, each with specific core topics. The first (1880–1950), largely based on unpublished archival material, deals with the establishment of the state laboratories and the first production and use of diphtheria antitoxin and smallpox vaccine. The second (1951–1993) includes the story of the Swedish polio vaccine. The third section discusses reorganizations and discussions on vaccine production from 1993 to 2020. Sweden is a geographically extended and thinly populated country. The character of and relations between the few persons in the small world of relevance here have always been of importance, which justifies a certain degree of naming.

Some questions regularly recur. First, would it be better for Sweden's serum and vaccines needs to be met within the country by a state laboratory or a private company, or would the country be better served by relying on imports? Whether a state laboratory should be subject to a higher medical authority has also been a recurring issue. It has provoked public debates and disputes about the right path to take regarding infectious disease protection and vaccine production. Should there be a separate production unit for serum and vaccine, or should production be combined with diagnostics and research and development work? Should bacteriological preparations be treated as pharmaceutical products or have a special status, and if so, on what grounds? Voices in the parliament and from animal welfare associations have questioned the housing and welfare of animals used for the bacteriological work, though this discussion played little or no role in discussions of the laboratory's organization or its serum production.

1880–1950

When the first Nobel Prize in medicine was awarded in 1901, the KI chose to give it to the German bacteriologist Emil Behring,

> for his work on serum therapy and especially its use against diphtheria, thereby breaking a new path in the field of medical science and giving the doctor a victorious weapon in the fight against disease and death.[1]

Especially in Germany, France, and the United States, industrial serum production grew, laying the foundation for many of today's large pharmaceutical companies. The approaches to serum preparation and the results were regularly published in medical journals, enabling several competing companies to enter the industry.[2] In Sweden, too, bacteriology began to be institutionalized, though on a more modest scale. There was no private company that could immediately start industrial-scale production of anti-diphtheria serum as in Germany, nor any scientific institute built around a prominent researcher, as in France. In the later years of the nineteenth century, several small laboratories were established at the medical and veterinary institutions, and the RMB inaugurated its own bacteriological laboratory. At KI a bacteriological section within the pathological-anatomical department opened in 1895.

Bacteriologists from Sweden, few in number, travelled to Germany and France to learn the methods of serum production. KI Associate Professor Edvard Selander paid study visits to the Pasteur Institute and to hospitals in Paris. In the autumn of 1894, together with the doctor and bacteriologist Ernst Levin, he purchased four horses that would be immunized with diphtheria toxin.[3] In the same year, Thure Hellström at the newly established Stockholm epidemic hospital, also tested the new treatment. He first used foreign serum, from, among others, Behring and Roux, but later obtained better results with Selander's serum.[4]

The creation of two state laboratories 1909 and 1911

In 1896, the medical professor and Swedish Member of Parliament Curt Wallis, one of the introducers of bacteriology to Sweden, suggested that a larger state institution, to produce serum against various infectious diseases, was needed.[5] The RMB proposed that the government should look into the question of a state medical facility for epidemiological studies, bacteriological diagnostic investigations, and the manufacture of therapeutic bacteriological agents and vaccines.[6] A state institution would be able to provide serum at a lower cost than private producers, and would be better able to control the funds involved.

The investigation and proposal from 1899 pointed out that research was primarily the task of universities and colleges, and that a state laboratory would primarily meet the practical needs of the RMB.[7] The importance of a state institution to produce bacteriological preparations was stressed, as was state control over the production.

However, it took 10 years before the proposal began to take form. Meanwhile, in 1902, the first regulations came into force regarding state control of all anti-diphtheria serum sold in the country, via a regulator appointed by the RMB, Professor Carl Sundberg.[8]

The long delay was due to differences of opinion among politicians about how it would be organized and what its tasks and governance would be, as well as between representatives of human and veterinary medicine. The two medical faculties in Lund and Uppsala (at this time the only universities in the country) as well as KI did not want to see the new institution subject to the RMB. They considered that such a 'relationship of subordination' was inconsistent with the authority that the institution needed, both given the importance of its functions and in relation to foreign countries.[9] It was also considered inappropriate for the director of the institution to be both manufacturer and regulator, which could jeopardize trust on the part of doctors and the public. From a medical point of view, there was also a risk of infection if the same personnel were to carry out both diagnostic examinations and serum manufacture. The veterinarians, on their part, wanted an independent position in relation to human medicine.

After parliamentary debate, the proposal was reduced to an institution with only two departments: one bacteriological and one forensic.[10] In April 1909, Alfred Pettersson was appointed as the director of the medical-bacteriological department together with an assistant and a veterinary assistant. The laboratory first occupied a few rooms on Regeringsgatan 18 in central Stockholm, and then in 1913 moved to five rooms at the top floor of the building on Vasagatan 15–17 near Stockholm Central Station. These were leased premises in privately owned apartment buildings, from the outset considered by the director to be too cramped and unsuitable for their purpose. Smaller animals such as mice, guinea pigs, and monkeys were kept there (on one occasion a monkey escaped into the town), while calves for vaccine production and horses for serum preparation were housed elsewhere.

In 1911, the Swedish parliament approved a veterinary bacteriological institute, the main focus of which would be diagnosis of bovine tuberculosis and the manufacture of tuberculin. The institution was a separate unit, not integrated with the state medical institution, though initially also subordinate to the RMB.[11]

Serum production questioned

When SBL was established, the first few horses were purchased for the production of anti-diphtheria serum, but it took several years before there was any serum for distribution. Meanwhile private serum production continued.

Carl Kling worked both at SBL and as a doctor at Stockholm epidemic hospital. In June 1916, he alerted the RMB that an infant at the hospital had died of tetanus after an injection of anti-diphtheria serum from the laboratory.[12] Shortly after four more children in other hospitals also fell ill, though they survived. RMB immediately terminated the use of the serum and requested an investigation of what happened and of the conditions in the laboratory.

In the spring of 1916, anti-diphtheria serum from only one horse had been available. The mare had been drained of blood only once before she fell ill and died of tetanus. According to manager Alfred Pettersson, serum had been tested on a guinea pig that survived, after which serum was distributed, even after the horse died.

After a very critical report by Inspector Sundberg, all production of anti-tetanus serum at the facility was terminated. Pettersson was sent to court on charges of misconduct and causing another's death by the RMB. The Board requested the government to allow the Veterinary bacteriological laboratory to take over the production of serum against tetanus. However, after strong protests from the medical community, SBL was able to resume production in 1917, whilst Pettersson was merely fined 100 SEK for misconduct. Once again a unified institution, to include the veterinary laboratory, was discussed but rejected by the veterinarians. Moreover, both veterinarians and the medical community wanted more independence from the RMB.

The years following the resolution of the 'serum scandal' remained turbulent for the laboratory. In 1917 the RMB issued new regulations for the laboratories and for inspection and control. Alfred Pettersson moved to a professorship at KI, Carl Kling became acting director, and the laboratory changed its name to SBL. Selander's private serum production was closed down – put out of business by the RMB that priced serum at well below the manufacturing costs.[13] His former colleague Ernst Levin saw possibilities however, and in 1917, he started his private Swedish Serum Institute.

Carl Kling characterized the period from 1919 to 1924 as 'a troublesome state of uncertainty, continuous worries and repeated moments of almost excruciating suspense'.[14] In 1919, new official inspections of SBL premises and stables once again resulted in severe criticism. The hygienic conditions of both animals and production were rejected. It was in effect the stable foreman who managed serum production from horse to bottle.[15] The RMB noted that in no single year from 1910 to 1918 had the laboratory been able to meet the country's need for serum.[16] Serum had had to be purchased from Germany, from Selander, and since the autumn 1918 from Levin's new Serum Institute. Kling held the laboratory's subordination to the RMB responsible for the problems and demanded better premises. The government and the head of the Ministry of Civil Affairs, Carl Svensson, also highlighted other measures as important in the fight against infectious diseases.[17] While bacteriologists and serologists focused on serum and vaccine, Svensson, in parliament in 1920, pointed to measures that would prevent diseases from entering the country and spreading. They included quarantine and observation facilities, ambulatory doctors, and equipment. During the 1918–1919 influenza epidemic (the 'Spanish flu'), when approximately 38,000

Swedes died, measures were taken to keep social distance, and theatres, schools, and cinemas were closed. Kling and SBL produced and tried vaccination material for prevention and treatment of the flu, but without decisive results. Kling wrote of his doubts on this very uncertain business but found it worth a try, due to the serious circumstances.[18]

In 1920, an investigation committee pointed out that Levin's private Serum Institute produced serum in larger quantities and of better quality than SBL.[19] The fact that it took so long to obtain anti-diphtheria serum from the state institution was attributed to both the manager and the staff lacking experience with serum production. Manufacturing had been a loss-making venture. The investigation suggested a split of SBL: education in bacteriology should be taken over by the colleges, and SBL could be absorbed into KI's bacteriological laboratory. However, the proposal to completely terminate state production of serum was strongly opposed by the medical community, and in 1924, the government formally decided against implementing the committee's proposals. SBL's premises were slightly expanded, the staff was increased, the equipment modernized, and Kling became the ordinary director.

Smallpox vaccine and mandatory vaccination

In 1816 Sweden became one of the first countries to implement mandatory smallpox vaccination for all children. Until the beginning of the twentieth century, arm-to-arm vaccination was conducted mainly by midwives, church bell-ringers, and other specially appointed inoculators.[20] In the 1900s, the disease was no longer endemic in the country, and occasional imported cases caused only minor outbreaks with few secondary cases.

In other countries the transfer of lymph from humans to cow to 'regenerate' the vaccination material had been tried much earlier. In Sweden it was only in 1884 that the city physician in Stockholm, Klas Linroth, tried to produce animal lymph with calf vaccine from the State Institute in Brussels.[21] One argument in favour of animal vaccine was that this inoculation material 'with complete certainty' could not transmit diseases such as syphilis and tuberculosis, now recognized as a risk when vaccinating with human material.[22]

In 1909, the new state laboratory took over responsibility for preparing animal inoculations. The serum 'scandal' of 1916 meant that the following year the Medical Board issued the first instructions regarding the production and also control of animal inoculation against smallpox. The vaccine would be produced with material from natural cowpox or real smallpox. After laboratory analyses, the strength of the inoculum would be tested – not on guinea pigs as for serum, but on 'arms'. These usually came from orphanage children at the *Allmänna barnhuset* or other children in Stockholm.[23]

As in 1916, a new law on smallpox vaccination replaced earlier provisions. Doctors were made responsible for the vaccination, which was not popular either among them or with the previous lay vaccinators.[24] A clause was introduced that allowed anyone who could demonstrate personal experience of adverse effects of vaccination, to be granted exemption by the RMB. This was not a 'conscience clause' like the one in England, introduced in two stages in 1898 and 1907, and used so diligently that vaccination coverage there declined radically.[25] In Sweden, 'conscientious objections' was not a valid reason for exemption. Peter Baldwin describes the Swedish modified vaccination act in 1916 as the abolition of the obligation.[26] In practice though, the RMB and the government did not grant any exceptions in the early years, and eventually only a few.[27]

Regulations for bacteriological preparations

The year 1914 can be taken as the starting point of Swedish drug control. The State pharmaceutical laboratory (SFL) was set up to control drug quality and carry out supervision under the Pharmacy goods charter. This law of 1913 defined pharmaceutical goods and controlled the goods that were manufactured at and dispensed through the pharmacies. In Sweden, serum and vaccines were defined as 'bacteriological preparations' until the 2000s, while, e.g., in the United States, they were included in the broader category of 'biological preparations' already at the beginning of the 1900s. The preparations continued to be treated on a side-track alongside other pharmaceuticals, produced from other types of raw materials. In 1925, new regulations were issued for the preparation and testing of serum and other bacteriological preparations.[28] They concerned control and trials in the laboratory, but there was still no regulatory framework for clinical trials. In 1927 SBL obtained exclusive rights on the sale of bacteriological preparations and in 1934 exclusive rights on the import of such preparations.[29] However, there was still no monopoly on production.

Tuberculosis and BCG vaccine

Anders Wassén was employed at SBL between 1921 and 1924, when he became director of the city of Gothenburg's bacteriological laboratory. After bringing home a BCG strain from Paris in 1926, he began to test the vaccine. At the same time, and continuing into the 1930s, Carl Naeslund conducted parallel vaccination attempts in the north of Sweden. Having noted reduced mortality rates among vaccinated compared to unvaccinated children, he noted that several possible explanations for this, including non-specific immunological effects, were conceivable.[30] Starting in 1927 Arvid Wallgren, senior physician at Gothenburg children's hospital from 1922 to 1942, vaccinated children from tubercular environments with vaccine produced in Gothenburg. His procedure differed from that used in France, involving a lower dose and intradermal instead of subcutaneous injection.

In 1930, 251 children in the German city of Lübeck were vaccinated with BCG. A total of 77 died and another 131 fell severely ill. Though BCG vaccination ended in Germany, Swedish doctors continued vaccinating, even though most of the Swedish medical profession was sceptical of the procedure and concerned by the risk of side effects. In 1942, however, Wallgren recommended vaccination of all new-borns, conscripts, and health workers, and in 1950, more than 90% of all new-borns were vaccinated. Sweden was then self-sufficient with BCG vaccine. Only five years later, however, Wallgren suggested that the mass vaccination should be discontinued in Scandinavia, as so few now benefited from it.[31] He felt that improved living standards, socio-economic improvements, early diagnosis, and more effective treatment were of greater importance. Nevertheless, infant vaccination – considered such a simple and inexpensive measure – continued until 1975. Pulmonary specialist Ingela Sjögren had then demonstrated several cases of osteitis (bone rot) and argued to end general BCG vaccination. Legal proceedings followed, with parental claims for damages. Since then, only children in families at risk have been vaccinated, now with vaccine based on another strain.

Problematic mass vaccination against smallpox in Malmö 1932

Around the turn of 1931–1932, a small smallpox epidemic that occurred in the city of Malmö in southern Sweden was traced to a worker who had returned from work in the Urals. The infection affected 10 people of whom one died.[32] The initial measures with attempts at contact tracing, vaccination, and isolation of contact cases proved insufficient. When the infection spread, a mass vaccination in the city and the surrounding area was carried out.

On 15 February 1932, the Royal Medical Board called off the vaccination campaign. At that time, a large part of the population was already vaccinated, many due to the earlier law on mandatory vaccination. However, the reason for halting vaccination was that several cases of encephalitis, brain inflammation, had been identified, and some of them were fatal. That smallpox vaccination could lead to post-vaccinal encephalitis that had been known since the 1920s, but was considered to be due to individual factors rather than the vaccine itself. In addition, a relatively large proportion of the inoculated showed other problems after vaccination, with swellings and large deep necrotic pox on the arm that could take weeks, and (as it turned out later) months to heal, in addition to work-inhibiting general symptoms of various kinds.

The vaccine from SBL became the focus of a deep conflict between various experts in bacteriology, pathology, and hygiene. Director Carl Kling at SBL and city doctor in Malmö, J. Axel Höjer, were not fully cooperative when the RMB tried to clarify how the vaccine was produced and what had caused the side effects. A veterinarian and bacteriologist in Malmö, Hilding Magnusson, pointed out that there was a large amount of pus bacteria, *Staphylococcus aureus*, in the vaccine. Kling argued that this was of no significance, that the vaccine was 'excellent', and that they obviously chose to send 'strong' vaccine when faced with epidemic threats. It was said to be made from calves, as was customary.

It has not been possible to determine exactly what kind of vaccine was used in Malmö. However, at the beginning of the epidemic, Kling had announced that a vaccine produced via the rabbit brain could be delivered at short notice. Rabbit vaccine, so-called neurovaccine (which was thereafter not mentioned in connection with the story of Malmö), had been tested elsewhere during the 1920s. Positive results had been reported from some countries, including Spain. Some other countries, including the Netherlands, had stopped using this kind of vaccine due to severe side effects, Kling reported years later.[33]

The question of the importance of the so-called 'Begleit'-bacteria was sent by the RMB to *l'Office International d'Hygiène Publique* (1907–1946, forerunner to WHO), which did not consider the complications in Malmö to be remarkable, given the number of vaccinations. However, where several countries set the maximum concentration of bacteria in the vaccine – at this time, for example, 5000 per cubic centimetre in England – the Swedish vaccine from SBL could contain up to several million bacteria.[34]

Aftermath

After the vaccination story in 1932, the vaccine manufacturing at SBL was inspected and once again found unsatisfactory. The Parliament now granted funds for a new laboratory. In 1937, newly built larger premises for the laboratory and its animals were inaugurated in Solna in the outskirts of Stockholm, and new regulations were issued for a rapidly expanding business.[35]

The debacle surrounding the Malmö vaccination resulted in a revision of the Vaccination Act. There were also reports from doctors around the country describing both vaccination side effects and extensive vaccination refusal. An investigation published in 1937 was not in agreement. A majority suggested that child vaccination should be voluntary. In order to combat epidemics, isolation, contact tracing, and vaccination of the contacts were considered as sufficient measures – only if one lost control of the contact cases would mass vaccination be needed. However, a minority proposed continued compulsion. The medical community was mobilized to advocate for continued mandatory vaccination, and few physicians dared to express a different opinion.[36] In 1939, with a very small majority in Parliament, it was decided to continue with mandatory vaccination.

Thereafter vaccination was transferred to the newly established maternity and childcare centres, where other voluntary vaccinations were soon introduced. This was considered both rational and psychologically correct, and maternal resistance to vaccination decreased. Nevertheless, in 1958, it was estimated that only about 10% of the population had sufficient protection against smallpox. From 1959, the possibility of exemption in the event of 'serious concerns' against vaccination was increased.

In 1943, the serum against diphtheria was succeeded by diphtheria toxoid – a modified version of diphtheria antitoxin inactivated with formalin and heat – and vaccination against diphtheria became general in the country. Three years later, the manufacture of tetanus toxoid began. In 1952, the bacterial triple vaccine was introduced – against diphtheria, tetanus, and whooping cough.

New activities and regulations

The veterinary bacteriological laboratory was never united with SBL. In 1944, it was transferred from the RMB to the Ministry of Agriculture, reorganized and changed its name to the State Veterinary Institute (*Statens Veterinärmedicinska Anstalt* [SVA]), still at work. On 1 July 1947, the Veterinary Board was established, which took over the supervisory role from the RMB.

An investigation in 1942 suggested (again) that domestic serum production could be discontinued and instead be purchased (though perhaps not under the current war and crisis conditions), and that the doctors in the laboratory could to some extent be replaced by (cheaper) pharmacists.[37] However, production continued.

In 1945, Kling was succeeded by Gunnar Olin as director of SBL, which expanded with new departments, research groups, and the production of new products. In 1946, a virological department was added, that manufactured influenza vaccines as well as other vaccines. Three years later a defence medical laboratory was also established.

1951–1992

Growing interest from the pharmaceutical companies

The emerging national pharmaceutical industry wanted a uniform pharmaceutical legislation and considered that special rules for bacteriological preparations thwarted such a development. To form a united force, the Pharmaceutical Industry Association was formed in 1951 by several companies, including Astra, Pharmacia, and Kabi. The Parliamentary State Committee of 1952 questioned the constant expansion of SBL.[38] Instead, to save money, parts of the production could be transferred to the pharmacies or the pharmaceutical industry. From a cost point of view, research should be better coordinated with similar activities elsewhere. Furthermore, the state's audit did not consider it justified that the similar production of human and veterinary medicinal products was divided between SBL and the SVA. The production of bacteriological serum and vaccines was once again investigated, and a reorganization was proposed, so that SBL would receive its own Supervisory Board.[39] SBL still did not want to separate diagnostics and manufacturing, nor did it want to release the research to the companies. This was not least because of the Swedish polio research. Sven Gard and co-workers were working on developing their own polio vaccine and were dependent on close relations with the hospitals.[40] The parliament approved the proposal, and in October 1954, the half-century old demand that the laboratory be emancipated from the RMB was finally realized. SBL became an independent authority with now more than 300 employees and new statutes.[41] Also, after a major outbreak of salmonella in Sweden in 1953, emanating from a slaughterhouse in Alvesta, an epidemiological department and a state epidemiologist were established at SBL in 1955.[42]

As the national child vaccination programme developed further, after the introduction of the bacterial triple vaccine, the laboratory was given a central role. SBL was almost the sole supplier of human bacteriological preparations, partly through its own production and partly through other manufacturers inside and outside the country. During the 1950s SBL produced among others; bacteriological vaccines against diphtheria, tetanus and whooping cough, dysentery, staphylococcal infections and typhoid/paratyphoid, as well as viral vaccines against influenza, smallpox, and polio.

The Swedish polio vaccine

Scandinavia was one of the first regions to suffer from polio epidemics in the late nineteenth century. In 1905, the first nationwide polio epidemic irrupted. The disease was little understood. The first comprehensive study of cases and spreading patterns was done by Ivar Wickman, who concluded that it was an infectious disease that was spread by contact. These conclusions were based on clinical observation and mapping.[43] Wickman admired the German orthopaedist Jacob von Heine and the Swedish researcher Oskar Medin and suggested that the disease should be called Heine-Medin's disease, which also had an international impact. During the next major polio epidemic in Sweden in 1911–1913, together with colleagues, Kling studied how the infection entered the human body, on the basis of among other things, experiments on monkeys. Together with Constantin Levaditi at the Pasteur Institute, Kling showed that viruses were present in and could spread through the secretions of the mouth, nose and throat, and the intestinal system, causing paralysis. Other scientists, including Simon Flexner of the Rockefeller Institute, dismissed the Swedish research and considered at this time that the virus was airborne. Kling continued with polio research in 1927 on behalf of *l'Office International d'Hygiene Publique*.[44] In 1952, professors Sven Gard, Gunnar Olin, and Tore Wesslén began work at SBL on developing their own vaccine together with the City of Stockholm's bacteriological laboratory and the Department of Viral Research at KI.

On 12 April 1955, Jonas Salk in the United States presented a vaccine with inactivated virus (IPV), and vaccinations started. A vaccine that was launched as effective and safe also raised high hopes in the Swedish media. However, the first more extensive vaccination in the United States led to some production problems, inadequate inactivation, and some deaths. Sven Gard had criticized Salk's methods for disabling viruses as inadequate at an earlier international polio conference in Rome, but not been heard.[45] After the 'Cutter incident', the American vaccination campaign was temporarily stopped.

Only seven days after Salk's vaccine was launched, Gard and Olin presented a Swedish IPV – inactivated at other temperatures, based on other viral strains, and cultured on human tissue. Most countries used monkey tissue for virus research, but at SBL, viruses were grown on lung tissue from legally aborted foetuses from Stockholm hospitals, aborted in the second trimester.[46] These foetuses were used for the first Swedish vaccine. In Sweden there was a reluctance also at ministerial level to use tissue from monkeys due to possible undesirable immunological effects, but in 1956, in order to increase production, SBL switched to kidney tissue from monkeys. But a foetus from Stockholm, sent to The Wistar Institute in 1962, became the cell line WI-38, which since has been used to produce several types of vaccine.[47]

After news of polio vaccine production failures in the United States reached Sweden, plans for a wider launch of the Swedish vaccine were paused. It wasn't until 1957 that polio vaccine was used for nationwide vaccination for all ages, with Swedish vaccine produced on tissue from monkeys. Because in the first year SBL couldn't produce enough vaccine, this was supplemented with imported vaccine from the American company Eli Lilly. The Swedish vaccination programme reached close to 100 percent coverage, excluding some regions with more sceptical populations. After 1963 there were very few cases of polio in the country. In 1965 polio vaccination was included in the national child immunization program.

Whilst in the 1960s most countries switched to Sabin's live attenuated vaccine (OPV), Sweden, like the Netherlands, chose to stick to IPV, and has done so ever since. As an explanation for Sweden's choice of IPV, polio historian Per Axelsson leans towards Stuart Blume's notion of path dependency and lock in – the Swedish researchers had invested both knowledge and finances in a particular production method, and in addition, the control of live vaccines is more tedious. The proud Swedish tradition of polio research may also have weighed in when one chose to stick to one's own method. An additional explanation may be that Sweden's well-developed drainage system spared the country from the spread of polio via live (vaccine-derived) viruses in faeces. Today, imported IPV vaccine from Sanofi Pasteur is used.

The last years of smallpox vaccination

In 1963, a smaller smallpox epidemic occurred in Stockholm via a previously multiply vaccinated person, whose disease was not detected before it had spread to several people. Vaccination of a six-digit number of inhabitants was quickly organized.

In 1953 SBL discontinued the production of calf lymph and tried other methods, but without success. Between 1955 and 1957, production had been suspended. In addition, it had become difficult to have vaccines tested on children, possibly, according to SBL, a result of the public smallpox vaccinations having been replaced by vaccination at childcare centres.[48] Nevertheless, in 1967, SBL sold both Variola calf vaccine and ditto egg vaccine. The Swedish research on smallpox vaccine continued until just a few years before mandatory vaccination ended in 1976.[49] Although the scientifically published statistics were unknown to the public at the time and there are figures lacking for several years, a compilation of available data shows that there were at least 126 cases of post-vaccinal encephalitis after smallpox vaccination in the years 1924–1975 of which 15 had a deadly outcome. In the same time span, 38 cases of smallpox occurred with 4 deaths.[50] However, a comparison of endpoints is misleading, as the disease would almost certainly have spread significantly more without vaccination.

Further proposals for the reorganization of vaccine production

Even though it was primarily SBL that manufactured bacteriological preparations in Sweden, there were no legal or principled obstacles for the private pharmaceutical industry to engage in such manufacturing. In the 1950s, Sahlgrenska hospital in Gothenburg produced BCG vaccine. Veterinary bacteriological preparations were produced at SVA and to some extent at a veterinary bacteriological laboratory in Malmö. However, the partly state-owned pharmaceutical industry began to show more interest in bacteriological and similar preparations.

In 1957, a study presented three different proposals concerning the location of the production of bacteriological and virological preparations. One was to have an enhanced cooperation between SBL and SVA to rationalize production. Another was to retain the status quo with production at both laboratories. The third proposal, from SBL, was for a separate unit for production methods that had left the first stage of trials.[51]

In 1960, a new study found that with a few exceptions (such as immunoglobulins) SBL had not for a long time contributed significantly to the development of the field. The resources of the 1950s had mainly been focused on polio vaccine. The investigators believed that other vaccines, such as against measles and mumps developed abroad, would not receive general use, but only be prescribed for certain groups or on certain indications.[52] The investigators, including the head of SBL, suggested that all manufacturing should be transferred to a single production department. This happened in 1962, with new premises five years later. The fact that SBL could maintain its own production was justified by economy and contingency reasons. The domestic pharmaceutical industry did not consider that it could produce competitively, given that there were no import restrictions. In 1966, an immunological department was also added to SBL.[53]

In the second half of the 1960s, plans for state pharmaceutical manufacturing were introduced. At the end of 1969 a critical report on SBL influenced the development of events. The report had first been classified 'confidential' by the Interior Ministry but was later released.[54] The assignment had been given to Bertil Åberg, professor of clinical chemistry and since 1969 head of research at the pharmaceutical company AB Kabi (and before that head of the clinical laboratories at the School of Veterinary Medicine). It concerned issues of common interest to SBL and Kabi.

The production conditions at SBL received scathing criticism. The immunological department suffered from 'outrageous difficult premises conditions', and Åberg suggested that the department 'urgently' build new and adequate premises. Of the department for viral vaccines, he wrote:

> that drug inspectors would never approve SBL as a supplier of vaccines. Some of the current animal houses that I visited are such that no farmer would dream of keeping their animals in such conditions. Countries requiring inspection by suppliers of medicinal products and vaccines would thus never be able to approve SBL's products before a complete re-equipment of SBLs premises.[55]

There were plans for provisional premises for virus vaccine production above an animal house, which would never be approved by, for example, FDA inspectors. The United States and other countries would thereby be excluded as export markets. Several pharmaceutical companies already were or would become joint stock companies, while SBL was an authority governed by the principle of public access, which meant that production methods and research results could not be kept secret. Åberg proposed that the production at SBL be transformed into a joint-stock company with its own board of directors, to include representatives of other companies of the (partly state-owned) pharmaceutical group. In the media debate that followed, SBL's director emphasized that the issue should not be viewed from a narrow business perspective. It had to be recognized that from a societal view SBL's responsibilities were broader. In addition to the production of bacteriological preparations, its tasks also included diagnostics and epidemic surveillance.[56] No measures were taken.

A proposed relocation of SBL to Umeå in northern Sweden was met by fierce resistance from the laboratory and was not pushed through. An investigation presented in 1978 once more proposed splitting the institution to create an independent production unit, a state vaccine institute. One justification given was that the state control of human bacteriological preparations was still considered insufficient.[57] The Parliament rejected this proposal. In 1984 another committee instead proposed that the production should remain mainly within SBL.

Pharmaceutical control including bacteriological preparations

In the 1960s, more careful regulation of Swedish drug manufacture began. Prior to 1962, there were no paragraphs concerning adverse reactions in Swedish pharmaceutical legislation. At that time the thalidomide tragedy raised serious concerns: pregnant women, having taken a prescribed relaxing drug (in some countries Softenon, in Sweden named Neurosedyn) gave birth to children with missing limbs. The Ministry of the Interior developed regulations that, among other things, stated that a medicinal product, under normal conditions of use, should not have harmful effects that were in disproportion to the intended effect.[58] Rules on clinical trials were not created until 1963, such as, among other things, requiring the manufacturer to perform adequate pharmacological and toxicological tests on animals before switching to humans. Two years later, a Drug Side Effect Board was added, which was later replaced by a permanent national side effect committee. A new pharmaceutical regulation came into force in 1964.[59] 'Bacteriological preparations' became a sub-group of pharmaceutical specialties with requirements for special control procedures. In 1966, WHO established regulations for national control of bacteriological preparations. The production method was to be approved by a National Control Authority, and each stage of the production process for each individual product was to be described in writing. The Swedish recommendations for production hygiene in pharmaceutical production shifted the focus from final control of the finished product to an emphasis on process control, a starting point for good manufacturing practice.

As proposed already in 1946, Sweden's pharmacies were nationalized in 1971, and the previous RMB, since 1968 the National Board of Health and Welfare (NBHW), received a pharmaceutical department. In 1972, an amendment to the Swedish pharmaceutical regulations meant that the bacteriological preparations were subject to virtually the same requirements as other pharmaceuticals. They must be registered with the NBHW, whose state inspector was responsible for control, and adverse reactions were to be reported to the committee on adverse drug reactions. In the same year, an inspection agreement was signed between the NBHW and the FDA in the United States, which included serum and vaccines. In his otherwise critical report, Åberg had stated that SBL still had a 'significant goodwill' abroad, including regarding hygiene in pharmaceutical production.

In 1990, the newly created Medical Products Agency (*Läkemedelsverket*) took over the control of pharmaceuticals from the NBHW, and in 1992, a new pharmaceutical act replaced the one from 1964, subsequently revised in 2015.[60]

New vaccines

Meanwhile vaccines against measles, mumps, and rubella had been developed abroad. As mentioned, there was initially scepticism among some paediatricians and microbiologists in Sweden regarding these becoming standard vaccinations for all children – measles was considered by some not to be sufficiently serious to justify universal vaccination. The debate became public. Doubts also concerned the preference for live or inactivated virus vaccine. Concerns were vented by Sven Gard who suggested that vaccination with live virus could contribute to the later development of multiple sclerosis (MS).[61] It was said that measles vaccine would be suitable for certain groups or in some cases, but not for all children. Nevertheless, after several years of discussions, the measles vaccine was incorporated into the child vaccination programme in 1971, and in 1982, along with rubella and mumps, the triple vaccine was introduced. Since then, measles has appeared only sporadically as imported cases, and extensive outbreaks have been avoided, thanks to high vaccination coverage.

The bacterial triple vaccine was introduced in the 1950s, but in 1979, the vaccination against whooping cough with whole bacterial cells was terminated, as the vaccine was considered too weak, and there had been adverse reaction reports from the United Kingdom. Stopping vaccination resulted in a steep increase in the number of cases, but also the possibility to carry out studies on pertussis vaccine, in a developed country with access to unvaccinated children who could constitute a control group.[62] SBL tested a Japanese acellular vaccine that would cause fewer side effects, and the U.S. authorities also wanted to cooperate with Sweden as they themselves could not carry out controlled tests. The tests also interested the WHO since as a government agency, independent of major commercial interests, SBL had high international status. A total of about 100,000 children were enrolled in studies led by Patrick Olin. Not until 1996 was general vaccination with pertussis vaccine reintroduced in Sweden.

In the 1970s and 1980s SBL and Swedish vaccinologists and epidemiologists were increasingly active in international work on infectious disease control. Among other things, the laboratory participated in the WHO's child vaccination programme, in the campaign against tuberculosis, and the smallpox eradication campaign, in which SBL manager Holger Lundbäck played an important role.

1993–2020

The end of SBL as SBL

The all-encompassing activities of SBL, including diagnostics and epidemiological surveillance, as well as the production of bacteriological preparations, were increasingly questioned. There was a conflict of interest if the same agency were advising the government on vaccination and at the same time manufacturing and marketing vaccines. Added to the long-lasting problems concerning capacity, hygiene, and security at the vaccine production sites, crisis was approaching.

The beginning of the end of SBL was not a result of neoliberal politics and globalization – these had an impact on later developments. Instead, it was a social democratic Minister of Social Affairs, Gertrud Sigurdsen, who in 1988 appointed a new director of SBL. The new director, Hans Wigzell, was some years later given the task of writing a report on future organization of disease control and vaccine production. Vaccine production had been losing money in recent years, new vaccines were in an introductory stage, and SBL was unable to adjust to the new developments and standards of production. For SBL to have a monopoly on sales and distribution of vaccines was viewed as no longer either fair or feasible. On the other hand, there did seem to be opportunities for successfully continuing with research and export at market prices, possibly through collaboration with other vaccine-producing companies. Director Wigzell proposed a separation of the vaccine production from other tasks.[63]

Although the process of division started during a social democratic government, it was the succeeding conservative government that carried it through. The policy pursued in the early 1990s aimed at the 'marketization' of the economy and the privatization of state enterprises. Private ownership was seen as a prerequisite for efficient business and successful entrepreneurship, and the conservative government talked about 'freeing' the state from the production of things to be marketed and sold. The production of vaccines (and decision-making processes) would in future be done most smoothly and effectively in the form of a joint-stock company.[64]

In 1992, the government decided that the production of vaccines was a task for industry. No bodies consulted objected to the corporatization of SBL, except the Swedish National Audit Office, which considered it unlikely that the company would be commercially viable on its own.[65]

Thus, in 1993, SBL was divided into on one hand an Infectious Disease Control Institute (*Smittskyddsinstitutet* [SMI]), a statutory body that in close cooperation with the NBHW was to monitor the epidemiological situation and promote the development of operational infectious disease prevention and control,[66] and on the other hand, the initially state-owned joint-stock company SBL Vaccin AB. Professors with previously shared positions between SBL and KI moved over to KI. Hans Wigzell became the first director of SMI as well as a board member of SBL Vaccin AB.[67]

National or international vaccine production

In 1997 SBL Vaccin AB was sold to a private Swedish company, Active Biotech, and has since then changed owners several times: in 2001 PowderJect, in 2003 Chiron, in 2004 the company was taken over by the Swedish bank SEB, 3i and Board Members of SBL vaccine, but was then in 2006 sold to Crucell, in 2009 itself taken over by Johnson & Johnson's company Janssen, and is today incorporated into Valneva. Through all these changes, SBL Vaccine has kept its name (though with an added 'e'). Vaccine production ceased during the years after the split, and was limited to a cholera vaccine, Dukoral, but the company also served as distributor of vaccines manufactured elsewhere. Dukoral was developed by Jan Holmgren and Ann-Marie Svennerholm at Sahlgrenska Academy, Gothenburg University, and registered in 1991 as the world's first oral cholera vaccine, now used in more than 70 countries.

For a medical historian, the shift from state-owned and public activities to private enterprise also means a shift in access to source material. The consequence of privatization for transparency became apparent when I contacted SBL Vaccine in the mid-2010s to ask about possible archival material regarding the company's vaccine production and was stopped already at the switchboard: 'But that is a trade secret!'.

Still, issues related to national or international vaccine production are closely related to the organization of the country's epidemic preparedness. When in 2006, the company became Crucell Sweden, the transfer of production to Spain and Switzerland was discussed, while the research department was to move to Leiden. The current state epidemiologist Anders Tegnell, then employed at the NBHW, felt that the move would not compromise the vaccine availability in a pandemic, arguing that the factory had no decisive role in Swedish crisis preparedness.[68]

The epidemics and pandemics of the 2000s returned the question of national vaccine production to the political agenda. In 2005–2006, avian 'bird influenza' A/H5N1 raised the issue of access to possible pandemic vaccines. Since 1997, influenza vaccine was no longer produced in Sweden. The NBHW considered it in 2007 best (but most expensive) if Sweden had its own production of vaccines – otherwise the vaccine availability would not be enough for a mass vaccination.[69] The alternative was Advance Purchase Agreements with existing manufacturers, which incur high annual fees. The then Minister of Public Health (a social democrat) was in favour of a Swedish factory in collaboration with a private international manufacturer. At that time there was a consortium in Kalmar in eastern Sweden with regional actors, in cooperation with the by-then privatized SBL Vaccine in Solna who wanted to start manufacturing. The Ministry of Social Affairs was hesitant regarding a new vaccine factory. A complication was the ongoing technology shift from egg-based vaccine to cell-based, as well as the issue of whether vaccine production should be purely a Swedish concern or rather a Nordic one. NBHW hesitated as well, and the government rejected a new Swedish vaccine factory. The then CEO of SBL Vaccine was disappointed that the state was unwilling to invest in the project on the grounds that the technology for ordinary influenza vaccine and pandemic vaccine was considered too risky.[70] In 2007, the NBHW instead signed an agreement with GlaxoSmithKline (GSK) for 18 million doses in the event of a pandemic, at a price of 1.3 billion SEK, corresponding to two doses for the entire population. In addition, the Swedish state paid an annual guarantee fee of SEK 82–83 million.

However, the question of a national vaccine factory lived on. GSK also considered a Swedish vaccine factory, but when they did not get a clear message from the Swedish state, they chose to expand their existing plants in Germany and Belgium.[71] A new inquiry calculated that a Swedish-made flu vaccine would be relatively cheap; the price of the vaccine supplied by GSK was several times higher. According to Anders Tegnell at the NBHW, the decision not to build the factory had been correct: the technology with cells instead of eggs was not as good as had been anticipated. However, according to SBL'S CEO, there were safer cell-based vaccines, and there would have been greater delivery security with their own vaccine.[72] The Swedish Civil Contingencies Agency (MSB) on the other hand, saw a Swedish vaccine factory as something based on the old

Cold War idea of large reserves. 'Today you want to build as flexible systems as possible because you do not know which is the next threat'.[73]

Swine flu 2009–2010

When the WHO in June 2009 upgraded swine flu (H1N1) to a pandemic, extensive vaccination programmes were triggered, and Sweden chose a different route from most other countries. Sweden had committed to buying Pandemrix and was the only country to decide on universal vaccination. The overall objective was to prevent the spread of infection and to achieve herd immunity. At the same time the autonomous decision-making process was emphasized. In the end, 10–12% of the population was affected by the disease, 60% allowed themselves to be vaccinated. Sweden had the most cases of narcolepsy attributed to vaccination with Pandemrix. By 2020, of the five million people vaccinated with Pandemrix in Sweden, 600 have reported narcolepsy as a side effect; the Medical Products Agency refers to 150–200 acknowledged cases.[74]

Reorganized infectious disease control

In 2009, a study on infectious disease control proposed a clearer division of responsibilities between state authorities, and between these and the level of operational responsibility, which lies with county councils and regions.[75] In a new Infectious Disease Protection Act (*Smittskyddslagen* 2004:168), the NBHW had been given a broadened mandate, but it was imprecise. SMI was the expert authority but with unclear responsibility. A new infectious disease control authority was proposed, with a main task being epidemiological surveillance and analysis, and NBHW would focus on coordination, supervision, standardization and regulation.

In 2010 vaccine issues came up once more. At that time, the child vaccination programme was controlled by the NBHW, and child vaccine was procured by county councils and municipalities directly and provided via, for example, SBL Vaccine. International comparison showed that in most countries, vaccine programmes were decided at government level, and such vaccines were paid and distributed through the state. A law on national vaccination programmes was proposed. And since 2013, in Sweden too the government determines what infectious diseases should be included in national vaccination programmes.[76]

In 2014, the Public Health Agency of Sweden (*Folkhälsomyndigheten* [FHM]) was formed by a merger of the Center for Disease Control (SMI) in Stockholm and the National Public Health Institute based in Östersund in northern Sweden. With the merger even more scientific competence was lost at the new agency – professors, their doctoral students, and laboratory workers had to leave. The NBHW was responsible for the national protection coordination under the Swedish Disease Protection Act until 1 July 2015, a task the new Public Health

Authority then took over. This lack of both scientific competence and 'hands' to do important work was criticized at the time, a criticism that flared up again in the pandemic year of 2020.

National policy in the year of Covid-19

Swedish pandemic management has attracted considerable attention, also from abroad. The lack of stock-piled protective material was obvious, with fatal consequences. The Public Health Agency's actions, or perceived lack of action, has been criticized. Researchers from outside the Agency have interpreted available scientific reports and recommendations from the WHO and the European Centre for Disease Prevention and Control (ECDC) differently from the Agency (ECDC is geographically situated in the outskirts of Stockholm not far from the Public Health Agency). In the context of these debates, some critics have referred to the earlier reorganizations of the country's infectious disease control that resulted in the fragmentation of competences and weakened cooperation between government-affiliated researchers and academic and more independent research. The Public Health Agency is not solely an infectious disease control authority – nowadays there is no such agency in Sweden – but also deals with sexually transmitted diseases, alcohol and drug abuse, food, environment, and mental health issues. That the Agency has been given the responsibility for both risk assessment and risk management has also been criticized, as has a lack of transparency regarding the decision-making basis for the chosen path.

Without joint EU procurement of pandemic vaccine, Sweden would have stood at the back of the queue for access to vaccines against Covid-19. The year 2021 has displayed protectionist measures all over the world to ensure access to vaccine. Although SBL provided ongoing vaccine supply for Sweden's needs from the 1950s, an upscaling of production in a pandemic with a new virus had nevertheless required dependence on foreign actors for access to materials, technology, skills, and likely supplementary vaccine. At the time of writing, several research groups in Sweden are engaged in trying to develop vaccines against Covid-19 and anti-virus treatments. Valneva, which includes SBL Vaccine, is working on developing a Covid-19 vaccine together with the UK government. The vaccine will be produced in Scotland, while 'fill and finish' will be done in Solna, in collaboration with KI. Other researchers in Sweden are working to develop new DNA vaccines against Covid-19. And independent researchers in the field have once more proposed national or Nordic vaccine production in collaboration with one of the major pharmaceutical manufacturers.

The Covid-19 pandemic has also shown that quickly switching gears, moving into an international cooperation, is relatively easy. Within Sweden, specialists in research and clinicians in hospitals have begun to communicate and collaborate in ways rarely seen in recent decades. Also, the benefits of cooperation between human and veterinary medicine have been clarified. The State Veterinary Institute SVA, with its roots in 1911, quickly offered its services in the spring of 2020, and has assisted with both test kits and laboratory capabilities.

Final comments

The issue of national vaccine production is complex. The 1960s saw the Swedish state increasingly committed to the pharmaceutical area. By the 1990s, this had been replaced by commitment to selling off vaccine production to private interests. The history of vaccine production at SBL displays achievements and successes as well as problems and backlashes. The areas of conflict have been numerous. The history of the Swedish SBL shows clearly that difficulties are created when government enforcement is combined with vaccine advocacy. Scientists and producers in the field of vaccinology do not necessarily have the same priorities as authorities in the field of infection protection. For their part governments need to take many more factors than access to vaccines into account. Among them are limits on financial resources, precautionary principles in times of uncertain knowledge, socioeconomic conditions and public health in a broader perspective, intergovernmental relations, and solidarity with countries with more limited resources. Rapidly developed and introduced vaccines from any company can display serious side effects – especially apparent with mass vaccinations. Among the lessons to be learned from this history is the importance of transparency, knowledge-sharing, and dialogue in ongoing work on pandemic management, and vaccinology.

Notes

1 *Les Prix Nobel* (Stockholm: Norstedt, 1904).
2 Axel C. Hüntelmann, 'Diphtheria serum and serotherapy: Development, production and regulation in *fin de siècle* Germany', *Dynamis,* 2007, 27, 107–131, 117.
3 *Betänkande av den för verkställande av en allsidig utredning och angivande av förslag beträffande riktlinjer för Statens bakteriologiska laboratoriums organisation och utveckling den 25 september 1917 tillsatta kommitté* (Stockholm, 1920), 9.
4 Thure Hellström, 'Fyra fall af difteri, behandlade med det nya difteri-antitoxinet', *Hygiea*, 1895, 57, 73–94; Thure Hellström, 'Mortaliteten vid Stockholms Epidemisjukhus 1895', *Hygiea*, 1896, 58, 479–492, 483; Derek S. Linton, *Emil von Behring: Infectious Disease, Immunology, Serum Therapy* (Philadelphia: American Philosophical Society, 2005), 186.
5 Ulrika Graninger, *Från osynligt till synligt: Bakteriologins etablering i sekelskiftets svenska medicin* (Stockholm: Carlssons, 1997).
6 *Underdånigt betänkande och förslag rörande inrättandet af en statsmedicinsk anstalt. Afgifvet den 30 november 1899 af därtill i nåder utsedde kommitterade* (Stockholm, 1899).
7 *Ibid.*
8 *Kongl. Maj:ts nådiga kungörelse angående kontroll å antidifteriserum samt angående handel med dylikt serum* (1 November 1901).
9 *Betänkande,* 18–19.
10 *Kungl. Maj:ts nådiga instruktion för Statsmedicinska anstalten* (98, 1908).
11 Henrik Björck, 'Institutionsbygge i gränsland: Om tillkomsten av Veterinärbakteriologiska anstalten', in Motzi Eklöf, ed, *Humanimalt: Oss djur emellan i medicin och samhälle förr och nu* (Malmköping: Exempla, 2020), 57–61.
12 The story is described in detail with references in Motzi Eklöf, *Fallet Blända: Statens serumtillverkning, en skandal och vetenskaplig krishantering* (Malmköping: Exempla, 2018), to a large extent based on archival material from RMB (*Kungl. Medicinalstyrelsen*) and SBL (*Statens bakteriologiska laboratorium*) at the Swedish National Archives (*Riksarkivet*) in Stockholm.

13 *Betänkande*, 9.
14 Carl Kling, *Minnesbilder från Alfred Petterssons liv och verk. Tecknade vid Svenska läkaresällskapets sammanträde den 22 januari 1952* (Lund, 1952), 15.
15 Handwritten report dated 24 January 1919; Report on visits to Norrtullsgatan 40, 28 January 1919, RMB archives.
16 RMB, 7 May 1919, RMB archives.
17 Parliamentary protocol No. 46 1920 of the Second Chamber, 27 April 1920; Carl Kling, 'Statens bakteriologiska laboratorium', *Allmänna Svenska läkartidningen*, 1920, 460.
18 Carl Kling, 'Statens bakteriologiska laboratorium', offprint from *Allmänna Svenska läkartidningen* (Stockholm, 1920).
19 *Betänkande*, 41.
20 Peter Sköld, *The two Faces of Smallpox: A Disease and its Prevention in Eighteenth- and Nineteenth-Century Sweden* (Umeå: Umeå University, 1996); Peter Sköld, 'The Key to Success: The Role of Local Government in the Organization of Smallpox Vaccination in Sweden', *Medical History*, 2000, 45, 201–226.
21 Klas Linroth, *Om animal vaccination* (Stockholm: Samson & Wallin, 1886), 465; Klas Linroth, *1886 års erfarenhet från ympanstalten för animal vaccin i Stockholm: Aftryck ur Hygiea 1887* (Stockholm: Isaac Marcus' Boktryckeri-Aktiebolag, 1887).
22 Linroth, *1886 års erfarenhet*, 8.
23 Motzi Eklöf, *Variola & Vaccinia: Om massvaccination och folkhälsopolitik, vaccinforskning och läkaretik* (Malmköping: Exempla, 2016), 173.
24 Lag (1916: 180) om skyddskoppympning [Law on protective pox inoculation].
25 Nadja Durbach, *Bodily Matters: The Anti-vaccination Movement in England, 1853–1907* (Durham: Duke University Press, 2005); Deborah Brunton, *The Politics of Vaccination: Practice and Policy in England, Wales, Ireland, and Scotland, 1800–1874* (Rochester: University of Rochester Press, 2008).
26 Peter Baldwin, *Contagion and the State in Europe, 1830–1930* (Cambridge: Cambridge University Press, 2005), 273, 312.
27 Motzi Eklöf, 'Preventionens vapenvägrare: Samvete, vetenskap och personliga erfarenheter – om (il)legitima grunder för samvetsbetänkligheter till obligatorisk smittkoppsvaccinering', *Socialmedicinsk tidskrift*, 2015, 92, 662–673.
28 RMBs Circular 30 December 1925, No. 59 1925.
29 RMBs Circular 1927; RMBs Decree No. 151 1934.
30 Carl Naeslund, 'Erfarenheter och rön beträffande BCG vaccinationen i Norrbotten 1927–1933', *Hygiea*, 1934, 23, 917–918.
31 Erik Rabo, 'Arvid Wallgrens framgångsrika kamp mot tuberkulosen', *Läkartidningen*, 1998, 95, 5788–5790.
32 The Malmö 1932 events are described in detail with references, to a large extent unpublished archival material from RMB and SBL, in Eklöf, *Variola & Vaccinia* and in Motzi Eklöf, 'Smallpox in Malmö, Sweden, 1932: Disputed Knowledge of Infection, Contagion, and Vaccination in the Baltic Sea Region', in Nils Hansson and Jonatan Wistrand, eds, *Explorations in Baltic Medical History, 1850–2015* (Rochester: University of Rochester Press, 2019), 87–112.
33 Carl Kling, 'Skyddskoppympningsproblemet i ljuset av senare årens forskningar och erfarenheter', Appendix F, in SOU 1937:28 *Betänkande med förslag till lag om skyddskoppympning m. m. avgivet av Vaccinationsutredningen* (Stockholm, 1937), 396.
34 Eklöf, *Variola & Vaccinia*, 71, 76.
35 Governmental Instruction No. 641, 1937.
36 Motzi Eklöf, 'Den obligatoriska smittkoppsvaccinationen ifrågasatt: Kättaren Israel Holmgren om kaninpassager, kårinstinkter och känsloskäl', *Svensk medicinhistorisk tidskrift*, 2015, 19, 157–180.
37 Torsten Thunberg, *Utredning rörande statens bakteriologiska laboratorium*, 1942. Kommittébetänkanden 1942, National Library of Sweden, Stockholm.

38 *Organisationen av den vid Statens bakteriologiska laboratorium bedrivna preparattillverkningen mm. Betänkande avgivet av SBL-utredningen* (Stockholm, 1960).
39 *Utredningen om bakteriologiska sera och ympämnen 1953*, RA 321952, Swedish National Archives; was later presented in Bill No. 128 to the 1954 Parliament.
40 Meeting minutes 30 October 1954, and PM 30 November 1954, by B. Malmgren in *Utredningen,* 1953.
41 Sveriges Författningssamling, SFS 1954:482 Instruktion för Statens bakteriologiska laboratorium; SFS 1955:475.
42 Cecilia Jernberg, 'När storskalig livsmedelsproduktion ledde till storskalig smitta', in Eklöf, ed., *Humanimalt,* 117–125.
43 Per Axelsson, *Höstens spöke: De svenska polioepidemiernas historia* (Stockholm: Carlssons, 2004), 79–81.
44 *Ibid.*, 133.
45 *Ibid.*, 152; Per Axelsson, 'The Cutter Incident and the Development of a Swedish Polio Vaccine, 1952–1957', *Dynamis*, 2012, 32, 311–328.
46 Since 1938, abortions were legal on certain indications.
47 Meredith Wadman, *The Vaccine Race: How Scientists Used Human Cells to Combat Killer Viruses* (London: Transworld Publishers Ltd, 2017), 78–94; Isabel Dussauge, 'Foster mot polio: Virusforskning, abort och tystnad i Sverige 1950–1970', in Motzi Eklöf, ed., *Medicinska moraler och skandaler: Vetenskapens (etiska) gränser* (Stockholm: Carlssons, 2019), 160–181.
48 SBLs Annual Report 1 July 1956 – 30 June 1957, SBL Archives.
49 Karl-Göran Hedström, *Studies on a Purified, Inactivated and Freeze-dried Vaccinia Virus Preparation grown on Chick Embryo Membranes* (Stockholm: The National Bacteriological Laboratory, 1973).
50 Eklöf, *Variola & Vaccinia*, 261.
51 *Tillverkningen av bakteriologiska och virologiska preparat. Betänkande* 1957-03-25, referred to in *Organisationen,* 1960, 12; *Arbetsuppgifter och organisation för Statens Bakteriologiska Laboratorium. Betänkande av SBL-utredningen* (Stockholm, 1984), 37.
52 *Organisationen,* 1960, 61.
53 Holger Lundbäck, 'SBL 1909–1982', in Carin Winter, ed, *Statens bakteriologiska laboratorium 1909–1993* (Stockholm: SBL, 1993), 17.
54 Bertil Åberg and A. B. Kabi, 'Angående frågan om gemensamt intresse för statens bakteriologiska laboratorium och Kabi', unpublished report, decided confidential at the Departement of Trade and Industry on 19 December 1969.
55 *Ibid.*
56 'Samhällsnyttan främst', *Svenska Dagbladet,* 12 February 1970.
57 *Produktionsavdelningen vid Statens Bakteriologiska Laboratorium. Betänkande av SBL 77-utredningen* (Stockholm, 1978).
58 Government bill 1962:184.
59 Läkemedelsförordningen 1962:701; Decree 1963:439.
60 Läkemedelslag 2015:315.
61 E. g. 'Ska mässlings-vaccineringen med levande virus stoppas?', *Aftonbladet*, 6 October 1968; Heng Österberg, 'Professorsbatalj: Levande eller dött vaccin? Bör vaccination uppskjutas?', *Svenska Dagbladet,* 5 December 1968; Heng Österberg, 'Kritik mot massympning', *Svenska Dagbladet,* 17 February 1972.
62 Lars-Olof Kallings, *Det passionerade sändebudet* (Stockholm: Carlssons, 2016), 164–168.
63 SBL, *Bolagisering av vaccinproduktion och försäljning.* Report February 1992.
64 Direktiv 1991:101 om ett nytt smittskyddsinstitut.
65 Government bill 1992/93:46.
66 Direktiv 1991:101; SOU 1992:29 *Betänkande av utredningen om ett nationellt smittskyddsinstitut mm.*; Government bill 1992/93:46 om ett nationellt smittskyddsinstitut mm.
67 Kallings, *Det passionerade sändebudet*, 44-46. Wigzell was thereafter in 1995 to 2003 Principle of KI.

68 Petra Hedbom, 'SBL Vaccin flyttar produktionen utomlands', *Läkemedelsvärlden*, 29 August 2008.
69 'SBL Vaccin föreslås få bygga dyr vaccinfabrik', *Dagens Medicin*, 17 January 2007.
70 Ewa Stenberg, 'Spelet om vaccinet', *Dagens Nyheter*, 29 August 2009.
71 *Ibid.*
72 *Ibid.*
73 Anna Nyman from MSB in *Ibid.*
74 Charles Olsson, 'Sökande efter kunskap och konklusioner efter vaccinationen mot svininfluensa', in Eklöf, ed, *Humanimalt*, 87–93; The Medical Products Agency, 'Svininfluensan, Pandemrix och narkolepsi', lakemedelsverket.se, 20 November 2020 [acc. 2021-04-13].
75 SOU 2009:55. *Ett effektivare smittskydd. Betänkande av smittskyddsutredningen* (Stockholm: Fritze, 2009).
76 SFS 2012: 452, Lag om ändring i smittskyddslagen (2004:168).

4

THE FAILED PROMISES OF A BRIGHTER FUTURE

The Institute of Immunology in Zagreb from a public asset to a privatized burden

Vedran Duančić, Snježana Ivčić, and Ana Vračar

Introduction

The centennial of the Institute of Immunology in Zagreb (IMZ) – and, in fact, of modern public health in Croatia in general – was marked in 1993.[1] The occasion called for reflection on the Institute's past achievements and its future prospects. A lot indeed was to be said about the former. The Institute could, and did, boast about its globally pioneering role in important research fields, renowned products, and financial success, manifested in a steady revenue – in hard currency, no less – coming from the export of vaccines, toxins, antitoxins, and sera across the world. Considerations about the Institute's future, however, were somewhat more restrained, though still largely optimistic. The centennial took place in extraordinary political and economic circumstances that were difficult to overlook, and which instilled a sense of caution in contemporary commentators. Croatia had proclaimed independence from Yugoslavia in 1991 and, until 1995, was engulfed in a war. The country was also undergoing a transition from the specifically Yugoslav self-managerial socialism in which companies were publicly owned (by the 'society', not by the state) and in which workers were supposed to have a say in running the companies, to liberal capitalism, where they did not. Plans to make the IMZ, out of the entire Croatian public health sector, into a joint stock company began already in the last days of the socialist period. Its extraction from the public health sector meant that the IMZ would get a new owner(s), but it was not clear just who or what they would be. With the market of the former Yugoslavia now largely gone and the new domestic market – that of Croatia alone – insufficient to maintain profitability, it was hoped that the Institute's global exports would make up for the difference. Highly skilled workers, infrastructure, know-how, and well-established global contacts seemed to be a healthy foundation for future growth.

DOI: 10.4324/9781003130345-5

The hopes and aspirations from the time of the centennial did not come true. Unlike some public vaccine production institutions examined in this volume, the IMZ survived the massive global reconfiguration of vaccine production and exists to this day, even if in name only. With a greatly reduced scope of production, having lost the vital World Health Organisation (WHO) export license in 1998 and accumulating significant losses, it filed for bankruptcy in 2013. Making a decision about its future has been postponed several times since. In the meanwhile, several models for restructuring have been discussed, and the Institute has occasionally occupied public attention – not least during the Covid-19 pandemic, when its loss was particularly bemoaned.

The 1993 centennial is an appropriate starting point for methodological reasons, too. The Institute has frequently been mentioned in the media, especially since 2009, when problems and irregularities became publicly known. However, although it is rightfully considered one of the most successful stories in the twentieth-century history of medicine in Croatia (and the former Yugoslavia), there have been few historical accounts of it. These were sometimes written by 'insiders', people personally acquainted with the structure, functioning, and daily work of the Institute, privy to its internal documentation.[2] To this day, the archival documentation pertaining to the Institute remains incomplete, scattered across various institutions, and occasionally inaccessible, which makes such first-hand insights invaluable.[3] 1993 was also the last time that relatively optimistic reflections on the situation at the Institute were published. The reports written since then, and especially since 2013, have been of a different kind: written by official financial inspectors, consultants, and journalists, they have been primarily concerned with restructuring and consolidating the Institute's finances, search for investments and potential buyers – and, in the case of a 2017 parliamentary investigation, with assigning responsibility for the Institute's predicament.[4] A wider picture and the awareness of the fact that the IMZ shared the fate of many similar public institutions across the world have been consistently absent from these reports.

A 1993 text by Vlatko Silobrčić, the Institute's director between 1992 and 1997, is particularly revealing and allows for observing the Institute against the backdrop of the global transformations in vaccine production that took place in the 1980s and 1990s.[5] The IMZ had flourished within the 'international health' paradigm and profited from the 'free' exchange of knowledge (though not equipment and technology) among various national institutions, especially during the 1960s. It fell victim not only to dubious management decisions and governmental neglect, as one could conclude from the recent public debates, but also to a paradigm shift that influenced many similar public institutions worldwide: the rise of 'global health' and the emergence of new dominant agents in the field – large multinational pharmaceutical companies that could commit to huge investments necessary for ever more demanding R&D in vaccinology, but which also ensured profitability by patenting their know-how and products.[6] Additionally, the WHO has implemented increasingly strict requirements for 'good manufacturing practice' (GMP), before accepting ('pre-qualifying') vaccines for its expanded programme on immunization (EPI). This required investments on an entirely new level, and of a new type, which exceeded IMZ's capabilities.

Were the specialists and policy-makers in the early 1990s Croatia aware of these far-reaching changes and did they take them into consideration when envisioning the future of the Institute? And did Croatia's (and Yugoslavia's) socialist heritage make a difference? The 1960s and 1970s were the Institute's 'golden era', and historians of medicine like, notably, Dóra Vargha have recently pointed to socialist countries as success stories in suppression and eradication of infectious diseases, including poliomyelitis.[7] (The swift vaccination of 18 out of 20.8 million citizens of socialist Yugoslavia against smallpox in response to the outbreak in the spring of 1972, the last outbreak in Europe, when 175 people were infected and 35 died, has been repeatedly brought up during the Covid-19 pandemic.)[8] Yet in the public discourse, the socialist period is also identified – not incorrectly – as the starting point of IMZ's downward trajectory. The Institute, however, was competitive in the global market and was a net contributor to the state budget, rather than dependent on it, during most of the socialist period. The inherited problems indeed came to the foreground during the post-socialist transition in the 1990s, but they were not specifically 'socialist' and, in any case, the Institute's 'socialist past' does not explain the financial difficulties, stagnation or eventual demise of comparable institutions in non-socialist countries such as Australia, Denmark, Netherlands, or Sweden, to name but a few.[9] In an attempt to explain IMZ's downward trajectory, we address both the structural and contingent developments, pointing to similar trajectories of public vaccine production institutions across the world and specifically Croatian phenomena.

The chapter offers a brief and selective institutional history of the Institute, with a stronger emphasis placed on the 1960s and the period since the 1990s, as we attempt to complicate the narrative of the 'rise and fall' of yet another national public vaccine production institution. As do other contributions to this volume, the chapter elaborates on the social, political, and economic contexts in which the Institute has operated and focuses on the Institute's most important efforts in the research and production of vaccines. Yet the chapter goes beyond a narrow institutional history and examines a larger set of issues, including, at a very fundamental level, the role of public health as 'a source of national pride and prestige, and a sign of modernity'.[10] Importantly, the chapter links the history of medicine with economic history. It also examines the labour issue, including union actions and public protests that took place in the mid-2010s, against the backdrop of privatization of public health in Croatia since the 1990s, as well as the recent public discourse concerning the Institute's role in maintaining national sovereignty and as a common good that should not be viewed in terms of profitability alone – or, in the opinion of others, should no longer be artificially kept alive through governmental financial interventions.

The beginnings of vaccine production in Croatia

The IMZ celebrated its centennial in 1993, although the Institute changed names, was assigned to various administrative bodies, grew and shrunk as a result of institutional merges and splits, changed its address, and R&D focus several times since the *Kraljevski zemaljski zavod za proizvadjanje animalnoga cjepiva protiv boginjam* (the Royal State Institute for the production of animal vaccine against smallpox) was established in 1893.[11] Nor did the history of vaccines in Croatia begin only in 1893. The first inoculation against smallpox in continental Croatia took place already in 1791, and more systematic efforts in Dalmatia started at the beginning of the nineteenth century, under the Habsburg and the brief French (during the Napoleonic wars) governments. In the 1870s, local physicians – trained abroad, primarily in Graz and Vienna, as the School of Medicine in Zagreb became operational only after 1917 – called for the use of animal lymph for vaccine material to replace arm-to-arm transmission, and for a domestic production facility to be established.[12] A legal framework mandating animal vaccines was introduced in the early 1890s. Production started soon after: at first not in Zagreb, but in Bjelovar, in northern Croatia, where in 1890, a local physician started a private production of smallpox vaccines, having procured the strain of cowpox from Vienna.[13] The 1891 law made vaccination (and revaccination) obligatory, and in 1893, the regional government took over the Bjelovar institute and moved it to Zagreb where it was (re)established as the *Kraljevski zemaljski zavod*, which became one of the 15 facilities for the production of vaccines in Austria-Hungary.[14]

As elsewhere, alongside smallpox, bacterial diseases were at the centre of vaccine production efforts in the early twentieth-century Croatia. Because the government failed to establish the planned bacteriological institute, bacteriologist Ljudevit Gutschy (1874–1961), who had studied in Graz and specialized at the Institut Pasteur in Paris, in Vienna, at Koch's Institute for Infectious Diseases in Berlin, in Cologne, and in Lübeck, opened a private bacteriological institute in Zagreb in 1907.[15] The two institutions at the very heart of modern public health in Croatia thus resulted from private initiatives, with the government stepping in and incorporating them into the nascent public health sector. Gutschy's Bacteriological Institute became a state institution in 1912 and proved to be of immense importance for fighting outbreaks of cholera and typhoid shortly before and during World War I.[16] In 1918–1919 Gutschy finally started the domestic production of anti-rabies vaccine, as he had long hoped to do, and the Zagreb Pasteur Institute became operational in 1919 as one of three departments of the Bacteriological Institute (alongside the bacteriological–serological and chemical departments), though for a long time without a permanent address.[17] This structure was kept after the Bacteriological Institute was transformed into the Epidemiological Institute in 1923 – until 1926, when the consolidated Institute of Hygiene with the School of Public Health was opened in Zagreb, which incorporated all public health institutions. In 1926–1927, the

Institute of Hygiene moved into representative new buildings largely paid for by the Rockefeller Foundation, which included modern laboratories for immunobiological research.

Local vaccine production proved to be cheaper and allowed for a quicker response. No longer was it necessary – or even possible – to send samples (in case of suspected rabies, actual patients) to Budapest, capital of the Hungarian part of Austria-Hungary, to which parts of Croatia had belonged. This concern became especially important following the break-up of Austria-Hungary and the establishment of a Yugoslav state in December 1918, when reliance on what were now foreign countries became politically problematic. Interwar Yugoslavia was one of the Europe's economically least developed countries, though there were great regional differences in economy, education, or health of the population. Notorious for political conflicts that sometimes obstructed the most basic functioning of the state, interwar Yugoslavia was nevertheless intent on comprehensive modernization, though it lacked resources (and stability) to realize ambitious plans. The Central Hygiene Institute in Belgrade was the nexus of a growing network of research facilities, outpatient clinics, rural field stations, sanatoria, and schools aiming at 'enlightening' the local population.[18] However, this infrastructure was in the first place built because the country profited from the resources of, notably, the Rockefeller Foundation and from the internationalization of public health under the banner of the League of Nations Health Organization following the World War I.[19]

Croatian physician Andrija Štampar (1888–1958) was the central figure of reformist public health efforts in interwar Yugoslavia and was exceptionally successful in utilizing the substantial resources made available through the Rockefeller Foundation. Štampar belonged to a group of physicians, including prominent figures such as Ludwik Rajchman (1881–1965), who emerged as prime ideologues and facilitators of international public health efforts in the interwar period. Despite his successes during the 1920s, Štampar fell out of favour with the government and was forced to retire in 1931. Because of that, he spent much of the 1930s on the move as a League of Nations representative across the world – most importantly in China, which he visited three times for longer periods – sharing his experiences from Yugoslavia.[20]

Important as they were, vaccines did not occupy a central place in the contemporary public health discourse or in the investments at municipal and state levels in interwar Yugoslavia. Štampar continuously spoke of the prevention of diseases, but not through vaccination. Improving the living conditions, he believed, was the fundamental prerequisite for suppression and eradication of infectious diseases. Sanitation, sewage, circulation of air and ample light in living quarters, balanced diet, abstention from alcohol, and personal hygiene were the ways to better living and 'modernity'.[21] This is the spirit he took to China, too, where he was far more enthusiastic about, and supportive of, rural clinics that offered basic treatment and 'enlightened people' than of the expensive, state-of-the-art research facilities that he believed were too often out of touch with the population they were meant to serve. The interwar period nevertheless saw a noticeable expansion of pharmaceutical R&D in Yugoslavia in general, both at the public institutions and in private companies, many of which were affiliated to, or owned by, foreign companies. The production at the Institute of Hygiene was representative for the 1930s: vaccines against smallpox, typhoid, cholera, and pertussis; antitoxins against scarlet fever and diphtheria (as well as their toxins), Dick toxoid for immunization against scarlet fever; and sera against diphtheria, tetanus, scarlet fever, dysentery, streptococcus, and anthrax.[22] The production of vaccines and vaccination rates declined during the World War II, though the production of smallpox vaccines had been ramped-up in anticipation of the war, which engulfed Yugoslavia only in 1941.[23]

Public health in Socialism

In 1945, after four years of war destruction, Yugoslavia was recreated as a federal republic governed by the Communist Party of Yugoslavia. The ambitious yet inadequate modernizing efforts of interwar Yugoslavia suddenly paled in comparison with the agenda laid down by the new government. Socialist Yugoslavia saw some of the earliest attempts at replicating the Soviet model of comprehensive, quick-paced modernization through state investments in industry, but it was also the first socialist country to abandon the model in the aftermath of the Soviet–Yugoslav split of 1948–1949, which prompted a search for an 'alternative path to socialism'. Like many parts of Europe, the country emerged from the war facing a bleak public health situation and lacking resources to address the issue on its own. However, between the early 1950s and 1980s, there was a massive increase in the share of the population covered by public health insurance – rising from 25 to more than 80 percent – and overall availability of healthcare.[24] This was also a time when the programme of mandatory vaccinations was established and gradually expanded to include BCG and diphtheria (both in 1948), tetanus (1955), pertussis (1959), poliomyelitis (1961), measles (1968), rubella (1975),[25] and mumps vaccine (in 1976, produced from the further attenuated Leningrad–Zagreb strain, part of the trivalent MMR).[26]

Like other countries in the emerging Soviet sphere of influence, Yugoslavia refused to take part in the Marshall Plan, though it received substantial US aid in the early 1950s, after the break with the Soviet Union. Yugoslavia was one of the main recipients of United Nations Relief and Rehabilitation Administration (UNRRA) aid in the immediate post-war period.[27] Various medicines, equipment, and inventories of entire hospitals comprised a significant portion of UNRRA aid. The history of Yugoslavia's first penicillin factory, though only tangentially related to vaccines, was symptomatic of difficulties with capital-intensive investments in the early socialist period. Together with Czechoslovakia, Poland, and the Soviet republics of Belarus and Ukraine, Yugoslavia was offered a penicillin factory through UNRRA. The offer, however, was rejected and Yugoslavia ended up overpaying (though in the end it was also paid for by UNRRA) for a heavily used facility from the pharmaceutical giant, Merck.[28] Reassembling the factory and starting the production took a long time, but the factory, once set up in 1949, remained in use until the 1970s.

The 1950s saw another cycle of expansion in vaccine production, aiming at satisfying growing domestic needs. Because various institutions were assigned to it and new units established within it, the Institute of Hygiene had outgrown not only its 1920s infrastructure but also its initial mandate in public health. It was organized in three sectors – epidemiological–microbiological, hygienic, and administrative – with the epidemiological–microbiological sector comprising two bacteriological, one parasitological, and epidemiological department each, and the department for the production of sera and vaccines, which had a separate division for sera and vaccines, and for smallpox vaccine.[29] In 1952, the Department for the Control of Sera and Vaccines was also established in order to ensure that the rising standards of the manufacturing process were met. The 1950s in most part saw research and production being conducted the 'old way', along the lines of interwar practices, even though the production was now 20 times bigger.[30] At the end of the 1950s, the Institute was producing vaccines against tetanus, cholera, smallpox; combined vaccines against diphtheria and tetanus; against diphtheria, tetanus, and pertussis; against tetanus, typhoid, and paratyphoid a and b; and against cholera, typhoid, and paratyphoid a and b; purified and concentrated sera against diphtheria, tetanus, and gas gangrene; antivenoms against snake and spider venoms; sera against anthrax and scarlet fever; equine sera (which were especially lucrative); serodiagnostics for syphilis; bacterial suspensions and agglutinating sera for diagnostics; diphtheria toxins for determining achieved immunity; and various allergens.[31]

Building foundations for the 'golden age'

A more strategic, longer-term planning of vaccine production was difficult to achieve because of institutional fragmentation, even though under one institutional roof, that of the Institute of Hygiene. This changed in 1956, when the Institute for the Production of Sera and Vaccines was established, first within the Institute of Hygiene, but soon as an independent institution, which in 1957 was renamed as the Serovaccinal Institute, and in 1961 would finally become the Institute of Immunology. The period that followed was beyond doubt the Institute's 'golden era' and is often associated with the figure of Drago Ikić (1917–2014), who led the Institute between 1958 and 1982. But the reasons for the successes that were to come should not be sought in institutional developments or leadership alone – though they helped – but in combination with other factors: the expansion of global vaccine markets and the intensification of international cooperation in vaccine production, with the IPV and OPV being the best-known cases.

The seeming fixation with export of antitoxins, sera, and vaccines might seem strange, but it was deeply embedded in the budgetary logic and attempts at geopolitical positioning of socialist Yugoslavia, as well as the prevalent perception of what successful public companies looked like. In 1956, the export did not yet reach pre-war levels, but already at that point, its structure and ambitious plans for the future clearly pointed to a new direction.[32] The Institute was planning to re-enter old and enter new markets, well beyond Europe. Yugoslavia's newly forged friendly relations with recently decolonized countries in Africa and Asia, which would lead to the establishment of the Non-Aligned Movement in 1961, promised a cooperation that would be both politically and economically advantageous. In 1963, for instance, domestic sales outweighed exports – 467–300 million dinars – but the value of export had risen spectacularly, around 300 percent, since 1956, and would continue to rise.[33] Exports never really reached the levels of domestic sales but were nevertheless hugely important. In the mid-1970s, the IMZ earned $600,000 through export and an equivalent of $4 million in dinars in the domestic market.[34] Whilst exports decreased at times of economic crisis, such as in the early 1980s, they consistently contributed to the fact that as much as 90 percent of the Institute's revenue came from sale of its products.[35] (Incidentally, the success of global vaccination programmes led to a decrease in sales of therapeutic sera, which had been a major source of revenue for the Institute.)[36]

A careful look into the global presence of the IMZ and its export successes, which have been a source of great pride, offers a more complex picture. In absolute terms and in comparison to other Yugoslav companies, the export of the IMZ was hardly noteworthy.[37] It has occupied such an important place in the perception of the IMZ for other reasons: export was not part of the IMZ's core mission, but a side-accomplishment; the IMZ was a rare example of a public health institution that contributed to the state budget; some of its products had high added value and could compete with products from economically and technologically far more developed countries; it positioned Yugoslavia, itself still a developing country, on a global map in a very competitive field; and finally, hard currency flowing into the country was always welcome. The IMZ exported to 14 European countries, one Central and one South American country, six Asian, and seven African countries.[38] An internal study from the 1950s suggested that IMZ's main products would be profitable in foreign markets because of cheap raw materials and relatively low production costs, including wages.[39] But problems that were first identified in the mid-1950s were never fully resolved: the high and ever-rising standards regarding vaccine production in the developed countries (primarily West Europe) threatened to undermine the achieved successes. In the developing country markets the IMZ suffered from the low prices its products could achieve and competition from other socialist countries which, unlike Yugoslavia, were part of the Eastern bloc.[40] The IMZ continuously did best financially in West European markets (West Germany, Italy, and Switzerland, for instance), where it initially sold unfinished products, while much of its vaccine production programme – including typhoid fever, diphtheria, and pertussis vaccines – was oriented to developing country markets, often in collaboration with the WHO and UNICEF.[41] Close working relations with the WHO were also manifested in the fact that between 1971 and 1997, the IMZ was a WHO Collaborating Centre for Research and Reference Services for Immunobiological Biological Products, as well as, between 1973 and 1995, a Reference Centre for References and Research on Bacterial Vaccines and Immunization Programmes.[42]

New research directions, new vaccines

In a matter of years, the IMZ was transformed into a modern production facility that conducted systematic research, especially – though not exclusively – on viral vaccines, which at the time were at the centre of researchers' attention worldwide. Between 1963 and 1979, the IMZ published a journal, *Radovi Imunološkog zavoda Zagreb*, which offers a comprehensive and detailed insight into the research directions and results, as well as into a broad network of international cooperation. In collaboration with the Yugoslav Academy of Sciences and Arts in Zagreb, between 1957 and 1979, the IMZ organized numerous international conferences, dedicated to biological and immunological standardization, use of human diploid cell strains, and different bacterial and virus vaccines. Financial success of the late 1950s at the same time called for further capital investments and made them possible. Much-needed new research and production facilities were opened in the early 1960s, and in 1962, a lyophiliser, a vital piece of equipment in modern virus vaccine production, was bought from France.[43]

Under Ikić's leadership, the IMZ intensively worked on the polio, measles, rubella, mumps, and influenza vaccines – all fairly standard research directions for the time. The thread connecting them, however, was something more avant-garde – research in human diploid cell strains as a virus propagation medium. The work of Leonard Hayflick and Paul Moorhead at the Wistar Institute in Philadelphia in the early 1960s first revealed the benefits of Human Diploid Cell Strains (HDCS).[44] Their WI-38 strain, derived from foetal lung tissue, and MRC-5, a parallel cell substrate developed by J.P. Jacobs at the Medical Research Council Laboratories in London, have been vital for vaccine production ever since. Because WI-38 could not have been patented in the United States, where law did not allow patenting living material, Hayflick 'delivered ampules of WI-38 worldwide, gratis, to virtually every virus vaccine manufacturer in the world'.[45] The IMZ was just one of the recipients of the WI-38 cell strain, but Ikić quickly took on a pioneering role in connecting researchers from all over the world and, most importantly, building the research, production, and control of vaccines using the HDCS. As Hayflick later observed,

> Ikić was a significant figure because he became so convinced that the use of these cells would replace primary monkey kidney and other primary cell populations, like primary chick[en] cell populations, also used for vaccine production, that he took it upon himself to promote this idea

> internationally, and one of the first things he did, which is critically important, was to organize [in 1963] a conference in a resort town in Yugoslavia, called Opatija [...] and that was a very important and, to some extent, a famous meeting in respect to all the events that occurred subsequently.[46]

Setting up research and production of polio and measles vaccines on WI-38 – licensed in 1967 and 1968, first in the world – by Ikić was a critical step in proving their efficiency and safety for mass production. Early on, researchers at the IMZ found advantages of the HDCS to be manyfold: the tissue did not contain latent or oncogenic viruses, it had a normal karyotype and a broad spectrum of sensitivity for human viruses, it could be closely controlled, and certified parent strains could be used for vaccine production.[47]

In the public discourse, the IMZ is most frequently associated with the Edmonston-Zagreb strain of measles and safe and highly efficacious measles vaccine.[48] In 1963, the IMZ acquired Edmonston-Musser strain, cultured on dog kidney, from the Philips-Roxane laboratory in Columbus, Ohio. By 1967 this had been developed into the Edmonston-Zagreb strain.[49] Systematic vaccination against measles began in 1969, and in 1975 vaccination started with a combined, live measles–rubella–mumps vaccine.[50] The Edmonston-Zagreb strain was lucrative for the IMZ, as production licences were sold to Belgium, France, India, Mexico, and Switzerland.[51] It has been 'the most commonly used measles vaccine in the Expanded Programme on Immunization (EPI) of the WHO'.[52]

Interestingly, in specialist circles, research in the HDCS and human leucocyte interferon production is strongly emphasized, while the polio vaccine seems to have been ascribed a secondary role in the grand narrative about the IMZ. As another chapter in this volume shows, Salk's IPV and, later, Sabin's OPV were prominently featured at the Torlak Institute in Belgrade, the capital of Yugoslavia. Ikić, on the other hand, established contacts with Hillary Koprowski from the Wistar Institute in Philadelphia – the two institutes cooperated throughout the 1960s and 1970s – and alongside Congo and Poland, Croatia was one of places where early large-scale trials of Koprowski's attenuated polio vaccine were undertaken.[53] Three types of Koprowski's attenuated vaccine were administered between 1961 and 1963, and type 1 (CHAT) and type 3 (W-Fox) were found to be safe and highly efficient, showing a seroconversion of 91.5 and 93.5 percent, respectively.[54] Such a delineation – Salk's and Sabin's vaccines in Serbia, Koprowski's in Croatia – was most probably a result of some kind of an agreement between the two institutes, though we have been unable to find sources confirming that. (It also might be connected to Sabin's distrust of the HDCS.)[55] In 1958, attempts were made to coordinate the work on the polio and influenza vaccines. The Zagreb Institute was supposed to cover one-third of the production of polio vaccine and two-thirds of influenza vaccine.[56] Logical as the attempt might seem, as it would avoid potentially wasteful duplication of work in a country with still limited resources and diversify available vaccines, coordination among institutions in different Yugoslav republics was infrequent in most scientific fields. This was, for instance, visible in conferences organized by the IMZ in the 1960s and 1970s, when foreign participants, often from the United States, India, or elsewhere, by far outnumbered fellow Yugoslav specialists. Besides maintaining a lively communication with virologists and immunologists in the United States, the IMZ hosted dozens of foreign researchers who came for specialization (57 of them, mostly from developing countries, between 1967 and 1983) through WHO, and more than 200 other short-term guests.[57]

Transformations again: towards privatization

In 1965, Drago Ikić could summarize the recent successes of the Institute by saying, 'Eight years ago we faced different problems. We had to catch up with the most advanced institutes in our field of work in the world. Today our problems are different. We have in our research programme everything that the most advanced institutes in the world have in their research programmes'.[58] Future R&D at the Institute was to be built on the foundations set in the 1960s; there were breakthroughs and refinements of products, but they would not have global impact. Despite an economic crisis that was spilling over into the sphere of politics, the 1980s saw a new round of investments in equipment and production facilities (that would again quickly prove to be inadequate), with WHO's GMP as a target.

If, genre-wise, the history of the Institute until the 1980s reads as a standard history of public health, biomedical sciences, and vaccinology, since the 1980s it has moved towards the legal genre. The spotlight was no longer on the R&D but, increasingly, on suspicious contracts, unprofitable investments, loss of revenue, deteriorating working conditions, and dissatisfaction among the workers.[59] In the mid-1980s, cooperation between the IMZ and the Serum Institute of India, from Pune, began, with the IMZ selling its know-how and licence for vaccine production using the Edmonston-Zagreb measles strain. During a 2017 parliamentary investigation into the 'fall' of the IMZ, this transaction was heavily criticized. The contract was unclear and favoured the Indian company, which would grow to become the world's largest vaccine producer. The Serum Institute paid tens of thousands of U.S. dollars for a product that would earn it tens or hundreds of millions in the coming decades. This was interpreted as the IMZ having created and helped its own 'disloyal competition'.[60]

Towards the end of the socialist period, new legislation on private property and enterprise (in 1988 and 1990) created conditions for abolishing self-management and replacing it with 'social', 'cooperative', 'mixed', and private enterprises. Besides focusing on the market economy, the legislation also assigned a greater role to the executive management. It was in this context that Miroslav Beck, the IMZ director between 1986 and 1992, in 1990 initiated a formal transformation of the Institute with the intention of creating a dual-ownership – part public, part private – model, though the authorities blocked and reversed his attempts. The changes announced during Beck's mandate evolved in the following period, although they were slightly delayed by the onset of the Croatian War of Independence. During this period, the domestic market contracted – though it seems the IMZ did lucrative business supplying the Yugoslav National Army, which would soon become an aggressor in the war, with vaccines – but it was followed by a slight growth in 1992 and 1993, when export was expected to reach $3 million. This was the reason behind reserved optimism in Silobrčić's 1993 anniversary text on the IMZ. He believed that the IMZ was 'large enough so it could produce competitive quantities of its products but also small enough so it could be easily and quickly redirected'.[61] But no mention was made, for instance, of recombinant DNA technology, which had already been put to use elsewhere. Silobrčić saw virus vaccines (especially the MMR), equine antitoxic sera, blood derivatives, interferon, and testing kits as a healthy foundation for future growth and export.

The highly skilled workforce was another factor allowing for mild optimism. Between the mid-1950s and 1990s, the number of workers at the Institute grew from 112 to 406. The late 1950s and then the 1980s saw the biggest increase in the number of workers (the number nearly doubled in both periods), while between 2000 and 2014 the number fell from 406 to 167. The share of college-educated workers and workers with advanced degrees rose in particular, though they never represented a majority of the workforce. In 1961, for instance, the Institute had 116 employees (of which only 7 with university degrees), and in 1969, there were 240 workers (of which 61 with university degrees).[62] The trend was important for the Institute's research and control capabilities. The focus on achieving an effective workforce mix was also reflected in the practice of organizing courses for the workers with no, primary, and lower-secondary education aimed at helping them complete exams and strengthen their position in the workplace. This contributed to a 100 percent increase in production in 1956 compared to the previous year.[63]

By the early 1990s, privatization trends had intensified all over Central and Eastern Europe and were clearly reflected in the approach of Croatia's government to the Institute.[64] At the end of the 1980s, the World Bank and the International Monetary Fund exerted great pressure on the healthcare systems of all East Central European countries, including Yugoslavia.[65] The proposed changes varied depending on the local context, but 'there [were] some common issues – most notably, the introduction of several market-based instruments, including introducing health insurance financing systems to replace general taxation-based models, privatization and the introduction of private payments and co-payments'. The health system in Croatia was exposed to gradual changes leading to privatization, particularly in the field of primary health care.[66] Such policies were intensified following a 1994 pro-privatization manifesto by Andrija Hebrang, the minister of health between 1990 and 1998.[67] His vision corresponded to the measures that the international financial institutions had previously pushed for, such as the concession of the public health centres, the privatization of gynaecological and dental care, or introduction of additional health insurance paid by patients. By the end of the 1990s, most primary healthcare was privatized through capitation-based and concession agreements with primary healthcare specialists. Hospitals acquired a new, market-oriented terminology and public health measures fell well behind on the Ministry's priority list.[68] As a result of a combination of these trends, public health institutions, including the IMZ, could not count on the regular upkeep and development of their infrastructure, crucial for the production of biotechnological products.

In 1994 the IMZ became a joint stock company under the name Institute of Immunology for Drug and Pharmaceutical Chemical Production and Scientific Research. The notion of 'privatization' through listing the IMZ at the stock market here requires a clarification: the state has continuously been the main shareholder through various institutions such as health insurance and pension funds or agencies managing state assets, which made the downward trajectory of the Institute a political issue not only because of its effects, but because of responsibility as well. Counterintuitively, it was the Ministry of Economy, not of Health, that oversaw the Institute. Current and former workers were given the option of buying shares (up to 49 percent of the total number), and 498 of them did so, though many quickly sold them on.[69] Two currents collided at the Institute during the 1990s: one represented by the workers who insisted on maintaining the public status of the institution, and the other, backed by government policies, favouring privatization. Successive governments paid little attention to the Institute after 1994, and it continued to suffer from the lack of investment in infrastructure and machinery. The position of the Institute as a nominally private company that depended on the state as a large shareholder, buyer of its products, legislator, but not as a financier, was recognized as unsustainable. In 1995 and 1997, the lack of investment led to the cancellation of the WHO collaborating centre status. The 1998 loss of the WHO license, vital for export of IMZ's products to most of its previous markets, severely impacted the revenue. WHO representatives had warned that improvements in production procedure were necessary, and the IMZ was given two years to implement upgrades – including 'clean rooms' – but, although the Institute at that point was still making a profit, this did not happen. (Part of the problem was the fact that over several decades, new buildings had been built next to each other, but were not necessarily connected; some were even separated by a street.) Following the loss of its license, a Canadian company, InterVax, which had a contract with the IMZ for global distribution of its products (the contract was also heavily criticized for unnecessarily favouring InterVax) since the 1980s, sued the IMZ for the loss of future profits and won $3 million.[70] In 2004, the Institute faced bankruptcy, but avoided it because of a last-minute government loan and because workers forfeited a part of their salaries.

The bankruptcy and beyond

When Croatia entered the European Union in 2013, the problems that had led to loss of the WHO licence could no longer be overlooked: the implementation of EU regulations led to the National Agency for Medicinal Products and

Medical Devices revoking the IMZ's production licences (of blood derivates in 2013; bacterial vaccines in 2014; and viral vaccines in 2015). The bankruptcy announcement was supposed to lead to the loss of about 200 working places and mark the end of the Institute's operations.[71] However, workers, mostly members of Autonomous Trade Union in Power Industry, Chemistry and Non-Metal Industry (EKN), objected to the management plans, went on strike, and took the case to court. The workers gained support of several civil society organizations and activist groups, including Red Action (*Crvena akcija*), a far-left organization dedicated to anti-imperialist direct action. Their most notable collaboration form were picket lines near the Institute and demonstrations in front of government buildings, which made the national media attentive to the Institute's fate throughout the legal and political processes. Within a month, the bankruptcy filing was retracted, and the government was now forced to act.

The next step was submitting a tender for IMZ's shares, thus further pursuing the privatization agenda.[72] The restructuring process was announced in May 2014, when 75 percent of the Institute's shares were offered for sale, in the hope that a strategic partner for the Institute would be found, willing and capable of making the investment needed for re-starting production. The announcement stirred interest among local and international companies, including Jadran Galenski Laboratoriji, Bilthoven Biologicals, the City of Zagreb, and the Croatian Health Insurance Fund. Eight letters of interest were submitted, including, unexpectedly, one from Visia Croatica, previously unknown to the public. Originally a small counselling company, Visia Croatica entered the tender process offering to take over the Institute through a limited partnership with a shares model operating on a 'one-person, one vote' principle. The model relied heavily on the concept of *Kommanditgesellschaft auf Aktien* (KGaA) used in Germany, although the initiators of Visia Croatica made a point of highlighting the differences between the KGaA and their vision of the Institute of Immunology, the main one being the approach to distribution of profit among shareholders: Visia Croatica announced that, were the initiative successful and it managed to buy the Institute, any profit generated through its operations would be reinvested in the Institute. According to the initiators, this would be possible thanks to a shared understanding among the financial backers of the initiative – citizens contributing to the collection of funds necessary to make an initial offer – that the key aim of Visia Croatica was not to make profit but to ensure that the Institute continued to operate in the public interest, contributing to the stability and functionality of the healthcare system.

The concept proposed by Visia Croatica has been a unique example in the recent history of privatization in Croatia, especially taking into consideration that it applied to an entity that was at the same time within and without the public sector. In fact, while there have been a few recorded cases of employee stock ownership plans in the shipbuilding industry and machine production, there were no experiments with democratic forms of ownership in the public sector. It was therefore surprising, in a way, to observe how the ideas presented by the core group comprising Visia Croatica spread widely in a very short time. In a matter of weeks, the initiative gained wide public recognition; the Trade Union of Medical Doctors, the Chamber of Physicians, and the Association of Hospital Physicians supported it, and it received donations for bidding in the tender process. It should also be noted that this initiative appeared during a time of other social mobilizations for the protection of public goods, including a very successful campaign against the monetization of public highways.[73] Visia Croatica appeared at a time, and in the context, that were particularly susceptive to its ideas, but it nevertheless attracted attention and support of an unusually wide array of individuals, organizations, and initiatives. These included progressive and left-leaning organizations such as Right to the City and Friends of the Earth, but also war veterans associations and right-wing and conservative groups. Over the course of a month, the core group of Visia Croatica managed to build up support through a combination of approaches – by relying on more mainstream PR techniques and liaising with the media, as well as by recognizing the importance of formats that target a more specific audience and allowed in-depth discussions. It managed to get its message heard and rallied support all over the country, strengthening its position ahead of the final phase of the process. In the end, it was the sole submitter of a binding proposal to purchase shares of the Institute in March 2015.[74]

Critics of the initiative, on the other hand, argued that only large companies had sufficient resources to restart the production and ensure adequate investment in production, and that an initiative basically relying on crowdfunding, such as Visia Croatica, stood no chance of building up enough capital to stop the Institute from eventually failing – again. They also argued that the limited partnership proposed by Visia Croatica was not a viable model. Even the original form of the KGaA in Germany was seldom used, which they took as evidence of its inherent impracticability. In the scenario of Visia Croatica, they argued, the situation was even worse because it declared that it would break with the model of distributing profit among shareholders, an approach that was supposedly doomed to fail in a market economy. The continuous emphases on the complexity of the proposed model did throw the shadow of a doubt over it.

Critique coming from the left argued that a more transparent and democratic model would have been better suited to achieving collective ownership and public control. Any kind of privatization, they argued, even by a benevolent group, would lead to additional reduction in access to key medical products. On several occasions, it seemed that the trade union (EKN) shared that belief, especially in open letters where the trade union leadership insisted that only a commitment to public ownership and management by the government would ensure the restarting of production.[75] However, whenever the privatization of the Institute became more probable, the trade union took on a more nuanced attitude, allowing the possibility of private ownership that would guarantee the quality and number of jobs at the Institute. Prompted by the impression that Visia Croatica would be more sympathetic towards the needs of the workers than a strictly commercial buyer, the EKN in the end supported its bid.

In retrospect, Visia Croatica put forward a proposal that in many ways fits in with current trends of rethinking ownership. If we look into the increasingly widespread wave of de-privatization and re-municipalization of public services around the world, some parallels with the approach of Visia Croatica are visible. A recent large-scale study of re-municipalization conducted by the Transnational Institute, which covered several examples in the field of healthcare shows that efforts to de-privatize are characterized by a strong drive to enable participation from different kinds of groups (e.g., workers and users of services), more transparent operations, and space for running key sectors or services in the interest of the common good, rather than profit.[76] These are all elements that Visia Croatica emphasized.

After other contenders backed out of the process, citing concerns related to the amount of investment expected, it seemed for a while that the initiative's bid could be successful. However, virtually overnight, the tender was cancelled, and it was announced that the state would keep the Institute in public ownership in order to protect public health interests. Although this sounded rather unconvincing, especially taking into consideration the continuous edging towards privatization of the Institute over the last decades, supporters of Visia Croatica rather graciously accepted the announcement. In fact, many of them said this outcome should be perceived as a success resulting from their effort, as the whole point of Visia Croatica was to prevent the acquisition of the Institute by a private company and an even stronger market orientation. On 30 July 2015, the Government of the Republic of Croatia adopted the decision on the initiation of the process of transformation of the company *Imunološki zavod d.d.* into a healthcare institution called *Imunološki zavod* (the decision was later reversed), and on 20 August 2015, the Government adopted the regulation on the establishment of *Imunološki zavod* as a public health institution of strategic and general economic interest for the Republic of Croatia.[77] The feeling that the Institute could be reinvigorated as public institution was further reinforced by a commitment of the mayor of Zagreb, who pledged to work with the government to restart production, and a strategic partnership agreement between the state and municipal government was signed in early 2018. Nevertheless, as signing of this agreement was delayed and was not followed by concrete action, the IMZ, unsurprisingly, has continued on its downward trajectory.

Although it is hard to disregard the fact that the efforts of Visia Croatica were stopped before its plan could have been judged in practice, the initiative should be recognized as a rare example of cross-sectoral mobilization for defending production of medicines. In fact, Visia Croatica managed to achieve a lot in a short period of time: in addition to having achieved widespread social mobilization in a field which had previously seen only limited popular participation, it was also responsible for introducing in the public discourse an alternative view of ownership in the production of vaccines and biomedical products. Even though this might not have taken material shape, it remains a possible base for imagining a different shape of the sector in the aftermath of the Covid-19 pandemic – in line with global trends and efforts to strengthen public production and ensure fair and equitable access to medical products.

The public perception of the Institute's fate, as far it can be discerned from the media, has revolved around several key notions, with the nominally 'right' and 'left' positions occasionally overlapping. Voices opposing the attempts to 'save' the Institute have been relatively few and far between. Rather than representing a political party or a movement, individuals opposing the restructuring attempts occasionally identified as libertarians or were connected to groups calling for small government. They were not alone in emphasizing the larger problems of economy and public finances over public health. The price of restarting production and further, much larger investments – likely in order of tens of millions of euros – indeed made most commentators cautious, but these oppositional voices went further. On various occasions they argued that large public companies were an inherently fertile ground for corruption; that this was yet another example of the 'real economy' (i.e., private sector) being forced to save the uncompetitive and unproductive public sector; or that the situation at the Institute was a manifestation of a 'socialist mentality' that favoured inefficient business at the expense of more adaptable, privately owned ones.

Knowingly or not, proponents of saving the Institute through public (governmental) investment revisited some of the motifs and arguments from the time of the establishment and early consolidation of public vaccine production in Croatia. Vaccine production was once again perceived as an issue closely connected to sovereignty – this time the perceived loss of it – and the long-term financial benefits of domestic production, not only of vaccines but of blood derivatives, too, were emphasized. The fact that the IMZ's bankruptcy captivated public attention at the time of Croatia's accession to the European Union in 2013, which in itself raised the issue of dependency in parts of the political spectrum, probably influenced the way the situation at the institute was perceived and interpreted by the public.

Unsurprisingly, the Covid-19 pandemic has once again brought the Institute to the centre of public attention. As in many other countries, the 'strategic importance' of public vaccine production institutions became less abstract when the global circulation of pharmaceutical products and medical equipment was interrupted by a combination of worldwide lockdowns and export restrictions, pointing to a long-neglected drawback of relying on a global market. Praises of the Institute's past glory have been combined with unrealistic musings on how it could have contributed to the global vaccine race – had it not been effectively ruined. No outcome of the protracted political, legal, and financial deliberations on the Institute's future can be ruled out, even if the developments over the last two decades seem to give little reason for optimism. A possible positive outcome is more likely to be a consequence of rethinking the role of such institutions on a global scale, or at least that of the European Union, than of visions of local politicians and policy-makers. Finally, thinking about the future of the IMZ through the lenses of Covid-19 might prove to be counterproductive, as it could emphasize a highly specific aspect of vaccine production and segment of public health mandate in general – one that requires immense resources – at the expense of numerous others that the IMZ could more readily engage in, and which would benefit the Croatian public just as much. In any case, the wider societal significance and impact of the IMZ, as well as the inherent intertwinement of science and medicine with the sphere of politics, remain clearly manifested.

Notes

1 For an overview of earlier public health policies, see Ivana Horbec, *Zdravlje naroda—Bogatstvo države: Prosvijećeni apsolutizam i počeci stvaranja sustava javnog zdravstva u Hrvatskoj* (Zagreb: Hrvatski institut za povijest, 2015).

2 Though by far not exhaustive, *Od 'Kraljevskog zemaljskog zavoda za proizvadjanje cjepiva protiv boginjam' do Imunološkog zavoda Zagreb 1893–1993* (Zagreb: Imunološki zavod, 1993) remains the best overview. The Institute has also been featured in volumes dedicated to other, similar institutions and overviews of the history of medicine in Croatia. See Živka Prebeg, *Mala knjiga o velikom nasljeđu hrvatske preventivne medicine* (Zagreb: Imunološki zavod, 1993); Berislav Borčić, *Hrvatski zavod za javno zdravstvo od osnutka do danas 1893–2003* (Zagreb: Hrvatski zavod za javno zdravstvo, 2003); Branko Vitale *et al.*, *Četiri stoljeća javnoga zdravstva i biomedicine u Hrvatkoj* (Zagreb: Medicinska naklada–Akademija medicinskih znanosti Hrvatske, 2007); Vlatko Silobrčić, *O Imunološkom zavodu, Zagreb* (Zagreb, 2017).

3 Our research relied on both categories of sources, as well as more recent governmental reports and media coverage.

4 *Izvješće o radu Istražnog povjerenstva za utvrđivanje odgovornosti za rezultate upravljanja i raspolaganja financijskim i drugim resursima Imunološkog zavoda*, Hrvatski sabor, 2017, https://www.sabor.hr/sites/default/files/uploads/sabor/2019-01-18/081348/IZVJESCE_ISTRAZ_POVJ_IMUNOLOSKI.pdf (Accessed 23/04/2021).

5 Vlatko Silobrčić, 'Imunološki zavod: Sadašnjost i pogled u budućnost', in *Od 'Kraljevskog zemaljskog zavoda za proizvadjanje cjepiva protiv boginjam' do Imunološkog zavoda Zagreb 1893–1993* (Zagreb: Imunološki zavod, 1993), 79–96.

6 Stuart Blume, 'Towards a History of "The Vaccine Innovation System," 1950–2000', in Caroline Hannaway, ed, *Biomedicine in the Twentieth Century: Practices, Policies, and Politics* (Amsterdam: IOS Press, 2008), 255–286.

7 Dóra Vargha, *Polio Across the Iron Curtain: Hungary's Cold War with an Epidemic* (Cambridge: Cambridge University Press, 2018); Dóra Vargha, 'Vaccination and the communist state: Polio in Eastern Europe', in Christine Holmberg, Stuart Blume, and Paul Greenough, eds, *The Politics of Vaccination: A Global History* (Manchester: Manchester University Press, 2017), 77–98.

8 S. Litvinjenko, B. Arsić, and S. Borjanović, 'Epidemiologic Aspects of Smallpox in Yugoslavia in 1972', World Health Organization WHO/SE/73.57, 1973; https://apps.who.int/iris/bitstream/handle/10665/67617/WHO_SE_73.57.pdf (Accessed 23/04/2021); Vesna Trifunović, 'Temporality and Discontinuity as Aspects of Smallpox Outbreak in Yugoslavia', *Glasnik Etnografskog instituta SANU*, 2017, 65, 127–145.

9 Clive Hamilton and John Quiggin, 'The Privatisation of CSL', The Australia Discussion Paper Number 4, 1995; Jan Hendriks, *Societal Vaccinology: The Netherlands Public Sector Vaccine Development, Production and Technology Transfer in the Context of Global Health*, PhD Thesis (University of Amsterdam, 2017), 1–162.

10 David Knight, *The Making of Modern Science: Science, Technology, Medicine and Modernity* (Cambridge: Polity Press, 2009), 195.

11 The terms 'animal' and 'human' vaccine in this context refers to the method of propagating the viral material, not the aimed recipients.

12 Biserka Belicza, 'Od proizvodnje animalnog cjepiva za zaštitu od velikih boginja do proizvodnje prvih humanih virusnih cjepiva, antibakterijskih preparata i antitoksičnih seruma, te osnivanje prvog odjela za proizvodnju lijekova biološkog podrijetla u Zagrebu', in *Od 'Kraljevskog zemaljskog zavoda za proizvadjanje cjepiva protiv boginjam' do Imunološkog zavoda* (Zagreb: Imunološki zavod, 1993), 8.
13 Dubravko Habek, *Iz povijest zdravstva Bjelovara* (Zagreb–Bjelovar: Hrvatska akademija znanosti i umjetnosti, Zavod za znanstveno-istraživački rad u Bjelovaru, 2015).
14 Belicza, 'Od proizvodnje animalnog cjepiva'; Josip Berlot, 'Razvitak mikrobiologije i imunologije u Hrvtskoj do 1923. godine', in Eugen Topolnik, ed, *I. simpozij o historiji mikrobiologije i imunologije u Hrvatskoj do 1923. godine* (Zagreb: Jugoslavenska akademija znanosti i umjetnosti, 1973), 31–45.
15 Belicza, 'Od proizvodnje animanog cjepiva', 39.
16 Ljudevit Gutschy, 'O protutifusnoj vakcinaciji', *Liječnički vjesnik*, 1918, 40, 1–9; Igor Despot, 'Kolera u Banskoj Hrvatskoj 1913. godine—mjere državne vlasti u prevenciji i suzbijanju epidemije', *Radovi Zavoda za hrvatsku povijest*, 2013, 45, 53–70.
17 Slavko Palmirovič, '50 godina rada Pasteurova zavoda u Zagrebu', *Liječnički vjesnik*, 1970, 92, 789–795.
18 Željko Dugac, '"Like Yeast in Fermentation": Public Health in Interwar Yugoslavia', in Christian Promitzer, Sevasti Trubeta, and Marius Turda, eds, *Health, Hygiene and Eugenics in Southeastern Europe to 1945* (Budapest and New York: Central European University, 2011), 193–232.
19 Željko Dugac, *Protiv bolesti i neznanja: Rockefellerova fondacija u međuratnoj Jugoslaviji* (Zagreb: Srednja Europa, 2005); Iris Borowy, *Coming to Terms with World Health: The League of Nations Health Organization 1921–1946* (Frankfurt am Main: Peter Lang, 2009).
20 Andrija Štampar, *Travel Diary 1931–1938*, Željko Dugac and Marko Pećina, eds (Zagreb: Srednja Europa, 2020); Sara Silverstein, 'The Periphery is the Center: Some Macedonian Origins of Social Medicine and Internationalism', *Contemporary European History*, 2019, 28, 220–233.
21 Željko Dugac, *Kako biti čist i zdrav: Zdravstveno prosvjećivanje u međuratnoj Hrvatskoj* (Zagreb: Srednja Europa, 2010).
22 Vojislav Milovanović, *Medicinski godišnjak Kraljevine Jugoslavije* (Belgrade: Jugoreklam, 1933).
23 *Godišnjak banske vlasti Banovine Hrvatske 1939* (Zagreb, 1940).
24 Branko Petranović, *Istorija Jugoslavije 1918–1988*, vol. 3, *Socijalistička Jugoslavija 1945–1988* (Belgrade: Nolit, 1988), 424.
25 Stanley A. Plotkin supplied the RA 27/3 rubella strain, which was used for a successful combined, attenuated MMR (measles, mumps, rubella) vaccine.
26 Bernard Kaić, 'Impact of vaccination on vaccine-preventable disease burden in Croatia', *Periodicum biologorum*, 2012, 114, 141–147. Hepatitis b was added in 1999 and *Haemophilus influenzae* type b in 2002.
27 George Woodward, *UNRRA: The History of the United Nations Relief and Rehabilitation Administration* (New York: Columbia University Press, 1950), vol. 1, 138–170.
28 Sławomir Łotysz, 'A Bargain or a "Mouse Trap"? A Reused Penicillin Plant and the Yugoslavians' Quest for a Healthier Life in the Early Post-war Era', in Stefan Krebs and Hieke Weber, eds, *Histories of Persistence: Repair, Reuse and Disposal* (Bielefeld: transcript, forthcoming).
29 Borčić, *Hrvatski zavod za javno zdravstvo*, 18.
30 Hrvatski državni Arhiv, Zagreb (HDA, Croatian State Archives), Fund 1692, Republički sekretarijat za financije Socijalističke republike Hrvatske 1956–1990, box 978, 'Obrazloženje završnog računa za 1956. godinu', 3.
31 HDA 1692, box 994, 'Proizvodi'.
32 Belicza, 'Od proizvodnje animalnog cjepiva'.

33 Drago Ikić, 'Razvitak i perspektive Imunološkog zavoda', *Radovi Imunološkog zavoda Zagreb*, 1965, 3/4, 3–8, 4.
34 Ikić, 'Razvitak i perspektive'; Silobrčić, 'Imunološki zavod', 86.
35 Silobrčić, 'Imunološki zavod', 85.
36 Ikić, 'Razvitak i perspektive', 5.
37 In the first half of the 1980s, which, admittedly, was a period of economic crisis, the IMZ was far from qualifying for a list of Yugoslavia's 333 most successful exporters. See '333 najveća izvoznika', *Direktor*, 1983, 15, 8–12; *Direktor*, 1984, 16, 22–44; and *Direktor*, 1985, 17, 37–45. Between 1980 and 1983, the value of exported good fell from $1,400,000 to $600,000, but it rebounded towards the end of the decade to $2,400,000 in 1989. However, Silobrčić warned the figure was by far exaggerated because of unrealistic exchange rates. See Silobrčić, 'Imunološki zavod', 85–86.
38 Drago Ikić, 'Izvještaj o Imunološkom Zavodu od 1960. do 1971', *unpublished document*, quoted in Silobrčić, 'Imunološki zavod', 81.
39 HDA 1692, box 978, 'Obrazloženje završnog računa za 1956. godinu', 2.
40 HDA 1692, box 1007, 'Izvještaj o poslovanju u 1961', unpaginated.
41 Berislav Pende, 'Prilog novijoj povijesti Imunološkog zavoda', in *Od 'Kraljevskog zemaljskog zavoda za proizvadjanje cjepiva protiv boginjam' do Imunološkog zavoda Zagreb 1893–1993* (Zagreb: Imunološki zavod, 1993), 63–77; HDA 1692, box 1007, 'Izvještaj o poslovanju za 1961'.
42 Renata Mažuran, 'Drago Ikić: Portait of a Renowned Croatian Vaccinonologist; Vision, Mission, Strategy and Goals', *Periodicum biologorum*, 2012, 114, 133–140, 138.
43 Pende, 'Prilog novijoj povijesti', 64.
44 L. Hayflick and P.S. Moorhead, 'The Serial Cultivation of Human Diploid Cell Strains', *Experimental Cell Research*, 1961, 25, 585–621.
45 Leonard Hayflick, 'Problems with patenting WI-38', video at Web of Stories, https://www.webofstories.com/play/leonard.hayflick/118 (Accessed 28/04/2021).
46 Transcript of Leonard Hayflick, 'Drago Ikić promotes the use of human cell culture', video at Web of Stories, https://www.webofstories.com/play/leonard.hayflick/129 (Accessed 28/04/2021).
47 Drago Ikić *et al.*, 'Postvakcinalne reakcije nakon primjene žive, oralne vakcine protiv poliomijelitisa priređene u sistemu humanih diploidnih stanica (soj WI-38)', *Radovi Imunološkog zavoda Zagreb*, 1964, 2, 22–28.
48 Felicity T. Cutts, *The Immunological Basis for Immunization Series, Module 7, Measles* (Geneva: World Health Organization, 2001).
49 Mažuran, 'Drago Ikić', 136; Pende, 'Pilog novijoj povijesti', 69.
50 Drago Ikić, 'Edmonston-Zagreb Strain of Measles Vaccine: Epidemiologic Evaluation in Yugoslavia', *Reviews of Infectious Diseases*, 1983, 5, 558–563.
51 Vitale, *Četiri stoljeća*, 249.
52 Aline Baldo *et al.*, 'Biosafety considerations for attenuated measles virus vectors used in virotherapy and vaccination', *Human Vaccines and Immunotherapeutics*, 2016, 12, 1102–1116.
53 Mažuran, 'Drago Ikić', 136.
54 Drago Ikić *et al.*, 'Preliminary Report on Vaccination in Croatia against Poliomyelitis with Type 1 (CHAT) and Type 3 (W-Fox) Attenuated Polioviruses of Koprowski', *Bulletin of the World Health Organization*, 1963, 28, 217–223; Drago Ikić, 'Our Experience with Live, Oral Poliomyelitis Vaccine Koprowski Type 1, 2, and 3', *Radovi Imunološkog zavoda Zagreb*, 1966, 5/6, 139–141; Hillary Koprowski and Stanley Plotkin, 'History of Koprowski Vaccine Against Poliomyelitis', in Stanley A. Plotkin, ed, *History of Vaccine Development* (New York: Springer, 2011), 155–166, 160. Both monkey kidney and HDCS were used as substrate cell. See B. Janičkić, D. Ćuk, and D. Ikić, 'Poliovakcinacija tipom 1 djece u prvim danima života i prevencija poliomijelitisa', *Radovi Imunološkog zavoda u Zagrebu*, 1967, 7, 3–22.

55 Stanley A. Plotkin, 'History of Rubella Vaccines and the Recent History of Cell Culture', in *History of Vaccine Development*, 219–231, 226.
56 Belicza, 'Od proizvodnje animalnog cjepiva'.
57 Pende, 'Prilog novijoj povijesti', 76–77.
58 Ikić, 'Razvitak i perspektive', 8.
59 The about-100-page-long 2017 report on the work of a parliamentary investigation dealing with the IMZ lists a fascinating list of complaints, accusations, and recriminations that are difficult to summarize. They should also be taken with caution because they partly refer to events from more than 20 years ago, and some depositions were based on hearsay evidence. See *Izvješće o radu Istražnog povjerenstva*.
60 *Izvješće o radu Istražnog povjerenstva*, 26–27.
61 Silobrčić, 'Imunološki zavod', 83.
62 *Ibid*., 81.
63 HDA 1692, box 978, 'Obrazloženje završnog računa za 1956. godinu', 2.
64 Juraj Nemec and Natalya Kolisnichenko, 'Market-based health care reforms in Central and Eastern Europe: lessons after ten years of change', *International Review of Administrative Sciences*, 2006, 72, 11–26; Stjepan Orešković, 'Postwelfare indikatori i reforma zdravstva u Hrvatkoj', *Revija za socijalnu politiku*, 1994, 1, 323–331.
65 Siniša Zrinšćak, 'Zdravstvena politika Hrvatske: u vrtlogu reformi i suvremenih društvenih izazova', *Revija za socijalnu politiku*, 2007, 14, 193–220.
66 Snježana Ivčić, Ana Vračar, and Lada Weygand, 'Primarna zdravstvena zaštita u Hrvatskoj od samoupravljanja do tranzicije: korijeni ideja privatizacije', in Chiara Bonfiglioli and Boris Koroman, eds, *Zbornik odabranih radova s Drugog međunarodnog znanstvenog skupa Socijalizam na klupi: Socijalizam; Izgradnja i razgradnja* (Zagreb: Srednja Europa, 2017), 99–128; Aleksandar Džakula *et al*., 'Decentralization and Healthcare Reform in Croatia 1980–2002', in G. Shakarishvili, ed, *Decentralization in Healthcare: Analyses and Experiences in Central and Eastern Europe in the 1990s* (Budapest: Open Society Institute, 2005), 133–191.
67 Andrija Hebrang, 'Reorganization of the Croatian Healthcare System', *Croatian Medical Journal*, 1994, 35, 130–136; Stjepan Orešković, 'Zdravstveni privatizacijski pendulum', *Društvena istraživanja*, 1999, 8, 601–621, 613.
68 Zrinšćak, 'Zdravstvena politika Hrvatske'.
69 *Izvješće o obavljenoj reviziji pretvorbe i privatizacije: Imunološki zavod, Zagreb*, May 2002, last accessed 10 October 2020.
70 *Izvješće o radu Istražnog povjerenstva*, 38–39.
71 'Imunološki zavod (The Institute of Immunology, Zagreb)', European Monitoring Centre on Change, https://www.eurofound.europa.eu/observatories/emcc/erm/factsheets/imunoloski-zavod-the-institute-of-immunology-zagreb-0 (Accessed 27/04/2021).
72 Ante Bajo and Marko Primorac, 'Croatian Institute of Immunology: Where have things got stuck?', Institute of Public Finance Institute – Press Releases 83, 10 June 2015, http://www.ijf.hr/upload/files/file/ENG/releases/83.pdf (Accessed 30/04/2021).
73 Tin Gazivoda, 'From Maribor Spring to Tuzla Revolt: Beyond the Protest Moments in Slovenia, Croatia, and Bosnia', *IEMed Mediterranean Yearbook*, 2015, 164–167.
74 Bajo and Primorac, 'Croatian Institute of Immunology'.
75 EKN, Pismo predsjedniku Vlade Republike Hrvatske, 22 April 2015.
76 Satoko Kishimoto, Lavinia Steinfort, and Olivier Petitjean, *The Future Is Public: Towards Democratic Ownership of Public Assets* (Amsterdam, 2020).
77 'Uredba o osnivanju Imunološkog zavoda kao javne zdravstvene ustanove koja je od strateškog i općeg gospodarskog interesa za Republiku Hrvatsku', *Narodne novine*, 91/2015, https://narodne-novine.nn.hr/eli/sluzbeni/2015/91/1762 (Accessed 29/04/2021).

5

WILFUL NEOLIBERAL INCAPACITATION OF INDIA'S PUBLIC SECTOR VACCINE INSTITUTIONS

Madhavi Yennapu

Introduction

India's public sector vaccine institutions (PSVIs) are over a century old. They did commendable service to the nation during both Worlds Wars, through epidemic outbreaks, and as key contributors to the country's routine national Universal Immunization Programme (UIP). The introduction of liberalization in India in 1990, however, led to the decline of the public sector and the increasing role of the private sector. This led to a vaccine shortage for the UIP, coupled with a surplus of expensive new vaccines produced and marketed by private sector companies.[1] Additionally, the Covid-19 pandemic has come at a time when India's PSVIs are struggling after receiving minimal state patronage as a result of neoliberal policies.[2] But the pandemic has also exposed the inadequacy of health systems around the world, forcing some rethinking of the relevance of the public sector in addressing health emergencies.[3,4] India's PSVIs are at a crossroads, with several lingering questions: Is this the right time to close down PSVIs? Will they be rejuvenated in order to play a legitimate role in maintaining vaccine affordability and spearheading national health security? Can the private vaccine sector deliver safe, efficacious, and affordable vaccines, as the PSVIs once did, especially when intellectual property rights are a barrier to affordability?

This chapter reviews the transformation of PSVIs in India under neoliberalism. It focuses mainly on the dramatic closure of three crucial PSVIs in 2008 – Central Research Institute (CRI), Kasauli; Pasteur Institute of India (PII), Coonoor; and BCG Vaccine Laboratories (BCGVL), Chennai – and their revival in 2010, as this case mirrors the current political economy of vaccines in India.

DOI: 10.4324/9781003130345-6

The emergence of PSVIs in India

In nineteenth century India, the prevailing infectious diseases specific to its tropical climate were poorly understood by British researchers, which caused high mortality in the British army compared to the local population. Three factors precipitated the emergence of PSVIs in India. (i) Medical officers (researchers) from the Indian Medical Services (IMS) and the local sanitary departments who did significant research on tropical diseases impressed on the British government the necessity of medical research institutions. (ii) In 1884 the Indian Medical Congress through its resolution urged the British government to set up vaccine R&D institutions.[5] (iii) The sudden outbreak of plague in 1896 in Bombay (now Mumbai) that swept rapidly through large parts of the country and threatened colonial economic interests. A promising field of microbiology for medical researchers in India was opening up. The first bacteriological institute was founded in 1892 in Agra, followed by the establishment of the King Institute of Preventive Medicine (KIPM) in 1889, the Haffkine Institute (HI) in 1898 following a plague epidemic, CRI (1905) and PII (1907). By the end of the first decade of the twentieth century, around 25 PSVIs had been established in different provinces throughout British India (Table 5.1).

R&D as the driving force of PSVIs in the pre-independence period

PSVIs carried out research on the prevailing diseases of the time (malaria, kala-azar, cholera, typhoid, polio, rabies, influenza, smallpox, tuberculosis, etc.) and developed vaccines, anti-toxins, sera and anti-venoms (Table 5.1). The main research in PSVIs was on trypanosomes, relapsing fever, leprosy, mycetoma infections, cholera, and snake and scorpion venom. There was also the discovery in 1898 by Haffkine and Simond of the aetiological agents of plague (demonstrating transmission by fleas); the identification of the vector of kala-azar by Short and Swaminathan at PII; work by Ross on malaria and Manson on cholera; while others looked at insect-transmitted diseases and their lifecycles.

The world's first plague vaccine was developed in India at the Haffkine Institute, Mumbai. Vaccine lymph for smallpox, as well as cholera, typhoid and TT (tetanus toxoid) vaccines were developed indigenously at KIPM, Chennai (then Madras). Import substitution policies during the two world wars boosted indigenous development of vaccines and sera, making PSVIs self-reliant.

The PSVI innovation model was an integrated one, where R&D, manufacture, and delivery systems were all under the same roof, with the necessary supporting facilities (reagents lab, blood banks, animal house, etc.). This favoured close coordination. The end of the Second World War left a void in the PSVIs' R&D activities, as many researchers and IMS officers who had left for war duties did not return. However, the routine manufacturing activities continued despite inadequate finance, manpower, and infrastructure.

TABLE 5.1 Vaccine R&D and production in Public Sector Vaccine Institutions (PSVIs) established since 1800

Name of the Vaccine PSVI	*Year of Establishment*	*Vaccines/Sera Produced*	*Operational Status*
		North India	
1. Pasteur Institute of India, Kasauli (Punjab province)	1900	Anti-rabies	Merged with CRI Kasauli 1939
2. Central Research Institute (CRI), Kasauli	1905	Typhoid, cholera, anti-snake venom, anti-rabies	Operational*
3. Provincial Hygiene Institute, Lucknow	1900	Cholera	Closed down Post-2000
4. Vaccine Lymph Department, Patwada Nagar, near Nainital (later State Vaccine Institute)	1903	Vaccine lymph, anti-rabies	Closed down 2003
5. Pasteur Institute Rangoon (currently Myanmar)	1915	Anti-rabies	Located in Myanmar
6. Vaccine Institute, Lahore (maintained by government of Punjab; after independence it became a part of Pakistan)	1910s	Vaccine lymph	Located in Pakistan
7. Bharat Immunologicals and Biologicals Ltd. (BIBCOL), Bulandshar, Delhi	1989	OPV formulations from imported bulk	Operational
8. Indian Vaccines Corporation Ltd. (IVCOL), Gurgaon	1989	Intended to produce measles vaccine, but could not due to the unavailability of the technology.	Closed down 2002
		South India	
9. Institute of Preventive Medicine, Hyderabad (formerly Plague Department)	1870	Plague, smallpox (since 1910), rabies (since 1976–1977), TT (since 1978)	Production of anti-rabies and TT stopped 2002; closed down 2005

10.	King Institute of Preventive Medicine, Guindy, Chennai (then Madras)	1898	Vaccine lymph, TT, typhoid, cholera	Operational Currently produces DT and DPT, anti-snake venom, anti-rabies, anti-tetanus serum; production of TT, typhoid, cholera vaccines suspended 2005
11.	Public Health Laboratory, Bangalore	1900	Cholera	Closed down Post-2000
12.	Vaccine Lymph Department, Belgaum	1904	Vaccine lymph	Production stopped and the department closed down 1980s
13.	Pasteur Institute of Southern India, Coonoor	1907	Anti-rabies, OPV (1967-1976), DTP, DT, TT (since 1978)	Operational*
14.	Public Health Laboratory, Thiruvananthapuram	1937	Anti-rabies; later functioned as immunology lab supplying yellow fever vaccine on demand	Closed down Post-2005
15.	BCG Vaccine Lab, Guindy, Chennai	1946	BCG vaccine	Operational*
16.	Indian Immunologicals Ltd., Hyderabad	1983	Main focus on veterinary vaccines; human vaccine production began 1998: tissue culture human rabies vaccine (1998), measles, MMR (2002), rDNA Hep B (2006), anti-rabies serum	Operational
			East India	
17.	Smithstrain Street Pharmaceuticals Ltd., Calcutta (established 1821 as a private company, became a PSVI1977)	1821	Vaccines/sera	Closed down 2000
18.	Vaccine Lymph Department, Calcutta	1890s	Vaccine lymph	Closed down 1980s
19.	Cholera Vaccine Lab, Calcutta	1890s	Cholera	Closed down 1980s
20.	Bengal Public Health Lab, Calcutta	1900	Cholera; later conducted sterility tests on other government labs	Closed down 1980s

(Continued)

TABLE 5.1 (Continued)

Name of the Vaccine PSVI	*Year of Establishment*	*Vaccines/Sera Produced*	*Operational Status*
21. Vaccine Institute, Ranchi	1900	Vaccine lymph, cholera, anti-rabies	Closed down 2008
22. Public Health Laboratory, Patna	1900	Cholera	Closed down 2008
23. Bengal Chemicals and Pharmaceuticals Ltd., Calcutta (established 1901 as a private company, became a PSVI in 1980)	1901	Chemicals, synthetics, dyes, vaccines/sera	Closed down 2000; recently being revived
24. Pasteur Institute, Calcutta	1910	Anti-rabies (unsatisfactory functioning); later a teaching institute	Closed down 1980s
25. Pasteur and Medical Research Institute, Shillong, Assam	1917	Typhoid, cholera, anti-rabies treatment	Closed down 2006
26. Bengal Immunity Ltd., Calcutta (became a PSVI 1980s)	1919	All vaccines required for EPI, cholera, typhoid, anti-rabies, anti-snake venoms, etc.	Closed down 2003
27. School of Tropical Medicine, Calcutta	1922	Epidemiological and other routine diagnostic services	No vaccine production since 1980s
28. West Bengal Lab, Calcutta (became a PSVI 1980)	1980	Sera/vaccines, synthetics and dyes	Closed down post-2005
		West India	
29. Haffkine Institute, Mumbai (formerly Bombay Bacteriological Laboratory)	1898	DT, TT, plague, cholera, typhoid, rabies, gas gangrene anti-toxins, anti-dysentery, anti-snake venom	Operational
30. Vaccine Institute, Nagpur (established 1959, became a PSVI in 1980)	1959	Smallpox, cholera (from 1968)	Production was stopped before it was closed down post-2005
31. Vaccine Institute, Vadodara (became a PSVI in 1973)	1973	Anti-rabies	Closed down 2009

* Production suspended in January 2008 and revived in 2010 on the recommendation of the GOI's Javid Chowdhury Committee report.

Source: Compiled from Health Information of India, MOHFW, Government of India (GOI), New Delhi, and Bhore et al., Medical Research, Chapter XIV (pages 161–197), Report of the Health Survey and Development Committee of the Survey, Vol.1, 1946. GOI, Manager of Publications, Delhi.

The fate of PSVIs in the post-independence period

Following independence, PSVIs received state funding to continue R&D and manufacture vaccines and sera. Twenty-five PSVIs were reduced to 23 as the institutes in Lahore and Rangoon were no longer part of independent India. BCGVL was set up in 1948 for the production of BCG vaccine. Vaccination against TB began in 1952. Vaccine lymph against smallpox was developed and manufactured in many PSVIs to combat smallpox epidemics in the 1960s, and until 1977, when India was declared smallpox-free. PSVIs manufacturing vaccine lymph/smallpox vaccine either closed down or diversified into other production activities (Table 5.1). Many PSVIs started to produce combined DPT (diphtheria, pertussis and tetanus), TT, DT (diphtheria and tetanus), BCG, typhoid vaccines, and OPV following the launch of the World Health Organisation's (WHO) Expanded Program on Immunization (EPI) in India in 1978.[1,6] After independence, six more PSVIs were founded: Vaccine Institute, Vadodara; Vaccine Institute, Nagpur; West Bengal Lab, Calcutta; Indian Immunologicals Ltd. (IIL), Hyderabad; Bharat Immunologicals and Biologicals Ltd. (BIBCOL), Bulandshar; and Indian Vaccines Corporation Ltd. (IVCOL), Gurgaon. The latter two were set up in the late 1980s, under the Department of Biotechnology (DBT), with the objective of achieving self-reliance in vaccine development and self-sufficiency in vaccine production using modern technologies.[6] This brought the total number of PSVIs to 29 (Table 5.1).

In the mid-1980s, India added the measles vaccine to its EPI (which has since been referred to as the UIP). However IVCOL, which was to manufacture the measles vaccine domestically, could not do so as the technology was unavailable.[6]

Of the total of 29 Indian PSVIs, 17 were closed down between the 1980s and 2005, despite their expertise in modern production technologies. By 2007, only seven remained operational. In 2008, three more PSVIs (CRI, PII, and BCGVL) were closed down, leaving only four. However, in 2010, the three PSVIs closed in 2008 were reopened, meaning that as of early 2021, seven PSVIs are in operation: two (HI, KIPM) under their respective state governments; three (CRI, PII, BCGVL) under the Union Health Ministry (UHM) or Ministry of Health and Family Welfare (MOHFW); one (BIBCOL) under DBT; and one (IIL, Hyderabad) under the National Dairy Development Board under the Ministry of Agriculture.

R&D contributions and services delivered by CRI, PII, and BCGVL

It is worth mentioning the significant research contributions and services delivered by CRI, PII, and BCGVL in their long histories – CRI and PII are both over 100 years old, while BCGVL is over 70 years old – before discussing their controversial closure in 2008.

The Central Research Institute (CRI), Kasauli was one of the pioneering institutions to develop and manufacture indigenous vaccines and serums: rabies (1911), typhoid (1906) and cholera vaccine (1914), diphtheria anti-toxin (1953), tetanus anti-toxin (1954), rabies serum (1955), yellow fever vaccine (1958), DPT (1978), Japanese Encephalitis (JE) vaccine (1982), vero cell–based JE vaccine (2007), and anti-snake venoms and sera (1906). According to its website, CRI Kasauli also serves as the Central Drugs Laboratory, a national quality control and certifying agency for all vaccines made in India.

The Pasteur Institute of India (PII), Coonoor, was set up with the aim of researching and developing an anti-rabies vaccine and is one of the leading institutes in India in the field. It was the first institute in the world to introduce anti-rabies serum vaccine therapy in human beings in 1917. During the 1918 flu pandemic, PII identified Asian flu strains in India through its epidemiological research, and in 1957 it developed a vaccine against the influenza virus. In 1979, PII was the first in India to develop a more economical tissue culture-based (betapropiolactone-inactivated) anti-rabies vaccine using sheep brain cells instead of mouse brain cells, and an affordable tissue culture-based JE vaccine. From 1967 to 1976, with support from the WHO and the government of India (GOI), it also manufactured OPV with seed virus obtained from Dr. Albert Sabin. PII also developed a DPT combination vaccine starting in 1978 and some years later a measles vaccine.[7]

The BCG Vaccine Laboratory (BCGVL), Chennai, was set up in 1948, soon after Indian independence, and was the sole institute manufacturing BCG vaccine for the entire country (for its UIP), initially from seed virus obtained from the State Serum Institute in Copenhagen. In 1993 BCGVL developed its own seed virus, named Madras Working Seed Lot (MWSL). By 2001 the laboratory produced all the BCG the UIP required and could also earn some revenue by selling the BCG vaccine to private suppliers. BCGVL also obtained a quality certification for its vaccine manufacturing process (ISO 9002) from M/s Bureau Veritas Quality International (BVQI), London. BCGVL claims that this is the first and the only Institute under the MOHFW that has been awarded an ISO 9002 certificate. BCGVL made several cost-effective incremental innovations to improve sterility and yield of its BCG vaccine. It also produces freeze-dried therapeutic vaccine for cancer chemotherapy. BCGVL serves as a National Quality Control Lab for BCG vaccine.

Dramatic closure in 2008

In January 2008, the Drugs Controller General of India (DCGI) took the surprising and bizarre decision to cancel the manufacturing licences of CRI, PII, and BCGVL, alleging that they were not compliant with the WHO's current good manufacturing practices (WHO-cGMP). Around 80% of the supply for the country's UIP came from these three institutions, and they were all self-sufficient in vaccine production with no complaints regarding the quality of the vaccines they manufactured.[8,9]

At the same time, the UHM announced the allocation of US$37.5 million to set up a centralized Integrated Vaccine Complex (IVC) in Chengalpattu near Chennai.[9] The public sector company Hindustan Latex Limited (HLL) was given the task of setting up the IVC (with help from international consultancy Ernst & Young Global Ltd.), even though it did not have any competence in developing or manufacturing vaccines, beyond having previously mediated the import of some vaccines by the GOI.[9,10]

The plan to create a centralized IVC in three years (by 2011), while abruptly suspending production in three PSVIs, raised several pertinent questions: How would the resultant huge shortfall of UIP vaccines be met until the new IVC became operational, given also the worldwide reduction in EPI vaccine manufacturers? Would it be through imports or from the private sector, and at what price? Would HLL be able to produce quality vaccines and remain WHO-cGMP compliant? What would guarantee that HLL's fate would not replicate that of the three PSVIs? What exactly is WHO-cGMP compliance, and is it really necessary for domestic production? What was the economic logic of spending over US$37.5 million on building a new IVC, when modernizing the existing PSVIs would have cost less than US$12.5 million? Would the companies involved in the IVC manufacture the vaccines locally or repackage vaccines imported in bulk? If they were to import vaccines, what would be the point in achieving WHO-cGMP compliance, at the cost of indigenous manufacturing ability? If dependence on private sector supply or import is inevitable, how would the government tackle issues relating to biosecurity and strategic national health security?

At the time, the UHM/MOHFW argued that UIP vaccine supply would be met by the private sector, and that WHO-cGMP compliance was important for the IVC, since WHO-cGMP non-compliance would lead to the de-recognition of India's National Regulatory Authority (NRA), which would in turn impact private vaccine manufacturers' exports. Furthermore, it claimed that there was not enough space to expand production facilities in the existing PSVIs, therefore a centralized IVC was necessary. In response to parliamentary questioning, the health minister informed parliament that a committee would be set up in April 2008 to look into upgrading existing vaccine production within WHO-cGMP compliant facilities. Later it was discovered that the terms of reference of the committee were not in fact for upgrading, but for converting the PSVIs into testing laboratories: their fate had been decided in advance.[9,10]

WHO-cGMP comes in handy to shut down three PSVIs

WHO-cGMP quality certification/compliance, certified through a country's NRA, is mandatory for pharmaceutical products that are sold to UN agencies or which will move in global markets, in order to ensure uniform standards.[11] WHO-cGMP compliance means conforming to certain basic standards for processes of production, infrastructure, technology, systems, methodology, protocols, and trained staff. Its objective is to avert any major risks involved in any pharmaceutical production and to ensure safe and effective pharmaceutical innovations/products for human consumption and public health. The GMP certification has been in operation since 1969 and many countries (around 100) have formulated requirements for GMP based on WHO-GMP in their national regulatory systems. Others have harmonized their requirements. The Indian GMP standards for vaccines/sera, comparable to WHO-GMP, came into force in 2005 (in Schedule 'M' under D&C Rules of the Drugs & Cosmetics Act 1945). WHO GMP certification in India is awarded by the Drug Controller General of India (DCGI) under MOHFW, who is the National Regulatory Authority (NRA).

India underwent its first inspection by a joint WHO NRA team in 2001. The NRA inspected PII, BCGVL, and CRI in 2001 and 2004, and they were instructed to comply with WHO-cGMP. The WHO team, which wanted to join the NRA team for the inspection of the PSVIs in 2002, was not permitted to do so by the GOI, on the grounds that it would interfere with Indian sovereignty. However, in May 2007, the MOHFW gave permission to the WHO to join its NRA team for an inspection which took place in August. In October 2007, the secretary of the MOHFW held a meeting in which the following decisions were taken:

> (i) Public Sector units should wind-down operations by stopping procurement of raw materials and production; (ii) the units [should] urgently prepare a plan for setting up new manufacturing facilities and (iii) efforts [should] be made by the UIP Div. to build up buffer stocks to meet possible shortages.[12]

PSVIs could rectify the deficiencies suggested by the joint WHO-NRA team following its inspection in 2001, but by 2004 they were no longer able to do so. Norms had become more stringent. In December 2007, all three institutions received notices requiring them to justify their continued functioning.[9,10,12] The three PSVIs responded that they were unable to meet WHO-cGMP compliance due to their limited funds, the result of inflexible government rules and regulations for running industrial units in the area of biologicals: an issue that had been raised on several earlier occasions.[9,10]

The PSVIs rectified some major shortcomings pointed out by the WHO-NRA team by 2007, with the exception of a few minor remaining infrastructure-related compliance issues, which could have been easily remedied given adequate time and finances. However, the PSVIs received neither.[10,12,13] Moreover, the joint WHO-NRA team that visited the three PSVIs in 2007 did not recommend the suspension of vaccine production or the PSVIs' closure, but rather offered to help upgrade the institutes' technologies. Instead of accepting the WHO's offer, on 16 January 2008, the then DCGI, Dr. P. Venkateswarlu, issued a notice suspending the manufacturing licenses of the three PSVIs, on the grounds that they were not WHO-cGMP compliant.[12] Interestingly, BCGVL was instructed to destroy all BCG vaccine samples in stock, alleging that they were WHO-cGMP non-compliant, despite no complaints from the WHO-NRA team regarding the quality of vaccines produced by the PSVIs.

Since WHO-cGMP certification is required only for exports, the UHM need not have succumbed to pressure to shut the PSVIs. They could have continued to meet domestic requirements until the new IVC was up and running and the PSVIs had been made fully WHO-cGMP compliant.[10] The 34th report of the Parliamentary Standing Committee on Health and Family Welfare noted that:

> there is no evidence to show that the vaccines produced by the three PSUs were unsafe for the children.... [Furthermore, the committee] cannot remain a mute spectator to a situation where in the name of exports, GMP compliance and new technology, the entire vaccine market is handed over to the private sector and an impending shortage of vaccines is allowed to loom large over the Universal Immunisation Programme.[10]

Shortages of UIP vaccines and high prices following the closures

The closure of the three PSVIs led to an acute shortage of UIP vaccines in 23 Indian states, as the private sector went back on its promise to supply UIP vaccines at public sector prices within six months.[12,14] A sharp decline in immunization coverage was noted in 2008-2009. Not only did incomplete immunization lead to greater morbidity and mortality in children, but a larger number of adverse effects following immunization (AEFI) were also reported.

The government procurement price for UIP vaccines from the private sector increased by 50–70% within two years. The procurement cost of DPT and BCG was US$16.07 million in 2008–2009, compared to US$8.05 million in 2007–2008.[15] Government procurement prices for vaccines from the private sector increased by 52% within a year and 250% within five years of the suspension of the three PSVIs, an increase that cannot be attributed to inflation.[15] In order to meet the resulting shortages the government was obliged to procure UIP vaccines stored by the very same suspended PSVIs. The procurement price for the last nine years (2013–2021) is currently not publicly available.

The private sector's vaccine prices have also increased; they are 10–600 times higher compared to PSVI prices (Table 5.2), in contrast to the claims of private companies that the UHM does not give a fair price (Table 5.2).[16]

Since CRI, BCGVL, and PII were under the UHM/MOHFW and functioned only according to its instructions, it was the UHM's responsibility to upgrade them to WHO-cGMP compliance, rather than blaming and axing them.[9,10,12,13] The irony is that while these three PSVIs were closed down for WHO-cGMP non-compliance, the UHM procured UIP vaccines from private companies that were also WHO-cGMP non-compliant at the time.[9,10] Nor did the government object to vaccine being imported from a WHO-cGMP non-compliant Chinese

TABLE 5.2 The difference in vaccine prices between the public sector (PSVIs) and private companies per dose (0.5 ml)

Vaccine	*Manufacturer*	*Brand Name*	*Price in US$*
DPT	**Private Sector**		
	Serum Institute of India	Triple Antigen (DTP)	0.22
	Serum Institute of India	Pentavac (DTP-HB-Hib)	6.60
	Chiron Panacea	Ecovac (DTP-Hepatitis B)	14.93
	Panacea	Easy Four (DTP-Hib)	7.06
	Chiron Panacea	Easy Five (DTP-HB-Hib)	7.80
	Aventis Pasteur	Tripacel (DTaP)	10.00
	Biological E Pvt. Ltd.	TRIPVAC	0.15
	GSK	Infanrix	9.32
	GSK	Tritanrix (DTP-HB)	3.00
	Public Sector		
	Haffkine Bio-Pharmaceutical Corporation Ltd.	DTP	0.022
	PII, Koonoor	DTP	0.04
	Central Research Institute	DTP	0.04
	Haffkine Bio-Pharmaceutical Corporation Ltd.	DT	0.02
	CRI, Kasaul	DT	0.02
DT	**Private Sector**		
	Serum Institute of India	Dual Antigen	0.18
	Public Sector		
	Bengal Chemicals and Pharmaceuticals Pvt. Ltd.	DT	0.04
	Bengal Immunity Ltd.	DT	0.07
	Pasteur Institute of India	DT	0.02
	Central Research Institute	DT	not available
TT	**Private Sector**		
	Serum Institute of India	TT	0.14
	Public Sector		
	Haffkine Bio-Pharmaceutical Corporation Ltd.	TT	0.018
	Central Research Institute	TT	0.02
BCG	**Private Sector**		
	Serum Institute of India	Tubervac	0.78
	Aventis Pasteur India Ltd.	BCG	0.33
	Green Signal Biopharma Ltd.	BCG	0.52
	Public Sector		
	BCGVL	Production has not yet started	0.17

Source: Compiled from www.drugsupdate.com/brand/generic/vaccineDTP/23518 and https://www.fiercepharma.com/r-d/india-s-vaccine-prices-soar-as-private-companies-gain-ground.

company! Questions were thus raised regarding the double standards applied by the UHM for the public and private sectors.[9,10]

This was not the first time that the 'quality' of a vaccine had been used to prevent the public sector from manufacturing vaccines, to the benefit of private companies. From 1967 to 1976, PII produced six batches of excellent quality OPV.

However, the seventh batch tested at NICD, Delhi, was found to be virulent. Instead of reviewing the case, domestic manufacture of OPV was halted. Given that OPV is required for the country's UIP, from 1978 it became one of India's major imports.[6,7] Later, Dr. S Archetti from the WHO confirmed that the seventh batch produced by PII was in fact of the same excellent quality as the earlier six batches.[9] After two decades, in 1997, domestic manufacture of OPV by Haffkine Bio-Pharmaceutical Corporation Ltd. was once more permitted.[6] In a similar case, BIBCOL was repackaging imported OPV bulk from a Russian company for domestic use and was also supplying to the UNICEF procurement system. Later, however, UNICEF refused the vaccine, alleging that the Russian provider was not WHO-cGMP regulated. It subsequently insisted that India should procure OPV from SmithKlineBeecham (now GSK).[6]

In 2008, when the Ukrainian government suspended its use of the MMR vaccine (supplied by the Serum Institute of India, SIIL) following the death of a 17-year-old and 92 hospitalizations, the WHO, UNICEF and the United States CDC stated that the halting of vaccination was regrettable while the investigation was still on-going.[17] In India, 237 deaths were reported following the pentavalent vaccine (protecting against diphtheria, tetanus, whooping cough, hepatitis B, and *Haemophilus influenzae* type B) during the period 2011–2016,[18] yet there was no review,[19] no halt to vaccination, and no cancellation of the production licenses of the private companies producing the vaccine. Instead, the vaccine's AEFI classification was revised.[20] In 2011, the WHO dropped the private company Panacea Biotech from its list of prequalified vaccine suppliers.[21] The US FDA served a warning letter to Panacea Biotech as recently as September 2020 regarding its non-compliance.[22] The above instances indicate that private vaccine companies have 'quality' issues that are underplayed, quite unlike with PSVIs.

Reinstating the manufacturing licenses of the three PSVIs in 2010

A public interest litigation admitted to the Indian Supreme Court in February 2009 sought to reverse the closure of the three PSVIs and bring about a resumption of production: essential to meeting the needs of the country's UIP.[23] The Supreme Court sent notices to the UHM, the DCGI, the secretaries of the respective state governments, and the directors of the three PSVIs on the legality and prudence of the original decision to close down the institutions.[24]

On 18 February 2009, a Parliamentary committee pointed out that: (1) the PSVIs did not produce sub-standard vaccines; (2) WHO-cGMP certification is required only for exports and for UN procuring agencies; and (3) many of the WHO-NRA team's recommendations had been addressed by the PSVIs and the few remaining points could have been easily achieved, given time and financial support.[10] In December 2009, the 38th report of the Parliamentary Standing Committee on Health and Family Welfare also called for reversal of the decision to close the PSVIs.[25]

In May 2009, the United Progressive Alliance (UPA) won the election and promised to reopen the PSVIs. In June 2009, the newly appointed Health Minister, Dr. Gulam Nabi Azad, set up an expert committee to form an action plan for the revival of the PSVIs. In September 2009, the Federal government established a three-member committee headed by Javid Chowdhury to enquire into the reasons behind their closure and to develop a roadmap for their revival. On 5 February 2010, the committee submitted its interim report, noting that it would submit its final report only after the three PSVIs' suspension orders had been revoked. On 26 February 2010, the UHM sent revival and upgrading orders to the three PSVIs.

In September 2010, the Chowdhury committee submitted its final report, concluding that the suspension of the three PSVIs, which had involved officials at the highest level, had been unwarranted, deliberate and malicious. The committee's main recommendations were (1) more funding for WHO-cGMP upgrading over the next three years; (2) urgent recruitment of staff to reach full production capacity; (3) functional autonomy for PSVIs; (4) replacement of the National Technical Advisory Group on Immunisation (NTAGI) with a National Vaccine Security Board with national vaccine regulatory authority, to advise the government on important issues relating to the National Vaccine Security policy; (5) development of modalities to strengthen R&D; (6) production of UIP vaccines in the public sector; (7) procurement of UIP vaccines based on price and opportunity parity; (8) no PSVI should be excluded from producing any vaccine or from government vaccine procurement, as long as quality and affordability are ensured; (9) the government may make advance market commitments with vaccine PSVIs, but not with private/foreign entities to the detriment of vaccine PSVI; (10) no private firm should be paid higher prices than their PSVI counterparts supplying to the UIP; (11) there should be legislation for monitoring AEFI; (12) the selection of vaccines for the UIP should be made on scientific grounds; (13) the unethical promotion of vaccines should be discouraged; (14) any private company that wishes to produce new (non-UIP) or combination vaccines must also produce some UIP vaccines (individually, not as combinations) to fill any shortfalls in PSVI production and government procurement; (15) there should be rigorous scrutiny of and public debate over the combination of UIP and non-UIP vaccines; (16) combinations must be proven to be equivalent to or more effective and safer than single vaccines before adoption; and (17) there should be a clear distinction between cocktail combinations and multivalent vaccines.[12]

The politics behind the closure of the three PSVIs that facilitated the growth of the private vaccine sector in India

Microbiologist Dr. Elangeswaran became director of BCGVL in 1998, and in 2005 he was given the additional charge of PII Coonoor. It was alleged that there were dubious dealings between Dr. Elangeswaran and some private firms, with the support of Health Minister Dr. Anbumani Ramadoss (appointed in 2005).

There were serious allegations of corruption, favouritism and mismanagement that underscored the need for a criminal investigation, as reported in a daily newspaper.[26] It was reported that Dr. Elangeswaran had facilitated the transfer of raw materials, seed virus, skilled manpower, and a bank loan worth US$6.3 million from Union Bank of India to a newly registered private company, Green Signal Biopharma Ltd. (GSBL), in 2005, then owned by Mr. Sundaraparipooranan, a close associate/party member (PMK) of Ramadoss. Another new company named Vatsan Biotech was registered in 2006; this was co-owned by the wife of Sundaraparipooranan, while the wife of Dr. Elangeswaran was a major shareholder. It was alleged that Dr. Elangeswaran also gave OPV and DPT seed virus to private companies such as Bharat Biotech Hyderabad, SIIL, Pune, and Sanofi Pasteur free of charge.[23,26]

PII then bought measles seed virus from GSBL at a highly inflated cost, US$8 million, which was otherwise available for free from other PSVIs, in order to enable Ramadoss' associate Sundaraparipooranan to earn US$35.75 million. It was a conspiracy to help a politically well-connected entrepreneur.[23,26] Sundaraparipooranan did not provide the original source of the measles seed that he sold to PII, and scientists did not rule out the possibility of theft from government laboratories. It was alleged that the deal was signed on 27 November 2006, in complete violation of government rules, since no tender was issued and it was agreed according to the one-sided terms dictated by Sundaraparipooranan. That the deal between GSBL and PII was illegal came to light when the integrated finance division of the UHM pointed out that any proposal for new activity (PII's suggested measles vaccine production plan) required prior approval from the Planning Commission and a related budget allocation.[23]

Dr. Elangeswaran was also a contender for the post of DCGI as well as for a prominent post in the upcoming IVC. Interestingly, Mr. Surinder Singh, former Additional Director of CRI, Kasauli, was appointed DCGI in February 2008. Singh was also a member of the committee that had inspected the PSVIs in 2007, prior to their closure. It is ironic that he did not seek to improve his own institute (CRI), upon becoming DCGI.[9,10] Unhappy with these developments, Dr. Elangeswaran is reported to have confessed to former DCGI Dr. Venkateswarlu and to senior bureaucrats in the UHM that he had been pressured by the UHM to close down the PSVIs in order to facilitate vaccine production in private companies. The UHM denied these allegations and declared that it would file a defamation case against Dr. Elangeswaran, though it was never implemented as it could have implicated even higher ministry officials, including the former DCGI and the then health secretary.[8,23]

On 12 August 2013, Dr. Elangeswaran submitted a letter to the UHM secretary seeking permission to join as co-petitioner in the public interest litigation filed at the Supreme Court; he also sent a letter on 10 September 2013 alleging a nexus between officials from DCGI office, some functionaries within the PSVIs and private vaccine manufactures, and UHM officials. He named eight people who had misled the UHM with the intention of closing the institutes in the name of WHO-cGMP non-compliance.

Dr. Elangeswaran alleges that Dr. Singh and Dr. Mani together hatched the plan to convert the PSVIs into testing labs for combination vaccines, and to close them in collusion with private vaccine manufacturers. According to Dr. Elangeswaran, Dr. Mani had been appointed director of CRI, Kasauli in 2006, even though he did not qualify for the post. Dr. Singh was posted as Additional Director for the Central Drug Laboratory (CDL) to CRI, from the National Institute of Biologicals, and was later appointed DCGI by the back door, before the date of the interview with the UPSC, India's central recruiting agency for public servants. A hefty amount was said to have been paid by private vaccine manufacturers to the selection committee members to select Dr. Singh. According to Dr. Elangeswaran, the WHO gave a deadline to private vaccine companies to become GMP compliant within 6 months, but not to PSVIs.[27]

Deliberate incapacitation of the PSVIs from 2010 till today

The latest trends show that the share of the public sector supply of UIP vaccines is negligible (ranging from 0.3% to 24%), while the private sector's share has increased (ranging from 33–100%) for all UIP vaccines. However, between 2014 and 2016 the share of public sector production for DPT was higher than the private sector. Thereafter no vaccine has been produced in the three PSVIs as approval for its commercial production is pending with the DCGI. All new and combination vaccines are produced by the private sector (Table 5.3).

After suspension of the three PSVI was revoked, in 2013–2015, the UHM issued supply orders only for DPT. DPT production was, however, far below the 2005–2006 level (with a capacity of 40 million doses prior to suspension), indicating that the government was under-utilizing the PSVI and diverting orders to private companies, including Biological Evans Pvt. Ltd. (which was then WHO-cGMP non-compliant), SIIL (Pune), SBL (Hyderabad), and even multinationals like Sanofi Pasteur India. Production of DPT in PII was terminated in April 2015, as the production facilities involved in filling, packing and formulation for retail supply were handed over to Hindustan Lifecare Limited for modernization/upgrading. The production in the revived PSVIs was thus not restored to pre-suspension levels.[28]

The declining orders from the UHM for UIP vaccines (Figures 5.1–5.7) support the view that the government is allowing the PSVIs to produce DPT and TT vaccines to be supplied to private companies, for them to make combination vaccines, which would then be sold back to the government at a high price or exported.

BCGVL once supplied all of the UIP's BCG vaccine. Since 2009 BCG has been supplied by SIIL, Pune, and GSBL, Chennai. In 2017–2018, the UHM procured 25 million doses from GSBL at a cost of US$0.60 per 10-dose vial (a total cost of US$24.68 million). BCGVL's procurement price was 13.0 (US$0.3) for a 10-dose vial supplied to the UIP in 2007–2008.[15] The UHM procured a total of 177 million doses from GSBL in eight years (from 2010–2011 to 2017–2018),

TABLE 5.3 Percentage share of vaccine production by private and public sector in India

		2014–2015		*2015–2016*		*2016–2017*		*2017–2018*	
Sn.	*Vaccine*	*Private Sector*	*Public Sector*	*Private Sector*	*Public Sector*	*Private Sector*	*Public Sector*	*Private Sector*	*Public Sector*
	UIP Vaccines								
1	BCG	99	1	100	0	100	0	100	0
2	DPT	33	66	44	56	100	0	100	0
3	DT	100	0	100	0	100	0	100	0
4	TT	75	25	74	24	98.8	1.2	99.7	0.3
5	OPV	96	4	93	7	92.7	7.3	100	0
6	moPV1	100	NA	NA	NA	100	NA	NA	NA
7	bOPV	0	100	0	100	0	100	NA	NA
8	Measles	100	0	100	0	100	0	100	0
9	Hepatitis B	92	8	95	5	95.3	4.7	99.8	0.2
10	Pentavalent (DTwP-HepB-Hib)	100	0	100	0	100	0	100	0
	Non-UIP Vaccines								
11	JEV	100	0	100	0	100	0	100	0
12	YEV	83	17	82	18	100	0	100	0
13	TCARV	83	17	82	18	61	39	17.4	82.6
14	Typhoid (Vi-Poly)	100	0	100	0	100	0	100	0
15	Typhoid (AKD)	100	0	100	0	100	0	100	0
16	Quadrivalent MMV	100	0	100	0	100	0	100	0
17	*Haemophilus influenzae* type b (Hib)	100	0	100	0	100	0	100	0
18	Quadruple vaccine (DtPw-HB)	100	0	0	0	100	0	100	0
19	Tetravalent (DTwP+Hib)	100	0	100	0	100	0	100	0
20	Measles Mums Rubella (MMR)	100	0	100	0	100	0	100	0
21	Measles Rubella (MR)	100		100	0	100	0	100	0
22	Rubella	100	0	100	0	100	0	100	0
23	Seasonal Influenza	100	0	100	0	100	0	100	0
24	Pneumococcal	100	0	100	0	100	0	100	0
25	Cholera	100	0	100	0	100	0	100	0
26	Anti-tetanus serum (ATS)	100	0	100	0	100	0	100	0
27	Anti-diphtheria serum (ADS)	0	100	50	50	0	100	0	100
28	Anti-snake venom serum (ASVS)	66	44	62	38	NA	NA	NA	NA
29	Anti-scorpion venom serum (AScVS)	NA	0.06	NA	0.03	0	100	90	10
30	Anti-rabies Serum (ARS)	NA	2.23	NA	0.82	0	100	99	1

Source: Compiled from National Health Profile 2017–2019.

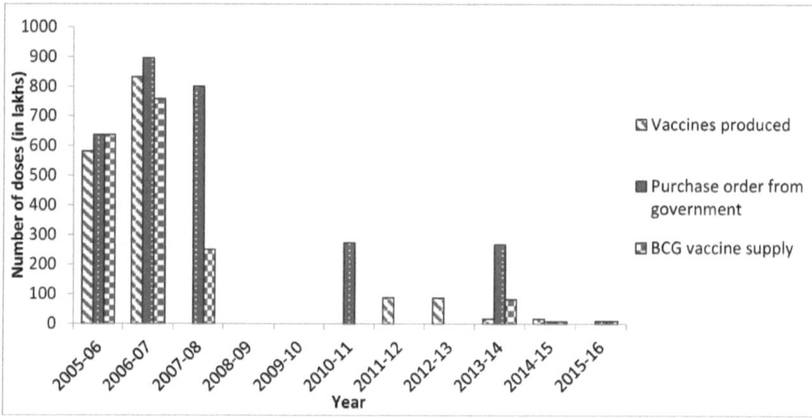

FIGURE 5.1 BCGVL Chennai: Production, purchase order from the government, and supply of vaccines to the UIP

Source: Compiled from NHP 2007–2019, MOHFW, GOI.

amounting to a total cost of US$88.63 million.[29] According to Dr. Elangeswaran, within six months of BCGVL's closure, Dr. Singh, the then DCGI, gave purchase orders to SIIL for the supply of 110 million doses of BCG at a rate of US$0.63 per 10 doses for the UIP.[27] Within two years of the public BCGVL having been closed, the private sector had completely captured the BCG UIP market.

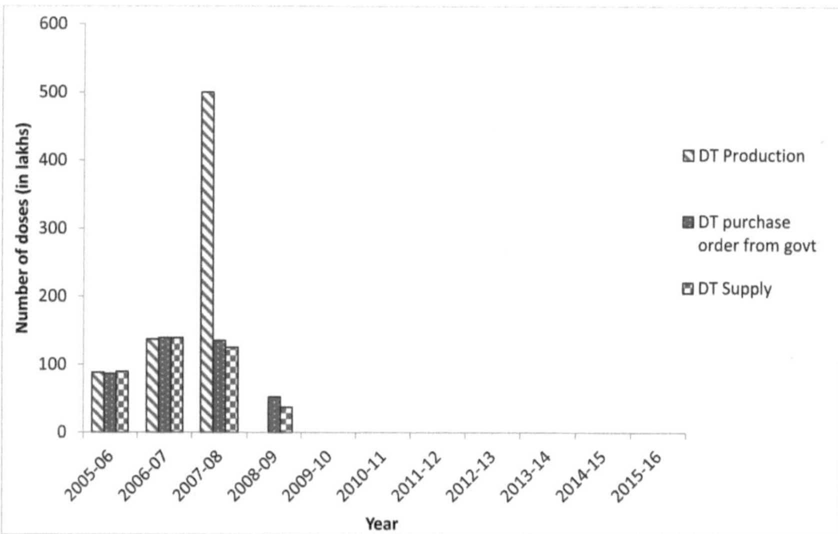

FIGURE 5.2 Central Research Institute (CRI) Kasauli: Production, purchase order from the government, and supply of DT vaccines to the UIP

Source: Compiled from NHP 2007–2019, MOHFW, GOI.

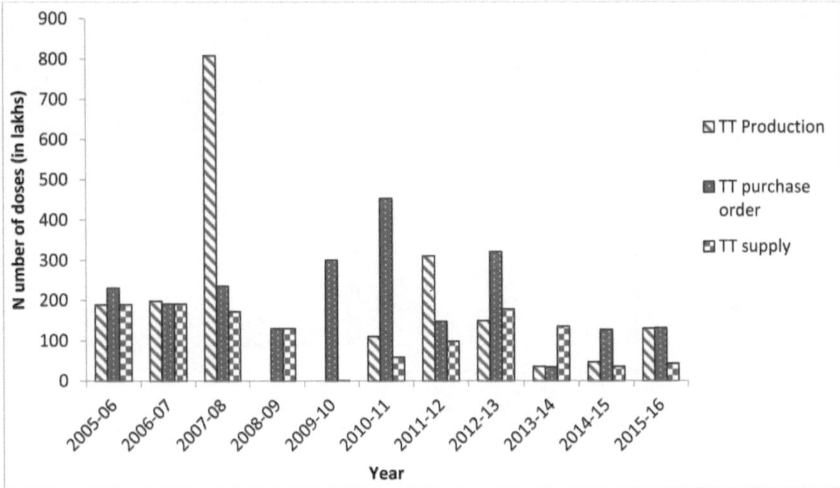

FIGURE 5.3 Central Research Institute (CRI) Kasauli: Production, purchase order from the government, and supply of TT vaccines to the UIP

Source: Compiled from NHP 2007–2019, MOHFW, GOI.

The immunization budget in India has increased seven times in the last five years.[30] The petitioners allege 'Union of India' (a legal parlance for the Federal government, GOI) is engaging in a practice of draining the public exchequer through the payment of high prices to the private sector for vaccines which

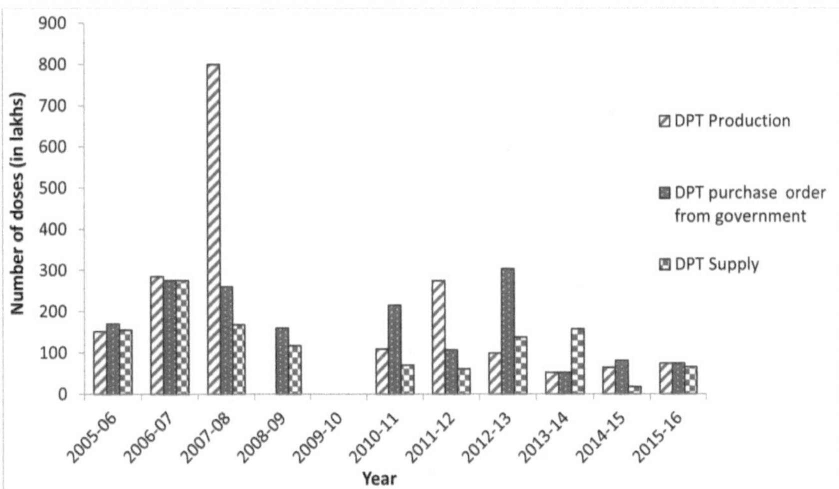

FIGURE 5.4 Central Research Institute (CRI) Kasauli: Production, purchase order from the government, and supply of DPT vaccines to the UIP

Source: Compiled from NHP 2007–2019, MOHFW, GOI.

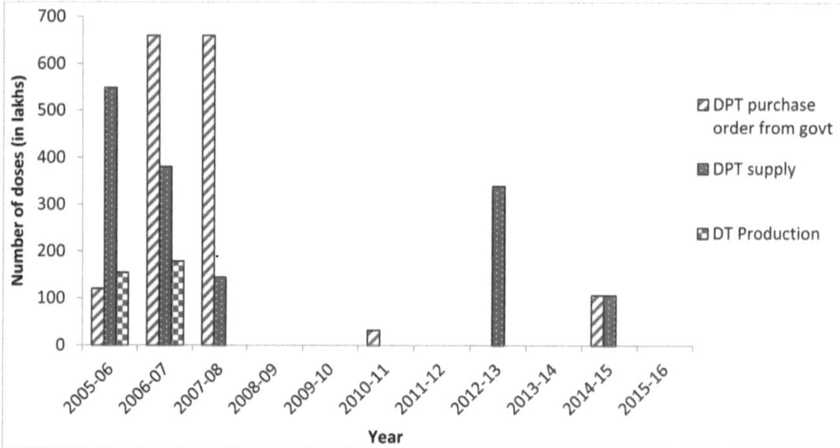

FIGURE 5.5 Pasteur Institute of India (PII) Coonoor: Production, purchase order from the government, and supply of DPT vaccines to the UIP

Source: Compiled from NHP 2007–2019, MOHFW, GOI.

could be produced in the public sector at less than half the cost (Table 3).[23] The Save Pasteur Institutes Association (SPIA) at PII has alleged that government-appointed officials deliberately set about suspending highly regarded PSVIs in order to help private vaccine manufacturers.[23]

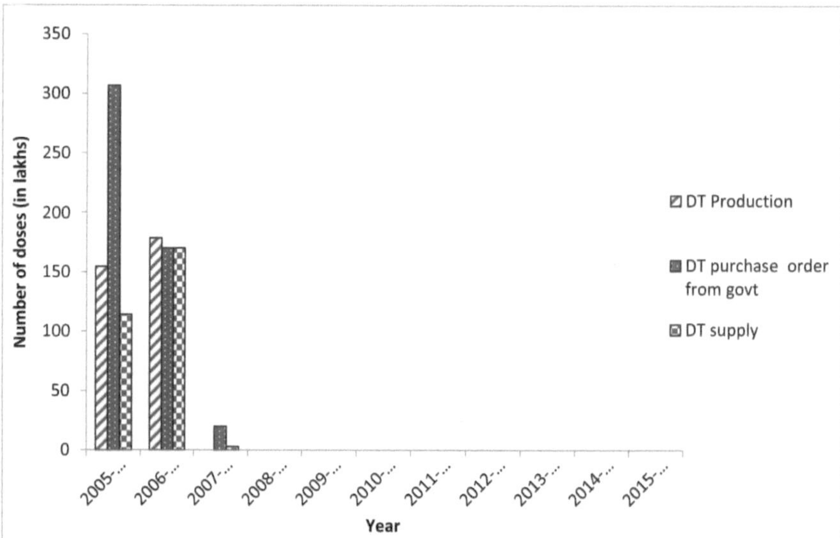

FIGURE 5.6 Pasteur Institute of India (PII) Coonoor: Production, purchase order from the government, and supply of DT vaccines to the UIP

Source: Compiled from NHP 2007–2019, MOHFW, GOI.

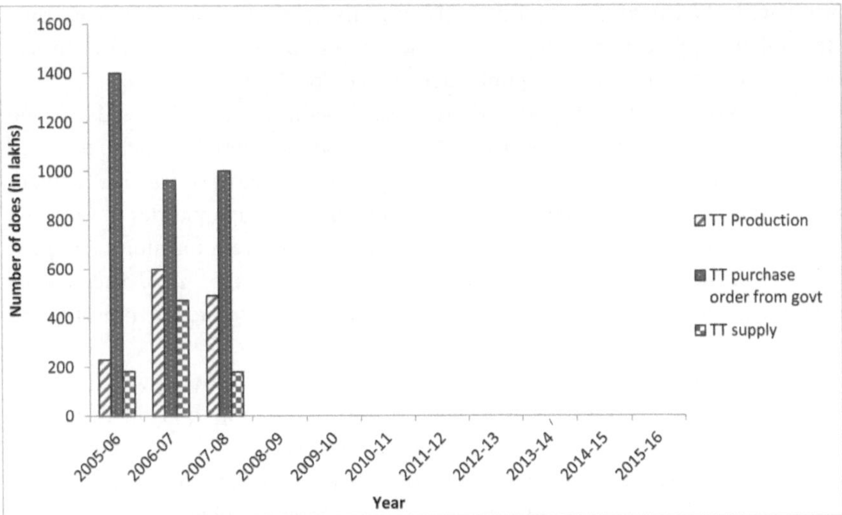

FIGURE 5.7 Pasteur Institute of India (PII) Coonoor: Production, purchase order from the government, and supply of TT vaccines to the UIP

Source: Compiled from NHP 2007–2019, MOHFW, GOI.

Government preference for pentavalent vaccine makes PSVIs redundant

In 2011, the GOI included pentavalent vaccine in its UIP, succumbing to pressure from the manufacturers and international funding organizations.[31] This move would essentially make the PSVIs redundant, as pentavalent vaccines are made only in the private sector and the UHM has not ordered its PSVIs to manufacture them. A petition led by former Health Secretary K.B. Saxena and others against the Union of India (GOI) was admitted to the Delhi High Court in 2009. It highlighted the GOI's arbitrary policy on the introduction of expensive vaccines (combination vaccines, pneumococcal vaccine) with doubtful utility, efficacy, and safety. The petition sought to quash any premature pentavalent vaccine requirement and formulate evidence-based policy. The High Court, in its interim order in April 2010, stated:[32]

> The main grievance of the Petitioners is that the pentavalent vaccines should not be introduced in the Universal Immunisation Programme without carrying out any proper studies of its economic impact, its need and efficacy and any other impact that may be relevant.

It went on to refer to a paper with a proposed draft of a national vaccine policy (ICMR-NISTADS), published in the *Indian Journal of Medical Research*, for the UHM to consult.[33] In response to the High Court's interim order, the UHM formulated a National Vaccine Policy (NVP)[34] in April 2011, launched with only a few officials present. Although ratification by parliament is mandatory, it had not been sought. Nor had any public debate been permitted.

The ICMR-NISTADS policy draft remains valid today.[35] It has drawn no criticism except for an opinion from a public health expert,[36] which resonated with the content of the GOI's NVP, which placed emphasis on vaccine delivery rather than on the non-mandatory selection criteria that qualifies a vaccine's introduction to the UIP. This expert recommended a system for monitoring the outcome of vaccination, administration, logistics, coverage, good vaccination practices, healthcare financing, etc. (a call echoed by private vaccine industry and the WHO, UNICEF, GAVI, BMGF, etc.).

The 2011 NVP was criticized as one man's policy, with mere guidelines that provide even more scope for evading the implementation of evidence-based policy.[37,38,39] According to its critics, it serves to justify spending public money through public–private partnerships or private vaccine production, in the name of protecting children, though on the basis of dubious incidence figures and public health statistics.[40]

The case of pentavalent vaccine in India is a reflection of how the 2011 NVP's lack of guidelines requiring robust epidemiological evidence puts healthy Indian children at risk, with no accountability for vaccine manufacturers. Notwithstanding the petition against pentavalent vaccine,[27] and the far greater number of post-vaccination deaths (compared to DPT vaccinees) the GOI went ahead with its introduction nationwide.[41] The UHM, which promised to study the vaccine's safety, revised its AEFI classification in a manner that makes it very difficult to establish a causal relation between the vaccine and any death or adverse reaction.[20] There is no consensus on the introduction of pentavalent vaccine in India's UIP.[42,43] Furthermore, even though PII has the capacity to make pentavalent vaccine, it has never received permission from the MOHFW to do so. Instead, it was asked to find its own vendors in order to supply DTP vaccine to private companies so that they could make pentavalent vaccine. There is no uniform policy on the use of acellular or whole cell pertussis vaccine in the pentavalent vaccine and companies are manufacturing both versions.[44,45] The pentavalent vaccine policy also became a gateway for the entry of dubious non-universal vaccines and their combinations into the UIP via the backdoor, riding piggyback on the universal vaccines.[46] This was substantiated by a former director of PII and BCGVL.[27]

The fate of the IVC

The IVC was conceived in 2008 by then Health Minister Anbumani Ramadoss. The MOHFW earmarked 100 acres of land at Chengalpattu, near Chennai, and appointed Hindustan Latex Limited (HLL, later Hindustan Lifecare Limited) to oversee the IVC's construction, with the aim of achieving national self-reliance and self-sufficiency in vaccines. HLL formed a wholly owned subsidiary company

HLL Biotech Limited (HBL) to execute the project. The IVC was intended to make pentavalent, BCG, measles, hepatitis B, human rabies, Hib, and Japanese Encephalitis (JE) vaccines in the first phase, with an annual capacity of 585 million doses.

Construction of the IVC started in 2012, four years after the closure of the three PSVIs, and was completed in 2018 with full WHO-cGMP compliance, though it was not yet operational. The GOI is currently planning to disinvest from both the IVC and its parent company HBL, as predicted by the then Health Minister Dr. Anbumani Ramadoss and the then DBT secretary Dr. Bhan, 10 years ago.[9] There are a yet no purchasers for the facility, after the government spent around US$81.46 million on it.[47] An executive of IVC, anonymously, stated that the facilities in IVC are not useable. Their poor design was said to be based on inadequate understanding of which technologies correspond to the production of which vaccines: itself due to lack of expertise within HLL Lifecare Limited. The company had relied completely on outside consultants.

Substantial bureaucratic delays in the project's execution entrenched it in debt, due to which HBL was unable to obtain more loans or pay the outstanding ones. Neither the state government nor the central government is willing to support the IVC, even through a public–private partnership. HBL's parent company HLL Lifecare Limited, also stopped funding in 2019. As a result, since August 2019 salaries have not been paid to around 275 HBL employees.[48]

In January 2020, Bharat Biotech International Ltd. (BBIL) showed an interest in investing US$44 million to revive the IVC, though this has not yet transpired. The Tamil Nadu Health Development Association (TNHDA), a body of doctors and health activists in Chennai, appealed to the UHM in January 2021 to expedite work on the IVC and made it ready to produce vaccines in collaboration with some other big vaccine manufacturers.[48,49] According to media reports, another problem with the IVC is that although all of the state-of-the-art machines were installed two years ago, the authorities could not conduct the building and machinery validation work to kickstart the production process. A world-class WHO-cGMP compliant vaccine manufacturing facility is now stuck making masks and sanitizers.[49] Sceptics believe that the news about the non-viability of IVC is intended to bring down (bargaining) the price of IVC for possible customers.

The way things have unfolded, it seems an ingenious ploy to create a manufacturing facility (the IVC) using public funds, and once it is ready with full WHO-cGMP compliance, to sell it on to the private sector. Even though BIBCOL and IVCOL (both public sector) are WHO-cGMP compliant, their fate is similar to the three revived PSVIs; their capacities are under-utilized, even in the midst of a pandemic, when there is dire need to fill shortages of the Covid-19 vaccine (currently only being manufactured in the private sector).

Discussion and conclusion

Indian PSVIs were global pioneers in the development of vaccines during the era of British India and enjoyed a near-monopoly on the production and supply of good quality, affordable vaccines, and sera. This continued for decades after independence, until, in the late 1980s, private industry began to take an interest in the vaccine business. The Indian public sector has suffered systematic neglect and closures ever since, while the private sector has grown at its expense. This has been particularly due to the GOI's favourable policies towards new vaccines and their combinations, rather than filling the supply gaps for existing UIP vaccines. Global policies such as trade agreements and intellectual property rights have also impacted PSVIs indirectly, with the introduction of economic reforms (through liberalization, privatization, globalization) in India courtesy of the IMF, World Bank, aid policies, and conditional loans. These have transformed the entire context of immunization, including decisions regarding which vaccines to include in the UIP.

The interest of the private sector in the vaccine business has also changed the perception of vaccines. They are no longer viewed as one of several tools to maintain public health based on epidemiological evidence, but as a magic bullet for the prevention of all diseases. This approach is increasingly driven by 'supply-push' rather than 'demand-pull' dynamics, even in the case of unproven and dubious vaccines whose need, safety, and efficacy have not been established. It is this vaccine-centric approach, rather than a public health approach, that is reflected in the WHO's recommended criteria for vaccine use,[50,51] as well as the revised AEFI definitions[52] in India and abroad, the latter of which render establishing a causal association of any adverse event with a vaccine virtually impossible.

A decade ago, the vaccine market in India was around US$150 million; this grew to US$900 million in 2016. Today, it is estimated to be around US$1 billion and is expected to grow by US$2 billion in the coming five years. In addition, no new drug molecules[53,54] have been produced in the last two decades, and so the pharmaceutical industry is looking to vaccines as a secure market where demand can be created and sustained through national immunization programmes. Since there is no demand for new expensive vaccines, however, the industry has turned to making combination vaccines (pentavalent, hexavalent, etc.), which include one UIP vaccine along with other non-UIP vaccines, thereby taking over a captive UIP market. Since UIP vaccines were predominantly made in the public sector in India, the domestic private industry, by lobbying actors in the GOI and the scientific/medical community, has managed to incapacitate the public sector and thus take over the UIP vaccine market.

To create sustainable vaccine markets, governments are encouraged by private industry to make advance market commitments and engage in innovative financing mechanisms (such as the International Finance Facility for Immunization [IFFIm], implemented by GAVI), even though they are unsustainable.[55,56,57] The nexus between vaccine manufacturers and paediatricians who promote unnecessary vaccines (through combination vaccines) for the UIP, and the gaps in vaccine decision making and immunization in India, are well documented.[58,59,60,61] Whatever vaccines are produced by private industry are aggressively advocated by paediatric academies/associations and industry-funded NGOs. Emphasis is placed more on the 'introduction' and 'coverage' of vaccines than on need or evidence-based vaccination, or how much protection is achieved following vaccination.

The experience of PSVIs in India reveals that neoliberal policies, privatization, and public–private partnerships enabled some stakeholders and domestic private industry to use WHO-cGMP compliance as an excuse to completely dismantle the existing and fully operational public sector. The PSVIs were effectively incapacitated for the profit of the private sector, through the diversion to the latter of all resources, facilities, technologies, and government purchase orders at ever-increasing prices. Thus, PSVIs were made to appear as incapable, and they were blamed and denied support by the UHM. Meanwhile, the private sector has become the sole determinant and driver of vaccines, immunization, and related policies. Only time will tell how the private sector will shape the dynamics of national and international public health.

The GOI adopted the slogan of self-reliance in combating the Covid-19 pandemic, but its favouritism towards the private sector is evident from its recent announcement of the privatization of 300 public sector companies across all sectors and their reduction to just 24. Given this, the likely fate of PSVIs is clear, including the fact that the publicly funded IVC is up for grabs for private vaccine enterprises, despite the Covid-19 pandemic. In view of growing Covid-19 vaccine shortages in the midst of an unrelenting second wave, GOI gave grants to two private companies – Serum Institute of India (US$400 million) and Bharat Biotech International (US$210 million) – for capacity building and production of Covid vaccines.[62] Such unprecedented expenditure on private companies is as stark as the starving of public sector for funds, administrative support, and government procurement. In addition, GOI gave permission to three PSVIs namely Bharat Immunologicals and Biologicals Ltd. (BIBCOL), Haffkine Biopharmaceuticals Corporation Ltd., and Mumbai and Indian Immunologicals Ltd., Hyderabad, to manufacture Bharat Biotech's Covaxin, thus making these three PSVIs into contract manufacturers for the private sector. This current situation is similar to the fate of CRI, PII, and BCGVL, reduced to component suppliers to the private sector for making pentavalent and combination vaccines. GOI letting these two private companies sell their Covid-19 vaccines with no price controls, making them unaffordable for the majority of the population, was criticized by experts.[63,64] Critics question the lack of public information on IPR issues between ICMR and Bharat Biotech and why PSVIs should make Covaxin for a private company rather than for the Government of India. Subjugation of the public sector to private sector profit has been ongoing for more than a decade in India. Surely this is the time to make use of the under-utilized capacities of India's PSVIs not only for the present pandemic but also for tackling future pandemics, and so to ensure access to affordable vaccines and India's biosecurity.

Notes

1 Madhavi Yennapu, 'Vaccine Policy in India', *PLOS Medicine*, 2005, 2, e127, 0387–0391.
2 Madhavi Yennapu, 'Liberalization: Its Impact on Indian Vaccine S & T and Implications for National Vaccine Policy', in Nadia Asheulova *et al.*, eds, *Liberalizing Research in Science and Technology: Studies in Science Policy* (Saint-Petersburg: Politechnika, Russian Academy of Sciences & IIT Kanpur, 2010).
3 Madhavi Yennapu, 'The Public Sector Is Crucial for Self-Reliance in Vaccines and Public Health', *The Wire Science*, 2020, https://science.thewire.in/health/covid-19-indian-psu-vaccines/ (Accessed 12/05/2021).
4 Belia Heilbron and Karlijn Kuijpers, 'How the Netherlands Largely Dismantled Its Vaccine Knowledge: "You're Not Going to Sell the Fire Brigade Either, Are You?"', *De Groene Amsterdammer*, 2020, Published in Dutch.
5 Mark Harrison, *Public Health in British India: Anglo-Indian Preventive Medicine 1859–1914* (Cambridge: Cambridge University Press, 1994).
6 Madhavi Yennapu, 'Transnational Factors and National Linkages: Indian Experience in Human Vaccines', *Asian Biotechnology and Development Review*, 2007, 9, 1–43.
7 Pasteur Institute of India, 'Golden Jubilee Souvenir, 1907–1957', 38; 'Diamond Jubilee Souvenir, 1907–1967'.
8 Madhavi Yennapu, 'Vaccine PSUs: Chronicle of an Attenuation Willfully Caused', *Medico Friend Circle Bulletin*, 2008, 329, 1–7.
9 R. Ramachandran, 'Vaccine Worries', *Frontline*, 11 April 2008, 4–27.
10 34th Parliamentary Standing Committee on Health and Family Welfare, Parliament of India, Rajya Sabha, Government of India, New Delhi; 18 February 2009: On the Functioning of three vaccine producing PSUs, namely – Central Research Institute (CRI), Kasauli, Pasteur Institute of India (PII), Coonoor, and BCG Vaccine Laboratory (BCGVL), Chennai. Notes: CRI met its UIP vaccines supply target for the first time in 2007; BCGVL achieved a peak production of 83.15 million doses against a demand of 89.49 million doses and supplied 75.87 million doses in 2006–2007.
11 https://www.who.int/medicines/areas/quality_safety/quality_assurance/production/en/ (Accessed 12/05/2021).
12 Javid Chowdhury Committee Report, 'Final Report of the Committee set up to determine the reasons for the suspension of the manufacturing license of CRI Kasauli, PII Coonoor, and BCGVL Guindy, and to draw the road-map for the revival of the three units', September 2010, http://www.mfcindia.org/main/bgpapers/bgpapers2011/am/bgpap2011s.pdf (Accessed 12/05/2021).
13 R. Ramachandran, 'Vaccine Fiasco', *Frontline,* 28 March 2009, 26, http://www.hinduonnet.com/fline/fl2607/stories/20090410260711400.htm (Accessed 12/05/2021).
14 V. Varshney, 'Get your Own Vaccine', *Down to Earth*, 2009, 26–32. Notes: From 2007 to 2008, BCG vaccine coverage fell from 100% to 52%, DPT from 81% to 43.8%, and OPV coverage from 81.4% to 43%.
15 43rd Parliamentary Standing Committee on Health and Family Welfare, Parliament of India, Rajya Sabha, Government of India, New Delhi, 4 August 2010.
16 V. Varshney, 'Vaccine Shortage to Continue', *Down to Earth*, 2009, https://www.downtoearth.org.in/news/vaccine-shortage-to-continue-2657 (Accessed 12/05/2021).
17 https://www.euro.who.int/en/media-centre/sections/press-releases/2008/05/who,-unicef-and-cdc-regret-the-government-of-ukraines-decision-to-suspend-the-national-measles-and-rubella-vaccination-campaign (Accessed 12/05/2021).

18 Jacob Puliyel *et al.*, 'Deaths reported after pentavalent vaccine compared with death reported after diphtheria-tetanus-pertussis vaccine: An exploratory analysis', *Medical Journal of DY Patil Vidyapeeth*, 2018, 11, 99–105.
19 Vaccine deaths in India have not been evaluated: Uppsala monitoring Center, Tuesday, 23 July 2019, http://www.pharmabiz.com/NewsDetails.aspx?aid=117094&sid=1 (Accessed 12/05/2021).
20 Jacob M. Puliyel and A. Phadke, 'Deaths following pentavalent vaccine and the revised AEFI classification', *LETTER*, 2017, http://ijme.in/articles/deaths-following-pentavalent-vaccine-and-the-revised-aefi-classification/?galley=html (Accessed 12/05/2021).
21 Nick Paul Taylor, 'Panacea Biotec accused of selling expired Vaccines', 2013, https://www.fiercepharma.com/r-d/panacea-biotec-accused-of-selling-expired-vaccines (Accessed 12/05/2021).
22 https://www.fda.gov/inspections-compliance-enforcement-and-criminal-investigations/warning-letters/panacea-biotec-limited-607837-09242020 (Accessed 12/05/2021).
23 *SP Shukla and others vs. Union of India*, petition no. 64 of 2009.
24 https://www.newindianexpress.com/states/tamil-nadu/2009/feb/21/supreme-court-issues-notices-on-writ-petition-27331.html (Accessed 12/05/2021).
25 38th Parliamentary Standing Committee on Health and Family Welfare, Parliament of India, Rajya Sabha, Government of India, New Delhi, 18 December 2009: The highlighted portion can be replaced with the following as this is how the report is titled. On the major issues concerning the three vaccines producing PSVIs, namely, the Central Research Institute (CRI), Kasauli; the Pasteur Institute of India (PII), Coonoor; and the BCG vaccine laboratory (BCGVL), Chennai.
26 J. Gopikrishnan, 'Ramadoss linked to vaccine scam', *The Pioneer, Daily Newspaper*, 2008, New Delhi, http://jgopikrishnan.blogspot.com/2009/03/vaccine-scam-sabotaging-vaccine.html (Accessed 12/05/2021).
27 *Dr. Yogesh Jain vs. Union of India & Ors.*, WP (C) 697/2013.
28 http://www.tribuneindia.com/news/himachal/community/kasauli-cri-fails-to-sell-dpt-vaccine-stock/179773.html (Accessed 12/05/2021).
29 https://www.iob.in/upload/CEDocuments/GSBPL%20RHP.pdf (Accessed 03/08/2021).
30 Susmita Chatterjee *et al.*, 'Current costs & projected financial needs of India's Universal Immunization Programme', *Indian Journal of Medical Research*, 2016, 143, 801–808.
31 https://economictimes.indiatimes.com/opinion/et-commentary/governments-uip-pressure-from-international-organizations-to-include-vaccines-for-other-diseases/articleshow/41280844.cms?from=mdr (Accessed 12/05/2021).
32 Interim Court Order WP (C) 13698/ 2009, dated 7 April 2010, on PIL against pentavalent vaccine by KB Saxena and others vs. Union of India and others, by Chief Justice Mukta Gupta, High Court, Delhi.
33 Madhavi Yennapu *et al.*, 'Evidence-based national vaccine policy', *Indian Journal of Medical Research*, 2010, 131, 617–628.
34 National Vaccine Policy (NVP), Ministry of Health and Family Welfare, New Delhi, April 2011.
35 Morgane Donadel *et al.*, 'National decision-making for the introduction of new vaccines: A systematic review 2010–2020', *Vaccine*, 2021, 39, 1897–1909.
36 Jacob John, 'Policy document: evidence-based national vaccine policy', *Indian Journal of Medical Research*, 2010, 132, 228–229.
37 Vidya Krishnan, 'Aid groups, experts criticize vaccine policy', *Live Mint News e-paper*, 24 February 2012, https://www.livemint.com/Politics/5BH6Ra4th-pvwRL6uSkRPUJ/Aid-groups-experts-criticize-vaccine-policy.html (Accessed 12/05/2021).
38 T. V. Padma, 'Critics indicate flaws in India's new vaccine policy', 1 September 2011, https://www.scidev.net/global/news/critics-indicate-flaws-in-india-s-new-vaccine-policy/ (Accessed 12/05/2021).

39 T. Jayakrishnan, 'National Vaccine Policy: ethical equity issues', *Indian Journal of Medical Ethics*, 2013, 10, 183–190.
40 Y. Madhavi and N. Raghuram, 'National vaccine policy in the era of vaccines seeking diseases and governments seeking public private partnerships', *Current Science*, 2012, 102, 557–558.
41 https://www.thehindu.com/sci-tech/health/medicine-and-research/pentavalent-vaccine-gets-clean-chit-set-for-national-scaleup/article5222381.ece (Accessed 12/05/2021).
42 S. Sreedhar, A. Antony, and N. Poulose, 'Study on the effectiveness and impact of pentavalent vaccination program in India and other south Asian countries', *Human Vaccines & Immunotherapeutics*, 2014, 10, 2062–2065.
43 https://blogs.bmj.com/bmj/2012/12/21/jacob-puliyel-on-the-pentavalent-study-in-kerala/ (Accessed 12/05/2021).
44 Joseph L. Mathew, 'Acellular Pertussis Vaccines: Pertinent Issues', *Indian Pediatrics*, 2008, 45, 727–729.
45 V. M. Vashishtha, C. P. Bansal, and S. G. Gupta, 'Pertussis Vaccines: Position Paper of Indian Academy of Pediatrics (IAP)', *Indian Pediatrics*, 2013, 50, 1001–1009.
46 Madhavi Yennapu, 'New combination vaccines: Backdoor entry into India's Universal Immunization Programme?', *Current Science*, 2006, 90, 1465–1469.
47 V. Pilla, 'Exclusive | 10 years on: How govt's Rs 600cr vaccine complex failed to take-off', 26 November 2019, https://www.moneycontrol.com/news/business/companies/exclusive-the-govts-fledgling-mega-vaccine-complex-in-tamil-nadu-may-soon-get-a-strategic-partner-4631991.html (Accessed 12/05/2021).
48 P. Kunnathoor, 'Centre unconcerned about PSU vaccine project in Chennai when country is in dire need of vaccines', Thursday 7 January 2021, http://pharmabiz.com/NewsDetails.aspx?aid=134623&sid=1 (Accessed 12/05/2021).
49 V. N. Kumar, 'COVID-19: How an Indian vaccine firm, HBL, ended up making sanitisers', 15 April 2020, https://thefederal.com/covid-19/covid-19-how-an-indian-vaccine-firm-hbl-ended-up-making-sanitisers/ (Accessed 12/05/2021).
50 WHO, 'Principles and considerations for adding a vaccine to a national immunization programme: from decision to implementation and monitoring', 2014, 1–140, http://apps.who.int/iris/bitstream/10665/111548/1/978924 1506892_eng.pdf (Accessed 12/05/2021).
51 WHO, 'Guidance for the Development of Evidence-Based Vaccine Related Recommendations Version 7', 2016, 1–53, http://www.who.int/immunization/sage/Guidelines_development_recommendations.pdf (Accessed 12/05/2021).
52 Alberto E. Tozzi *et al.*, 'Assessment of causality of individual adverse events following immunization (AEFI): a WHO tool for global use', *Vaccine*, 2013, 31, 5041–5046.
53 Edmond Differding, 'The Drug Discovery and Development Industry in India—Two Decades of Proprietary Small-Molecule R&D', *ChemMedChem*, 2017, 12, 786–818.
54 Emily H. Jung *et al.*, 'Do large pharma companies provide drug development innovation? Our analysis says no', *First opinion*, 2019, https://www.statnews.com/2019/12/10/large-pharma-companies-provide-little-new-drug-development-innovation/ (Accessed 12/05/2021).
55 Jacob Puliyel, 'Vaccine Policy and Advance Market Commitments', *Economic and Political Weekly*, 2011, 46, 18–19.
56 Y. Madhavi and N. Raghuram, 'Pentavalent and other new combination vaccines: Solutions in search of problems', *Indian Journal of Medical Research*, 2010, 131, 456–457.
57 Y. Madhavi and N. Raghuram, 'Crisis of speculation: Donors should fund only proven vaccine needs and local capacity-building', *British Medical Journal*, 2010, Response (www. bmj.com/cgi/eletters/340/may 12_3/c2576).
58 R. Lodha and A. Bhargava, 'Financial incentives and the prescription of newer vaccines by doctors in India', *Indian Journal of Medical Ethics*, 2010, VII, 28–30.

59 A. Bedi, 'Vaccine Vendors Greed gone Viral', *OutLookIndia Magazine*, 17 April 2017, 32–42, https://www.outlookindia.com/magazine/story/vaccine-vendors-greed-gone-viral/298718 (Accessed 12/05/2021).
60 R. Nagarajan, 'Many health ministry consultants paid by foreign aid agencies', *Times of India, Daily Newspaper*, 24 June 2015, http:// timesofindia.indiatimes.com/india/Many-health-ministry-consultantspaid-by-foreign-aid-agencies/articleshow/47794054.cms? (Accessed 12/05/2021).
61 Madhavi Yennapu, 'How many Vaccines does a child need?', *Medico Friend Circle Bulletin*, 2016, 371/372, 1–3.
62 Approves $610 million grant for Serum Institute, Bharat Biotech to boost vaccine production capacity, 20 April 2021, Express Pharma, https://www.expresspharma.in/covid19-updates/india-approves-610-million-grant-for-serum-institute-bharat-biotech-to-boost-vaccine-production-capacity/ (Accessed 12/05/2021).
63 Subhayan Chakraborty, 'Explained why government's funding of 3 PSEs won't raise overall vaccine production anytime soon', 2021, https://www.moneycontrol.com/news/business/economy/explained-why-governments-funding-of-3-pses-wont-raise-overall-vaccine-production-anytime-soon-6787271.html (Accessed 12/05/2021).
64 K. V. Balasubramaniam and N. K. Mehra, 'Reducing the cost of Covid-19 vaccines is desirable and possible, opinion', 2021, *Hindustan Times, Daily Newspaper*, Delhi, India.

6

START WITH THE WORLD AND CONTINUE IN ISOLATION

The Pasteur and Razi Institutes' Vaccine Legacy in Iran

Payam Roshanfekr and Parisa Roshanfekr

Vaccination in Iran dates back to the nineteenth century, which coincided with the reign of the Ghajar Dynasty. At that time, most of the population of Iran inhabited rural areas and general health was poor due to a lack of public health measures, poor transportation infrastructure, and general malnutrition among peasants of low social status. Life expectancy was therefore low, child mortality was as high as 50%, and epidemics such as typhus, smallpox, cholera, measles, plague, tuberculosis, trachoma, and malaria all took a toll on the population.[1]

At the time, there was no such concept as public health, so vaccination was a privilege mostly held by the king and his court, with the help of foreign missionary doctors. For example, the British doctor John Cormick vaccinated the family of then Crown Prince Abbas Mirza, who is noted as having been an early modernizer of Iran's armed forces and for establishing institutions against smallpox. Cormick was the crown prince's personal physician and wrote a treatise on smallpox inoculation, which was later translated into Persian and was published at the first printing house established by Abbas Mirza in Tabriz. It is said to be the first modern medical book in Iran. Abbas Mirza then attempted to inoculate people in villages in Azerbaijan, though his efforts faced public opposition. In 1806, his older brother, Prince Mohammad Ali Mirza Dowlatshah, the governor of Kermanshah, inoculated 25 princes in the region, using the Jenner method in both arms.[2]

Amir Kabir, Naseredin-Shah's prime minister and known as 'Iran's first reformer', made smallpox inoculation obligatory for all people in early 1848.[3] According to the newly established official newspaper of the government at that time, *Waghaye Etfaghyeh*, Amir Kabir dispatched health officials to different provinces, ordering them to perform the vaccination. The programme initially faced public resistance, but eventually it succeeded in inoculating a large number of children in Tehran, Rasht, Yazd, and other major cities. The parents of children

DOI: 10.4324/9781003130345-7

who were not vaccinated were fined by the government. Amir Kabir was assassinated after three years in office, and like most of his reforms the public inoculation programme was halted after his death.[4]

Amir Kabir also introduced several major reforms – simultaneously with other countries in the region, including the Ottoman Empire – which included licensing requirements for practicing physicians and dentists. He founded the *Dar al-Fonun* School, where, among other disciplines, modern medicine and pharmacology were taught to upper class Iranian youth. Shortly thereafter, the first three large state hospitals of Iran were founded in Tehran.

In between Amir Kabir's reforms and until the Mashrouteh Revolution (1905–1911), which was the first attempt to form a state based on the rule of law, the foundation of the *Majles-e Hefz al-Sehheh* (Council for Preservation of Health) in 1881 by Dr. Joseph Desiré Tholozan was another major health-related improvement made by Naseredin-Shah.[5] At the time, cholera posed a serious threat and the need for quarantine measures to impede its spread, as mandated by the International Sanitary Commission Meetings of Istanbul (1866) and Vienna (1874), were an important trigger for the formation of the council.[6]

During the Mashrouteh Revolution and with the formation of a national parliament, a smallpox vaccination code was ratified by the parliament in 1910, and in 1911, the *Majles-e Hefz al-Sehheh*, which was only a consultative council, was given a specific budget – secured from the tax placed on transportation vehicles – therefore transforming it into an established institute in charge of public health. This is considered as a turning point in the history of public health in Iran and the move accelerated vaccination in Tehran and the surrounding rural areas. The same budget ensured the free distribution of diphtheria serum and smallpox inoculation.[7] Also in 1911, Amir Kabir's former decree on licensing requirements for practicing physicians and dentists was legislated as the Code of Physicians.

Hand-in-hand with the World

Through the formation of a nation state during the last years of the Ghajar Dynasty and after the Mashrouteh Revolution, two public sector vaccine institutes (PSVIs) were founded – the Pasteur Institute of Iran and the Razi Vaccine and Serum Research Institute – as a step towards modernizing healthcare and improving public health in the country. With the formation of these institutes, Iran succeeded in moving from a vaccination-only programme to vaccine production.

Vaccine production by itself however is not enough for the successful immunization of the population. There was therefore a need to lay the foundations for the distribution of vaccines, along with a comprehensive immunization programme. The latter was formed many years later through the establishment of the primary health care (PHC) network, which merged with the Expanded Programme on Immunization (EPI), both within the framework of the WHO, with some innovations and revisions made by Iranian experts.

Pasteur Institute of Iran

After the great famine of 1917–1919 caused by aftermath of World War I and the outbreak of cholera, flu, plague, typhoid, and typhus epidemics, there was a dire need for public health and vaccine institutions. During the Paris Peace Conference, a group of Iranian delegates consisting of doctors and diplomats, on behalf of the Iranian government, held a meeting in the Pasteur Institute of Paris with Dr. Pierre Paul Émile Roux and discussed the establishment of a Pasteur Institute in Iran. The final agreement was signed between the Pasteur Institute of Paris and the Iranian Ministry of Foreign Affairs on 20 January 1920, thereby establishing the tenth Pasteur Institute in its international network. In July 1920, Dr. Joseph Mesnard travelled from France to Tehran to set up and manage the new institute, which was soon embraced by several Iranian nobles, including Abdol Hossein Farmanfarma, an influential Ghajar prince and the governor of Fars province. Concerned about the dependency of Iranian people on medicine provided by foreign governments and the inaccessibility of such medicine at times, he donated a large property to the institute where 'smallpox inoculum could be produced, where rabid animal bitten people could be treated, where sexually transmitted diseases were treated, and finally where inocula were prepared for all human and animal diseases'. The institute is still located there to this day.[8]

In the institute's first two years, until the launch of the Iranian institute's vaccine production line, a large amount of inoculum for cholera and smallpox, and other sera and vaccines, were imported from the Pasteur Institute of Paris.[9] During the first 50 years of the institute, there were five cholera outbreaks, which led to the mass production of anti-cholera inoculum to meet the country's needs. The volume of production was so high that during the outbreak of 1960, Afghanistan, Pakistan, India, Iraq, Georgia, and Azerbaijan all ordered cholera vaccines from Iran.[10]

In early 1922, Dr. Abolghasem Bahrami, a professor at *Dar al-Fonun* and then vice-president of the Pasteur Institute of Iran, visited the Paris institute, and upon his return, he set up a rabies department at the institute. The concurrent method of injecting serum and vaccine, demonstrated by the Pasteur Institute of Iran, was soon included in the WHO's guidelines for the treatment and prevention of rabies, which introduced Iran as one of the saviours of humanity.[11]

In 1953, the Iranian parliament passed the Vaccination Act and the Ministry of Health managed the public vaccination programme with the launch of the National Committee for a Rapid Response for eradication of smallpox, through which 120 healthcare groups travelled to every region of the country. Two years later, this model was also implemented by the WHO in neighbouring countries.[12] The Pasteur Institute, under the supervision of Dr. Mansour Shamsa as a consultant epidemiologist, participated in the smallpox eradication programme in Pakistan in 1971, and in Syria in 1976.[13] Finally, in November 1978, the Ministry of Health reported the eradication of smallpox in Iran; thereafter, the production of the smallpox vaccine at the Pasteur Institute of Iran was ended.

Due to the outbreak of World War II in 1939, relations between the Pasteur Institute of Iran and its parent institute were severed, and during this time, the institute was managed by Iranians, including Dr. Bahrami and later Dr. Mehdi Ghodsi. After the war, Iran's Health Secretary, Dr. Manouchehr Eghbal, invited a party from the Paris institute in order to revise the organizational structure and set new strategies for the Iran institute, which resulted in the signing of a new agreement, making the Pasteur Institute of Iran financially and administratively independent, and placing it under the supervision of the Ministry of Health. In 1946, Dr. Marcel Baltazard was appointed as the institute's fourth French president. Under his presidency, Iran succeeded in exporting smallpox vaccine to Iraq, Egypt, and Afghanistan, and the country also launched BCG vaccine production under the chairmanship of Dr. Ghodsi.[14]

It is interesting to note that the Pasteur Institute of Iran produced all its main vaccines – namely cholera, smallpox, tuberculosis, rabies, gonorrhoea, anthrax, typhoid, BCG, and typhus – in the first fifty years of its activities. Since then, however, the only addition to the collection has been the recombinant hepatitis B vaccine in 2008, produced in cooperation with Cuba.

Razi Vaccine and Serum Research Institute

Four years after the establishment of the Pasteur Institute of Iran and following agreements made by the Health Committee of the League of Nations, ratified by the fifth National Council of Iran (the parliament) in response to an outbreak of plague, the Institute of Animal Pest Control and Serum Production was created in 1924, operating under the Ministry of Agriculture, with the task of preventing animal and zoonotic diseases and producing related sera and vaccines. It was later re-named as the Razi Vaccine and Serum Research Institute.[15] The Razi Institute is still active as the second largest vaccine production institute in Iran, producing DTP, MMR, and polio vaccines.

At its founding, the scope of the institute's activities, according to the bill presented in the National Council, was as follows:

- Preventing zoonotic diseases using prevalent international scientific approaches;
- Making sera and vaccines to prevent all diseases for which a serum or vaccine has been discovered;
- Studying plant diseases and discovering useful and harmful insects; also finding a scientific approach to eliminate pests and vermin such as locust sand *Eurygaster integriceps*;
- Increasing the number of domesticated animals and useful plants; and
- Expanding the institute and its activities throughout the country.

During the first six years, with a staff of 22, the institute was run by Iranian doctors: first Dr. Abdullah Hamedi and later Dr. Morteza Kaveh. In the years 1926–1931, due to agricultural losses caused by locusts and the decline of rinderpest, the institute turned its focus to the production of anti-locust poisons. In the spring of 1924, however, rinderpest outbreaks re-emerged in some central regions. In 1932, in order to bring rinderpest under control, a French veterinary microbiologist, Dr. Louis-Pierre Delpy, came to preside over the institute. He and his team succeeded in producing a set of rinderpest vaccines; additionally, they also performed immunization studies to prepare various vaccines against bovine hemorrhagic septicaemia, pasteurellosis, sheep pox, anthrax, foot and mouth disease, cholera, and aphtha. In 20 years, the institute thus made a considerable contribution to vaccine and serum production in Iran.[16]

The Razi Institute has been producing sera and vaccines for anthrax, sheep pox, livestock gangrene, cattle pasteurellosis, diphtheria and tetanus, polio, rubella, measles, and Aleppo boil (cutaneous leishmaniasis). The institute's current mandate includes inactivated polio vaccine (IPV), foot and mouth disease oil emulsion vaccine, Peste des petits ruminants (PRP) vaccine, and also Pappataci fever vaccines.

For more than 100 years, the Pasteur and Razi Institutes, as Iran's two PSVIs, have been producing the necessary vaccines to control the major contagious diseases threatening the country's population, and have been successfully able to produce the necessary vaccines for Iran's national immunization programme.

Setting up an accessible immunization programme

For Iran, one of the major benefits of international cooperation has been its involvement with the WHO's PHC programme, which dates back to the early 1960s with a successful experiment in west Azerbaijan in 1971.[17] This aimed to evaluate the status of healthcare services and provide a model of healthcare service provision by community health workers in villages. Official implementation of the programme at the national level was not to start, however, until after its official endorsement as a major healthcare delivery strategy at the International Conference of Alma Ata in 1978; this was then interrupted by the Revolution of 1979.

A few years later, in 1983, the Ministry of Health revived the PHC programme and developed a partially modified version of the original plan. This resulted in the formation of a vast PHC network founded on the principles of maternal and child care and communicable disease control and consisting of a rural and an urban branch. The programme was implemented so successfully that only four years after it started more than 7,900 'health houses' had been built and staffed throughout the country.[18]

A major event was the integration of the WHO's EPI – which began in early 1984 – into the PHC network, which provided considerable coverage for major contagious diseases in the country. By implementing the EPI, immunization coverage among one-year-olds increased dramatically between 1980 and 2015: for diphtheria, tetanus toxoid and pertussis (DTP3), coverage increased from

32.0% to 98.0%; for polio (Pol3), immunization coverage increased from 38.0% to 98.0%; and for the measles-containing vaccine first-dose, immunization coverage improved from 39.0% to 99.0%. Furthermore, the country succeeded in eliminating measles, congenital rubella syndrome, and neonatal tetanus, and further sustained its polio-free status.[19] Successful implementation of the EPI, in line with the PHC network, helped Iran to reach Millennium Development Goals 4 and 5 (reducing maternal and child mortality rates) by 2015.[20]

Having achieved great success in terms of coverage and implementation, Iran's EPI is currently facing challenges to adapt to new health threats. According to the strategic plan of disease preventable by vaccine (2012–2016) prepared by the Centers for Disease Control (CDC) of the Ministry of Health, some of the challenges are as follows:

- A low budget, which limits the PSVIs' ability to purchase new vaccines, to improve their cold chains and transportation means, and to update their equipment and facilities to be able to produce new vaccines;
- Insufficient human resources;
- The non-cooperative approach of private sector doctors in the health care system;
- The low EPI coverage in neighbouring countries, which poses the risk of the re-entry of polio and measles viruses;
- The unpredictable mobility of immigrants due to social, economic or political reasons;
- Economic sanctions; and
- Anti-immunization beliefs, especially among immigrants.

Another factor that may impact the country's EPI as an accessible immunization programme for all, which is not mentioned in the CDC's report, is the threat of the privatization of primary healthcare. In 2008, the Ministry of Health started an initiative to offer the possibility for private sector companies to purchase the country's existing health houses or to set up new ones; it also looked at outsourcing the health houses' services to the private sector. Through this initiative, a small percentage of the country's health houses have been assigned to the private sector. The justification that the Ministry of Health gave for this was, *inter alia*, poor management by the public sector, general privatization policies in all sectors, and the chance for better overall performance and quality of services by private service providers. Meanwhile, according to a study conducted in 2010, vaccination coverage in privately owned health houses for under one-year-olds was less than that of the public health houses.[21]

Seeking independence

With the Revolution of 1979, religious, anti-colonial and pro-poor and -oppressed sentiments, and the yearning for a free, independent country governed by a welfare system, triggered a process of mass nationalization and the confiscation of major industries. From the very beginning, however, there was a lasting debate among the revolutionaries over the pros and cons of a state-centric economy; this debate later played an important role in the future of the healthcare system in general, and vaccination and vaccine production in particular. The nationalization of major companies, including pharmaceutical companies (mostly owned by foreign investors), was one of the first actions taken by the revolutionary forces. It should be mentioned, however, that the confiscation of private properties, including those of major industries, started with the workers and students, not the revolutionary government – which was not yet fully structured and in place. These confiscated industries were then later owned and managed by the new government and revolutionary foundations.[22]

Modern pharmacology in Iran had started with the establishment of a pharmacology faculty in 1934. The manufacture of drugs, such as ointments, pills, and syrups in local pharmacies, started shortly after the Mashrouteh Revolution, but the first drug manufacturing laboratory in Iran (the Gol Company), which produced herbal extracts, was founded during World War II. Dr. Abidi Laboratory – which is still one of the major pharmaceutical companies in Iran – was the first company in the field to acquire a license from the Ministry of Health.[23]

Especially after 1954 and after ratification of the code of Pharmaceutical, Medical, Food and Beverages Regulations by the parliament foreign investors from the United States, Germany, France, the United Kingdom, Switzerland, and the Netherlands started showing an interest in Iran's drug manufacturing market, which led to local production and small companies fading away and the market coming to be dominated by multinational companies. The Iranian market thus witnessed the foundation and proliferation of pharmaceutical companies working under the license of, or with investments from, foreign companies, which supplied the country mostly through importation, with around 30% local production.[24] At this time, drug production was mostly branded, while generic drugs had a weak presence.[25]

During the 1979 Revolution and faced with political and social turbulence, some of the foreign pharmaceutical companies left the country and later raised claims or settled cases regarding the transfer of ownership with the government via the selling of shares or other forms through the Iran United States Claims Tribunal.[26] In total, 28 out of 40 active pharmaceutical companies were confiscated by the revolutionary government and revolutionary foundations, and transformed into governmental entities, which for a long time dominated the supply market in terms of the importation and production of drugs and other pharmaceutical products.

As mentioned earlier, the pre-Revolution drug and vaccine market, being dominated by multinational and foreign pharmaceutical companies, was made up largely of brand name drugs. After the Revolution, however, through the transfer of ownership of the pharmaceutical companies to the government, Iran's new generic drug system was founded, though there is no documented evidence regarding the how and why behind the formation of such a system. Its legal foundation came only years later, in 1989, through the revision of the 1956 drug regulations. Nevertheless, aside from using generic names for manufactured and imported drugs, some of the key pillars of this new system included:

- Codifying the country's drug list and limiting the approved drugs to the list;
- Concentrating drug distribution in the hands of specific companies; and
- Nationalizing the pharmaceutical companies.[27]

Soon after the Revolution, it became clear that there were some differences of opinion regarding the best economic model for the country and there were rival positions on that front that were marked, *inter alia*, by their position towards privatization.[28] Nevertheless, for the first decade, the state-centric economy approach prevailed in the drafting of the Constitution, especially the famous Article 44, which is still a point of debate regarding the country's economic model.

Article 44 of the Iranian Constitution outlines the economic system of the Islamic Republic of Iran and defines three sectors – state, cooperative, and private – each of which has a role to play. In the article, major industries and foreign trade are categorized under the state sector, which is 'publicly owned and under the state's control'. This was in line with the anti-capitalist and pro-poor slogans of the 1979 Revolution and the mass nationalizations of major industries that resulted in the state (the government and revolutionary foundations) owning almost 70% of the nation's capital in the first years after the Revolution.[29] Gradually, the low performance of the government companies, along with the crippling effects of an eight-year war with Iraq (1980–1988) as well as US sanctions, led the government to reconsider its economic model and turn to the private sector for help.[30]

Moving towards privatization

Supporting the private sector in order to invest in production to create jobs and help reduce inflation was a policy adopted by the Iranian government in the aftermath of the Iran–Iraq War. It was reflected in Article 192 of the First Development Plan of 1989–1993. It was not until the Third Development Plan of 2001–2005, however, that the private sector was, for the first time, given the authorization to cooperate with the government in the governing of health services. This was later confirmed in the Fourth Development Plan 2005–2009. More detailed was the code on 'Financial Regulations of the Government' ratified in 2002, where '... in order to reduce the state's size and [the] gradual decrease of [its] expenses budget...', the governmental and public organization's in charge of social services were given the authority to delegate their services via public–private partnerships, outsourcing or assigning their management to the private sector.[31]

The most serious attempts at privatization were taken after the issuance of the General Policies of Article 44 of the Constitution by Iran's Supreme Leader in 2005, which has since formed a guideline when conducting privatization strategies throughout all areas. The general policies for privatization, as outlined by the decree, are in fact an interpretation of Article 44 of the Constitution in order to:

- Increase the pace of national economic growth;
- Expand ownership among the general public in order to provide for social justice;
- Enhance the efficiency of economic entities and effectively utilize monetary, human and technological resources;
- Increase the share of the private and cooperative sectors in the national economy;
- Decrease the financial and managerial responsibilities of the government in managing economic activity;
- Increase the public employment rate; and
- Encourage savings and investment by the public and enhance family income.

The General Policies refer to the expansion of non-governmental sectors, including through the transfer of government activities and businesses, prevention of the expansion of the governmental sector, and guidelines for the cooperative sector and for enforcing the law and preventing monopolies. According to the decree, the government '… is required to transfer any kind of activity (including the continuation and profiting from pre-existing [business] activities) that is not covered by Principle 44 to the cooperative, private, or public non-governmental sectors, at the latest by the end of the fourth 5-year development plan'. It is also stated that the 'transfer of 80% of shares of government businesses listed in the beginning of Principle 44 to the private sector, cooperative LLP's, and public, non-governmental businesses is permissible'.[32]

It has been argued that the General Policies for implementing Article 44 are in fact an implicit revision of the original article.[33] Despite such comments, Iran's desire to join the WTO required many changes in economic policy, one of which was to bolster the presence of a private sector that can compete with foreign counterparts. To achieve this, privatization is inescapable. Furthermore, these privatization policies have resulted in changes to regulations and strategic plans that have impacted vaccine supply in different ways.

Moving towards patent recognition

One of the manifestations of the tendency towards privatization has been a growing need to encourage and protect knowledge enterprises. This tendency was especially echoed in Iran's Fourth Development Plan 2005–2009. In this document, the government was assigned different tasks, including designing and implementing a comprehensive intellectual property system in order to expand the market for knowledge enterprises and to commercialize R&D achievements. In the Fifth Development Plan 2010–2014, the government's authority – and obligation – to support and encourage knowledge enterprises was amplified. For example, it was stated that the government was obliged to provide research facilities and laboratories to support privately established knowledge enterprises at a lower cost. Supporting knowledge enterprises in the health sector was also specifically mentioned. Subsequently, different knowledge enterprises that were authorized to become involved in the R&D of vaccine production were incubated in the Razi and Pasteur Institutes. There are currently 15 knowledge enterprises housed in the Razi Institute and 40 in the Pasteur Institute. They fully enjoy the institutes' support and have access to their facilities, laboratories, and experts.

Since Iran has not (yet) fully joined the WTO, it has not signed the TRIPS (Trade-Related Aspects of Intellectual Property Rights) Agreement, though the country did adopt the World Intellectual Property Organization's (WIPO) constitution in 2001, and in 2007, it ratified the Patents, Industrial Designs, and Trademarks Registration Act. The year 2001 was also marked by an interesting shift in the Iranian pharmaceutical industry. After the confiscation of pharmaceutical companies during the Revolution, Iran had a strict rule of producing only generic drugs; but from 2001, the Ministry of Health loosened these rules, and in order to promote competition and innovation, it authorized pharmaceutical companies to produce patent drugs.[34] Although some experts believe that Iran should not commit to strong patent laws in order to allow related players to increase their capabilities to conduct fundamental research and to use reverse engineering and other techniques to produce branded products,[35] it seems that the formation of patent companies and attempts to strengthen patent laws are among other measures that the country has taken in line with its aspirations to join the WTO.

It has also been argued that due to the outdated technology and facilities of both the Pasteur and especially the Razi Institutes, Iran faces some challenges in complying with the WHO's current Good Manufacturing Practice (cGMP) guidelines and thus in acquiring the WHO's pre-qualifications. Furthermore, the two PSVIs' current production lines do not seem to be able to compete with foreign and multinational companies, which will claim their market shares in the event that the country does join the WTO.[36] Such concerns have led some experts to believe that in order to enjoy new technologies and be able to produce new vaccines, the Pasteur and Razi Institutes should be assigned to the private sector, or should at least form a partnership with private sector actors.[37] In a study published in 2012, interviews with 16 opinion leaders in Iran's vaccine production industry revealed that most of them blamed government ownership and the public structure of the industry for its inadequacies, revealing an internal tendency towards privatization. It is also worth mentioning that in a visit from the WHO's Polio Eradication Department in August 2016, which was arranged to discuss technology transfer options of IPV production to Iran (to the Pasteur Institute), the need for a private investor was mentioned as a barrier to concluding the negotiations.[38] Despite such remarks, thus far the Iranian government has not shown any interest in losing control over the two PSVIs, so their privatization does not seem imminent.

Before the onset of the Covid-19 pandemic, the private sector was absent from the country's vaccine production system. This new pandemic context has, however, raised a strong show of interest from the private sector – or better said, semi-private companies and corporations – to enter the vaccine production market. This has been welcomed by the government. In other words, it appears that instead of fully delegating the market to the private sector, semi-governmental foundations and governmental sectors have formed private companies or enterprises that are strongly privileged in terms of financing and government support, and have even influenced regulations and measures. At times, this has led to exclusive market domination and the exclusion of independent private players.

As mentioned above, one of the areas in which such domination is visible is vaccine production. Barekat Pharmaceutical Group, registered as a private company but linked to the Execution of Imam Khomeini's Order (EIKO) Headquarters and in collaboration with Shafa Daru Holding, is one of the main players in the pharmaceutical industry and vaccine R&D. Especially since the onset of the Covid-19 pandemic, it has been highlighted as an important player in local vaccine production. Barekat's Covid-19 vaccine, named COV Iran Barekat, is based on an inactivated virus approach. In July 2020, the Barekat Foundation (one of the Barekat Pharmaceutical Group's main investors) announced that the first round of animal trials for their vaccine had been passed successfully. Later, in February 2021, they claimed success in the first round of human trials and promised the introduction of an Iranian vaccine to the market in the near future.

The Ministry of Defence is also supporting one of its dependent companies (Milad-e-Noor) to produce the Fakhra vaccine,[39] using an inactivated virus approach. The appointed project manager has stated that R&D for the vaccine began in March 2020 and has finally passed its first round of human trials. The Ministry of Defence claims that it will be able to mass produce the Fakhra vaccine by July 2021.[40]

The Pasteur and Razi Institutes have not been neglected in Covid-19 vaccine production. Using a genetic approach (mRNA), the Razi Institute is mid-way through human trials of COV Pars and was expected to report its test results to the Food and Drug Department of the Ministry of Health in the first half of May 2021. The Pasteur Institute is also working on a joint project with the Finlay Vaccine Institute of Cuba to produce the Soberana 2 vaccine, using the whole-microbe approach (viral vector), which, at this time of writing, is in its final stage of human trials. The Pasteur Institute is also supporting six knowledge enterprises resident in the institute on their testing and trials to produce a Covid-19 vaccine, using all three known approaches.

Struggling for independence

Iran's relationship with the world following the 1979 Revolution has been a complicated one, and these complications have affected all aspects of the nation's life, from policy-making to the implementation of strategic plans, from the military arena to education and health. Among the most important slogans of the Revolution were 'independence' and 'rejection of foreign domination', which later led to the confiscation of multinational companies, the expulsion of foreigners, and the drafting of many articles of the Constitution based on the concept. The infamous incident at the US Embassy on 4 November 1979,[41] was a symbolic manifestation of anti-capitalist and anti-foreign intervention sentiment, which triggered a set of sanctions against the country that have persisted and accumulated during the existence of the Islamic Republic of Iran. At first, economic sanctions were only imposed by the United States, but later on, with the rise of human rights issues, claims of supporting terrorism and finally concern about Iran's nuclear plans, not only did US sanctions grow and become more complicated and more severe, but European countries and the UN Security Council joined in and imposed various sanctions on different areas, which have had grave and sometimes devastating effects on many different areas of Iranian people's lives.

Since 2012, unilateral, multilateral, and especially secondary sanctions have been imposed – mostly by the United States – though these were without a UN mandate and went beyond the scope of UN sanctions since they targeted all sectors of Iran's economy and imposed an array of restrictions on banking, shipping, insurance, ports, trade, commodities and energy transactions, and ventures. This limited the country's ability to sell oil, which resulted in a decrease in its financial ability to import raw materials and other necessary supplies. Freezing the Central Bank's assets, cutting off Iranian banks from the international banking system, limiting payment channels, the sharp devaluation of the national currency, and the declining oil revenues and industrial production have all led to a high rate of inflation, a decrease in GDP and purchasing power parity (PPP), and a diminished industry and economy.[42] Some studies show adverse effects on the country's welfare system in terms of deteriorating mental health, and Social Determinants of Health (SDH) attesting to a widening health gap between income groups and impaired access to healthcare.[43] The government has faced great difficulty in purchasing raw materials for drug synthesis, as well as equipment for health centres such as CCU and ICU equipment.[44] Sanctions on opening letters of credit for Iranian banks and the shipment of imported goods have also caused a shortage of medicines, and it is said that humanitarian exemptions and the provision of supplementary aid are inadequate to ensure people's access to food and healthcare.[45]

The struggle to keep the economy from crumbling and intensified confrontation with the West have played into the increased securitization of critical sectors such as health, where the ability to fend for the nation without external dependency seems crucial to survival. In this context, Covid-19 has played an important role in highlighting the need for a more sophisticated and updated domestic vaccine production line. Restrictions on the country's banking system have posed a great challenge to the allocation and transfer of the funds necessary to purchase testing and hospital equipment such as Real Time PCR and X-ray machines. Facing the pandemic, the Ministry of Health has been forced to allocate most of its budget to fight Covid-19, hence leaving patients with chronic diseases with great difficulties in procuring their medications. The cost of cancer treatment has reportedly risen 30 times since the onset of the pandemic.[46] Even in terms of supplying Covid-19 vaccines, Iran has struggled to make the necessary purchase payments. After lengthy negotiations with South Korea, and even as Tehran insisted that the money could be transferred in South Korean currency and would be used exclusively for the purchase of sanction-exempt food and medicines, Seoul was hesitant to deliver the vaccines on the grounds of not receiving the necessary US Treasury assurances that the payments would not lead to fines.

Delays in supplying vaccines have had a very negative impact on the implementation of the National Development and Vaccination Plan (NDVP), codified in January 2021. According to the plan, which was prepared in line with the WHO Strategic Advisory Group of Experts' (SAGE) values of prioritizing Covid-19 vaccines and the equitable allocation of vaccines worldwide via the COVAX initiative and other direct purchasing methods, the Iranian government is supposed to vaccinate people based on the following prioritization categories and according to the timeline set by National Implementation Committee:

1. Frontline healthcare personnel plus high-risk people likely to face hospitalization and death due to Covid-19 (February and March 2021);
2. Elderly people and those with pre-existing conditions (April to July 2021);
3. Children in orphanages, soldiers in garrisons, and people in collective centres (August to November 2021); and
4. Other groups prioritized based on age (December 2021 to March 2022).[47]

In reality, at the time of writing this chapter (mid-April 2021), less than 30% of frontline healthcare personnel have been administered with a first dose of the COVID-19 vaccine, which is a considerable gap in the implementation of the plan.[48]

Dr. Alireza Biglari, Head of the Pasteur Institute, in his announcement of the successful testing of the Iran-Cuba vaccine, emphasized that 'COVID showed us that we can in no circumstances depend on foreign help… in such global shortage, no one will provide us with the needed vaccine… so let's support our scientists… vaccine is a matter of sovereignty and is linked to the country's biosecurity… as much as it is worth spending on defense system, it is worth spending on vaccine'.[49] The Iranian Foreign Minister Mohammad Javad Zarif also stated that 'Just as we were forced to manufacture missiles ourselves, we produced a coronavirus vaccine'.[50]

Mistrust of the West has added to the struggle for independent Iranian vaccine production. Iran's Supreme Leader, in an address on national television, announced a ban on the importation of the US and British vaccines, calling them completely untrustworthy. 'Given our experience with France's HIV-tainted blood supplies, French vaccines aren't trustworthy either', he added, referring to a scandal from the 1980s and 1990s.[51]

In such circumstances, the Iranian government has turned to its trusted semi-private players and has shared the financial burden of providing public health with them in order to find a permanent solution for a crucial problem. Economic shortage and the grave social and political pressures of controlling the ever-growing pandemic have even led to extreme measures, such as the President's call on all private sector players – health-related or otherwise – to import the much-needed vaccines through a governmental currency allocation and to administer them in locations approved by the Ministry of Health. Following this announcement, Alireza Raeesi, spokesperson of the National Anti-COVID Headquarters, declared that '… people who cannot wait to receive their vaccine per NDVP, could receive vaccines from the private entities who are given authorisation to import vaccines and pay for it'.[52]

Concluding remarks

A century-old vaccine production industry, along with a well-established public healthcare network and EPI, laid the foundation for a successful public immunization programme in Iran, which was able to resist opposing conservative voices and different political and economic situations. Nevertheless, long-lasting and intense economic pressures have weakened the state and therefore limited its capabilities to support the country's healthcare system. On the one hand, the limitations of the state's economic capabilities have impacted the functionality of its public healthcare network; and on the other hand, they have impeded the country's two PSVIs from replacing or updating their technological facilities and improving or expanding their R&D competencies. Additionally, the heavy burden on public healthcare, especially when faced with a devastating pandemic along with a securitized health attitude, has led the government to turn to private or semi-private players to help carry the weight of vaccine importation and recently also of production.

Notwithstanding the sanctions, Iran's intension to join the global market (particularly through the WTO) has been a matter of concern for the two PSVIs, which in their current state would not be able to compete with the major multinational pharmaceutical companies that would come to occupy the domestic market. The pro-privatization approach that has been dominant since 1990 was also delayed from entering the health sector, and the private sector's contribution to vaccine supply was for a long time limited to importation. In recent years, however, increasing calls to privatize the PSVIs, or require them to enter them into partnerships with the private sector, have been voiced. This is visible in recent collaborations with knowledge enterprises and might threaten the public nature of the PSVIs in the future.

Notes

1 Willem M. Floor, *Public Health in Qajar Iran* (Washington: Mage Publishers, 2004).
2 Aghazadeh Jafar and Farzad Khoshab, 'Mohammad Ali Mirza Dowlatshah measures to create a modern army in Kermanshah', *Policing History Studies*, 2016, 3, 19–38.
3 Azizi Mohammad Hossein, 'History of contemporary medicine: A brief history of smallpox eradication in Iran', *Archives of Iranian Medicine*, 2010, 13, 69–73.
4 *Ibid.*, 71.
5 Azizi Mohammad Hossein, 'The historical backgrounds of the ministry of health foundation in Iran', *Archives of Iranian Medicine*, 2007, 10, 119–123.
6 Floor, *Public Health in Qajar Iran*.
7 Saadat Ebrahim, *The Progress of Medicine in Iran in Recent Seventy Years* (Tehran: Golastan Publication, 1999), 154–159 (in Farsi).
8 S. Maslehat and D. Doroud, 'Pasteur Institute of Iran; a Leading Institute in the Production and Development of Vaccines in Iran', *Vaccine Research*, 2019, 6, 33–42.
9 *Ibid.*, 33.
10 Azizi Mohammad Hossein and F. Azizi, 'History of Cholera Outbreaks in Iran during the 19th and 20th Centuries', *Middle East Journal of Digestive Diseases*, 2010, 2, 51–55, 51.
11 M. Enayatrad and E. Mostafavi, 'Pasteur Institute of Iran: History and Services', *Journal of Research on History of Medicine*, 2017, 6, 209–226.
12 M. Baltazard, A. Boué, and H. Siadat, 'Study of the Behaviour of Variola Virus in Tissue Culture', *Annales de l'Institut Pasteur*, 1958, 94, 560–570.
13 Ehsan Mostafavi and Marjan Keypour, 'The life and career of Dr. Mansour Shamsa, A pioneer in public health', *Archives of Iranian medicine*, 20, 2017, 326–328, 326.
14 Marjan Keypour, Manijeh Yousefi Behzadi and Ehsan Mostafavi, 'Remembering Marcel Baltazard, Great Researcher and the French President of Pasteur Institute of Iran', *Archives of Iranian Medicine*, 2017, 20, 553–557.
15 Muhammad ibn Zakariya al-Razi (854–925 CE) was a Persian physician, alchemist and important figure in the history of medicine. He wrote a pioneering book about smallpox and measles, providing a clinical characterisation of the diseases.
16 A. Hosseini Chegeni and E. Mostafavi, 'Louis-Pierre Delpy: A French scholar and former director of the Razi Institute of Iran (1931–1951)', *Archives of Iranian Medicine*, 2019, 22, 675–679.
17 K. Nasseri *et al.*, 'Primary health care and immunisation in Iran', *Public Health*, 1991, 105, 229–238.
18 Leila Doshmangir, Esmaeil Moshiri, and Farshad Farzadfar, 'Seven decades of primary healthcare during various development plans in Iran: a historical review', *Archives of Iranian medicine*, 2020, 23, 338–352.
19 Global Health Observatory (GHO) data, https://www.who.int/gho/en/ (Accessed 20/01/2019).
20 Haniye Sadat Sajadi and Reza Majdzadeh, 'From primary health care to universal health coverage in the Islamic Republic of Iran: a journey of four decades', *Archives of Iranian Medicine*, 2019, 22, 262–268.
21 Irvan Masoudi-Asl, Mohammad Reza Maleki, and Ameneh Imani, 'Comparison of the health indicators of the state health sites and health indicators which have been outsourced to private sector health facility south of Tehran, Iran in 2009', *Journal of Shahrekord University of Medical Sciences*, 2012, 13.
22 Assef Bayat, *Workers and Revolution in Iran: A Third World Experience of Workers' Control* (London: Zed Books, 1987).

23 Morteza Azarnoosh, 'The evolution of the Iranian pharmaceutical system: Documenting the Iranian pharmaceutical system, examining the trend of drug imports in Iran from 1976 to 2011 and its influential factors in the health system', *Academy of Medical Sciences of the Islamic Republic of Iran*, 2017 (in Farsi).
24 Kavoos Basmenji, 'Pharmaceuticals in Iran: an overview', *Archives of Iranian Medicine*, 2004, 7, 158–164.
25 Documenting the New Drug System in Iran, Iranian Academy of Medical Sciences, http://www.ams.ac.ir/images/tarh1/66.pdf (Accessed 23/04/2021).
26 Abdol Majid Cheraghali, 'Trends in Iran pharmaceutical market', *Iranian Journal of Pharmaceutical Research*, 2017, 16, 1–7, 1.
27 'Iran Generic Drug System Over Time. 3', 2018, 2, 105–112, http://ijhp.ir/article-1-56-fa.html (Accessed 05/05/2021).
28 Eva Rakel, *Power, Islam, and Political Elite in Iran: A Study on the Iranian Political Elite from Khomeini to Ahmadinejad* (Leiden: Brill, 2008).
29 Shirzad Azad, 'The politics of privatization in Iran', *Middle East Review of International Affairs*, 2010, 14, 60–71.
30 *Ibid.*, 68.
31 The code on 'Financial Regulations of the Government', 2002, https://rc.majlis.ir/fa/law/show/93730 (Accessed 05/05/2021).
32 The General Policies pertaining to Principle 44 of the Constitution of the Islamic Republic of Iran, https://irandataportal.syr.edu/the-general-policies-pertaining-to-principle-44-of-the-constitution-of-the-islamic-republic-of-iran (Accessed 23/04/2021).
33 Seyyed Mohammadmehdi Ghamami and Mohsen Esmaeili, 'A Comparative Study of Competition Law in Iran and France', *Islamic Law Research Journal*, 2011, 11, 153–188.
34 Cheraghali, 'Trends in Iran pharmaceutical market', 1.
35 Hossein Safari *et al.*, 'A Comparative Study on Different Pharmaceutical Industries and Proposing a Model for the Context of Iran', *Iranian Journal of Pharmaceutical Research*, 2018, 17, 1593–1603, 1593.
36 Amir Hashemi Meshkini *et al.*, 'Assessment of the vaccine industry in Iran in context of accession to WTO: a survey study', *DARU Journal of Pharmaceutical Sciences*, 2012, 20, 1–7.
37 *Ibid.*, 4.
38 Note for the Record, Visit to Iran, 8–10 August 2016, WHO Polio Eradication Department.
39 Mohsen Fakhrizadeh Mahabadi (1958–2020) was a brigadier general in the Islamic Revolutionary Guard Corps, an academic physicist, and a senior official in the nuclear program of Iran. Likely due to his connections to Iran's alleged nuclear weapons program, Fakhrizadeh was assassinated in a road ambush in 2020.
40 Islamic Republic News Agency (IRNA), www.irna.ir/news/84318351/ (Accessed 05/05/2021).
41 Latest Developments | United States Diplomatic and Consular Staff in Tehran (United States of America V. Iran) International Court of Justice, 2021, https://www.icj-cij.org/en/case/64 (Accessed 23/04/2021).
42 Fatemeh Kokabisaghi, 'Assessment of the Effects of Economic Sanctions on Iranians' Right to Health by Using Human Rights Impact Assessment Tool: A Systematic Review', *International Journal of Health Policy and Management*, 2018, 7, 374–393, 374.
43 M. Aloosh, A. Salavati and A. Aloosh, 'Economic sanctions threaten population health: the case of Iran', *Public Health*, 2019, 169, 10–13.
44 Amir Abdoli, 'Iran, sanctions, and the COVID-19 crisis', *Journal of Medical Economics*, 2020, 23, 1461–1465.
45 Kokabisaghi, 'Assessment of the effects of economic sanctions', 374.
46 Abdoli, 'Iran, sanctions, and the COVID-19 crisis'.
47 National Development and Vaccination Plan (NDVP), MoHME, https://behdasht.gov.ir/inc/ajax.ashx?action=download&id=c662277f-b51b-462c-bb19-52ff2ee886e1&md5=2984B46119CBC2EF8E499EC4E55E097B (Accessed 18/04/2021).

48 Tasnim News Agency, https://www.tasnimnews.com/fa/news/1400/01/30/2487411/%D9%88%D8%A7%DA%A9%D8%B3%D9%86-%D9%81%D9%82%D8%B7-%D8%B1%D8%A7%DB%8C%DA%AF%D8%A7%D9%86-%D9%88-%D9%86%D9%88%D8%A8%D8%AA%DB% (Accessed 18/04/2021).

49 Iranian Students' News Agency (ISNA), https://www.isna.ir/news/99111511389/ (Accessed 05/05/2021).

50 Iranian Students' News Agency (ISNA), https://www.isna.ir/news/99122519012/ (Accessed 05/05/2021).

51 'Iran Bans Importation of Covid Vaccines from the US and UK', *The Guardian*, 2021, https://www.theguardian.com/world/2021/jan/08/untrustworthy-covid-vaccines-from-us-and-uk-banned-by-iran (Accessed 23/04/2021).

52 https://tejaratnews.com/%D9%88%D8%A7%DA%A9%D8%B3%DB%8C%D9%86%D8%A7%D8%B3%DB%8C%D9%88%D9%86-%D9%BE%D9%88%D9%84%DB%8C (Accessed 18/04/2021).

7

TRANSLATING PASTEUR'S VISION IN EASTERN EUROPE

The role of the Cantacuzino Institute in Romanian vaccination policies and vaccine production

Valentin-Veron Toma

Introduction

Until very recently, Romania was classified by the World Bank as an upper middle-income economy with a GNI per capita in 2018 of less than US$12,375.[1] In 2019, however, Romania was reclassified as a high-income economy.[2] In 1990 Romania had achieved self-sufficiency in vaccine production and the Cantacuzino Institute, the country's main public vaccine institute, had been able to cover all vaccines in the WHO's extensive expanded program on immunization (EPI). However today, like many other countries, Romania is completely dependent on large pharmaceutical companies for obtaining vaccine against Covid-19. Moreover, Romania has been integrated into the EU mechanism for distributing Covid-19 vaccines according to certain algorithms and not depending on the specific needs of the local population. The country has lost its autonomy in terms of decision making related to vaccination strategy during the pandemic. According to official documents, the Romanian government has concluded a collective purchasing agreement for 10.7 million doses,[3] together with other EU countries, and (at this time of writing) is waiting for the vaccine to be delivered by one or more of the manufacturing companies with which agreements were signed by the European Commission.

Without sufficient research infrastructure and lacking competitive production infrastructure, Romania is currently behaving on the world market like a country that has never had the capacity to produce the vaccines it needs. However, this is not the case. In fact, Romania has a long history of scientific research in the field of vaccines (from the first studies on the rabies vaccine from 1887–1888[4] to the last pandemic influenza vaccine in 2009), a long history of domestic vaccine production (1888–2013), a national vaccine production institute with a hundred-year history (1921–2021), and it has made important

DOI: 10.4324/9781003130345-8

contributions to the eradication or control of epidemics at the national, European, and global levels. How is it possible that these significant achievements have, for the most part, been consigned to history? What were the main factors that contributed to the increase, and later to the decrease, of the country's capacity to discover, produce, and develop vaccines locally for the needs of its population?

The present chapter discusses how the Romanian state built up its vaccine research and development (R&D) infrastructure; how it developed a state monopoly on vaccine production and distribution for the domestic market; its control of imports and exports; on national vaccination capacity, and quality control of vaccines administered on a mass scale. As will be shown, an essential role in consolidating this position of the Romanian state was played by Professor Ion Cantacuzino (1863–1934), one of the founders of microbiology in Romania, who was trained as a researcher at the Pasteur Institute in Paris, under the supervision of Ilya I. Metchnikoff. Cantacuzino was part of the first generation of young doctors who, under the influence of Pasteurian doctrines and the organizational philosophy of the Pasteur Institutes, founded a series of medical research institutes in Romania which played an important role in the production of vaccines at the national level, both for human and for veterinary use.

The chapter also briefly discusses some key elements of the strategy whereby the Cantacuzino Institute positioned itself on the domestic market, as well as the manner in which it positioned itself internationally, including: (1) within the international network of Pasteur Institutes and associated institutes; (2) in the Health Committee and Health Section of the League of Nations (1922–1948) and later of the WHO; and (3) within the European Centre for Disease Prevention and Control (ECDC). It will also examine the main stages of the process by which, after 1990, the Cantacuzino Institute went into decline and was finally eliminated from the domestic vaccine production market in 2013. Finally, it turns to the Romanian state's 'rescue' of the Cantacuzino Institute, which in 2017 was transferred from the Ministry of Health to the Ministry of National Defence to operate as a militarized strategic research and production resource.

Ion Cantacuzino and the laboratory of experimental medicine (1901–1921)

The beginning of the twentieth century brought important changes that left distinct marks on Romanian vaccinology. On 21 December 1901, the young Romanian doctor Ion Cantacuzino returned from Paris, where he had studied both medicine and biology and had trained as a researcher. He was called to take over the leadership of both the Department of Experimental Medicine at the Faculty of Medicine in Bucharest and the Laboratory of Experimental Medicine.[5] The Laboratory of Experimental Medicine was established in 1901, through the allocation of a special fund from the Ministry of Public Education, and was installed in one of the wings of the building of the Institute of Pathology and Bacteriology led by Professor Victor Babeş.[6] Many young doctors who wanted to pursue a scientific career in this new medical research centre were trained there. They formed the nucleus of what was later called the 'Cantacuzino School'.[7] Many of these scholars were sent to study at the Pasteur Institute in Paris as well as at other centres in Europe.[8] The laboratory would go on to play an important role in spreading the concepts of experimental medicine, but especially in putting into practice the theoretical concepts and methods of modern bacteriology, following the model of the French school. Moreover, from the very beginning, the Laboratory of Experimental Medicine was intended not only for education and scientific research, but also for practical activities for students and future researchers.[9] In fact, the organization of this modest laboratory was directly influenced by the organization of the Pasteur Institute, as Ion Mesrobeanu mentions, quoting Louis Pasteur, who famously said, at the inauguration of his new institute in Paris, on 14 November 1888: 'Our institute will also be a dispensary for the treatment of rabies, a research centre for infectious diseases, and an educational centre for microbial studies'.[10]

For the purposes of this chapter, the most important function of the Laboratory of Experimental Medicine was the production of sera and vaccines. Throughout its existence, it managed to offer solutions to problems faced by the Romanian state related to communicable diseases within the civilian population as well as in the army, in times both of war and of peace. The choice of Cantacuzino to position the newly formed laboratory in relation to the specific needs of the population and the capabilities of the public health system to deal with epidemics or pandemics was a strategic one, as we will see later. Indeed, he had a long-term vision of what had to be done in the fight against infectious diseases in Romania. It is therefore no coincidence that many authors have noted the continuity of the institutional project conceived by Cantacuzino, which began with the Laboratory of Experimental Medicine and culminated in the founding and development of the first national Institute of Sera and Vaccines.[11]

As mentioned in the monograph *Institut de Serologie de Bucarest: 1902–1932* (Bucharest Institute of Serology: 1902–1932), published by the Cantacuzino Institute in 1932, the transition from the small-scale experimental production of sera and vaccines for human use to a large-scale production took place relatively early on, soon after the laboratory's founding. Initially, the production of sera and vaccines for use in medical practice was carried out in the laboratories of the Faculty of Medicine in Bucharest, first in the Institute of Pathology and Bacteriology led by Professor Victor Babeş (from 1888 to 1904) and later in the Laboratory of Experimental Medicine of Professor Ion Cantacuzino (1904–1921). Although the main functions of these university laboratories were, initially, medical education and scientific research, they also ensured the domestic production of sera and vaccines, thus exceeding their original objectives.[12]

Due to the limited production capacity of the laboratory at the Institute of Pathology and Bacteriology, it focused more on the production of diphtheria antitoxin serum and anti-tetanus serum. The Sanitary Directorate of the Ministry of the Interior thus sought other solutions. The government then approached the Laboratory of Experimental Medicine in 1904 and 1905 to 'study the preparation and also the effectiveness of anti-streptococcal and anti-dysenteric sera' (Ibid.). Given the extremely promising results, the laboratory 'quickly moved from the purely experimental phase to large-scale preparation for application in current practice'.[13] Just a few years later, the Laboratory of Experimental Medicine was appointed by the Sanitary Directorate, to produce, on an experimental scale, vaccines against typhoid fever (in 1910) and Asian cholera (in 1913). After positive results were obtained in these experimental stages, the Directorate of the Romanian Health Service decided to pursue the mass production and systematic use of these vaccines in epidemics of typhoid fever and cholera (Ibid.). Immediately following this, the Army Sanitary Directorate reached the same conclusions. The vaccination and revaccination of all recruits in the Romanian Army led to the 'almost complete disappearance of typhoid fever in the army'.[14]

The year 1912 was a turning point in the history of Romanian medicine, as a method for scaling up the domestic production of antimicrobial vaccines was first developed. This had special significance, because it was the basis for the further development of the capacity of the future national institute to produce the necessary vaccines to meet the needs of the Romanian population. Referring to the entire volume of production during the pioneering period, in report no. 68 of 1 June 1921, addressed to the Council of Ministers, Cantacuzino reported that during the pioneering period of 1904–1921, the entire volume of production amounted to 44,000,000 cc of vaccines and 257,800 doses of sera.[15] This method of scaling up the production of sera and vaccines is probably one of the main achievements of Cantacuzino and his team during the operation of the Laboratory of Experimental Medicine between 1901 and 1921.

Ion Cantacuzino and the project of a national institute for the research and production of vaccines

Over time, production activities within the Laboratory of Experimental Medicine became increasingly difficult due to the lack of space and facilities to meet the new demands.[16] Thus the idea arose to create a research institute capable of ensuring the production of sera and vaccines according to the new needs of the population of the Romanian state, whose borders had expanded after the Great Union of 1918. As Cerbu states, it was envisioned that this new institute would be located in the vicinity of the building of the Institute of Pathology and Bacteriology led by Victor Babeş, and would include the institute itself (the central building, with one floor for laboratories, a library and a lecture hall), a vaccinogenic institute for the preparation of the smallpox vaccine, the domestic housing for the director and staff, and pavilions for large laboratory animals and farms for small animals.[17] However, this project was not approved by the government.[18]

Immediately after his return from Paris, where together with Nicolae Titulescu (1882–1941), he represented Romania at the signing of the Treaty of

Trianon, Cantacuzino began a systematic process of convincing state authorities of the need to establish a new institute. On 1 June 1921, addressing the Council of Ministers, he laid out on the one hand the important achievements of the Laboratory of Experimental Medicine, from its establishment in 1901 until 1921, and on the other hand, the discrepancy between local market needs and the laboratory's production capacities.[19]

His appeal was successful. A law establishing the Institute of Sera and Vaccines 'Dr. Cantacuzino' (Cantacuzino Institute) was published on 1 June 1921. This law, which was drafted and proposed by the founder himself, promoted 'an integrative vision in the field of public health that is similar to other prestigious international institutions such as CDC-Atlanta, SSI-Denmark or Robert Koch Institute in Germany'.[20] The law also outlined how the Institute would be financed, through: (1) an annual subsidy from the state, (2) a subsidy granted by different authorities or private companies, (3) the sale of sera and vaccines prepared in the institute, (4) the sale of various laboratory products necessary for biological reactions in relation to the diagnosis of contagious diseases, (5) fees for the various analyses performed in the institute for private clients, and (6) donations and bequests.[21]

Although the institution existed from a legal point of view, it did not yet have its own building, and thus for a while it had to operate from the headquarters of the old Laboratory of Experimental Medicine at the Institute 'Victor Babeş'. In 1924, however, the Cantacuzino Institute moved to its new premises built on a land ceded by the Bucharest City Hall. It was organized and run according to a model inspired by the Pasteur Institute in Paris, which was structured according to the criteria of the main etio-epidemiological groups. According to the decree regulating the organization and functioning of the Cantacuzino Institute, issued on 1 July 1924, its structure should be composed of the following sections: (1) serotherapy, (2) vaccines, (3) laboratory analyses, (4) parasitology, (5) scientific research, and (6) a general administration and accounting service.[22] Another important component of the Cantacuzino Institute was the animal farm in Băneasa founded by Prof. Alexandru Ciucă, in 1923, following the model of the Remoulin farm at the Pasteur Institute in Paris.[23] The land on which the farm was located was donated by the Royal House of Romania and over 80% of the buildings were erected between 1923 and 1925. To this would later be added the Dârvari farm, situated in Ilfov county.[24]

Cantacuzino's strategy for positioning the institute internationally

Cantacuzino's international orientation was visible early on, from the time when he coordinated the Laboratory of Experimental Medicine. His early strategic measures had the character of 'military epidemiological missions' and included establishing a relationship with the countries of the Balkan region, by conducting vaccination campaigns in Bulgaria and Serbia during the Second Balkan War (1913);

and by establishing missions to help France during World War I (1918–1919) under the auspices of the Red Cross.[25] There followed a period of intense activity at the Cantacuzino Institute, after its establishment in 1921. Relevant here were the steps taken by Cantacuzino and his team on several levels: (1) to establish a close relationship with the Pasteur Institutes in Paris and elsewhere,[26] including the Roscoff research station; (2) to establish sporadic vaccination campaigns for the population through exchanges of information and pathogenic strains (e.g., in 1926 BCG vaccination campaigns for newborns in collaboration with Albert Calmette)[27] and comparative studies of vaccines produced in Romania and France (e.g., the Moreni Study published in 1924, in which two types of typhoid-paratyphoid vaccine were administered in the middle of an epidemic outbreak in a community of crude oil extraction workers)[28]; and (3) the participation of Cantacuzino and his collaborators as experts in the specialized commissions within the Hygiene Commission of the League of Nations. A few years after Cantacuzino's death, Professor Mihai Ciucă became a member of the WHO Malaria Commission and later its secretary.[29] Professor Gheorghe O. Lupaşcu, a former disciple and collaborator of Ciucă, also became an international expert and was appointed advisor on malaria issues at WHO.[30]

The relationship with the League of Nations allowed the Cantacuzino Institute to adopt and assimilate methods standardized at the international level and to apply them at the national level, in the control and prevention of communicable diseases. The compilation of medical statistics and epidemiological reports was modernized, as was the elaboration of intervention and control plans for tuberculosis and malaria, among other diseases. Additionally, measures established at the international level were adopted for the control at the border of exotic epidemics and pandemics that affected Romania and neighbouring states. This consolidated the regulations on horizontal germ governance[31] established decades prior, through Romania's participation in the Dresden and Venice Conventions.[32] At the same time, as an institution representing the Romanian state, the Cantacuzino Institute began to report on the epidemiological situation at the national level in specialized sessions organized periodically by the Hygiene Committee of the League of Nations.

Cantacuzino's strategy for the national positioning of the institute

The national component of Cantacuzino's strategy included several measures that proved to be extremely effective in achieving a monopoly on vaccine production and for several decades maintaining the institute's central position on the domestic vaccine market. Of these measures, greatest importance must be given to the fact that basic scientific research was linked from the outset to applied research, in particular on vaccines and vaccination. Many of these key elements of the Cantacuzino Institute's national positioning strategy were maintained long after its founder's death, even during the communist period.

The first and most important objective of the Cantacuzino Institute's national positioning strategy was essentially economic in nature. It consisted of the establishment of a monopoly on the national production of sera and vaccines, and control over their imports and exports. The economic argument for this was based on the calculation of the amounts of money that could be saved if the entire production was made domestically, thus completely eliminating foreign imports. Moreover, these products had to be manufactured and marketed by public institutions, under the authority of the state, in order to allow for better control over production costs and, ultimately, savings to the state budget. However, for this to be achieved legislation would have to be amended. The national regulations for vaccination and revaccination published in 1893 prohibited the import of raw materials (i.e., lymph of animal origin), though it allowed the domestic production of the smallpox vaccine to take place on the free market, by competing public and private institutes.

The health law of 1910 – also called the 'Cantacuzino-Sion law', after the names of its two promoters Ion Cantacuzino and Vasile Sion – established for the first time the Ministry of the Interior's monopoly over the preparation of all vaccines. Article 84 of this law was a step forward in the Romanian state's efforts to control the production and marketing of domestic vaccines. The import of vaccines was allowed, but it became the exclusive right of the Ministry of the Interior, which controlled all imports and exports. Anyone who wanted to import vaccines had to obtain prior authorization from the Ministry of the Interior. For the first time, moreover, the export of vaccines produced in Romania was banned. The same article (art. 84) stipulated that production be provided by laboratories under the leadership of the Ministry of the Interior or be transferred to one or more university laboratories or veterinary school laboratories with an annual subsidy from the state budget. All marketing had to be done using only State control labels. This created a barrier to entry for any foreign or Romanian private company that might have wanted to enter the Romanian vaccine market.

The health law of 1930 pushed things further in favour of the Cantacuzino Institute. Article 161 reaffirmed the Institute's central position on the Romanian vaccine market, through which the state had a monopoly on both the production and sale of vaccines in Romania. This monopoly position for the institute was maintained in the health act of 1943.

Diversification of the portfolio of sera and vaccines made by the Cantacuzino Institute: 1921–1989

This component of the strategy – diversification – had begun long before the Cantacuzino Institute was established, during the operation of the Laboratory of Experimental Medicine, and it continued long after Cantacuzino's death. By covering as many diseases as possible, the need to import from abroad was reduced to almost zero. How did this process of continuous portfolio diversification evolve? Between 1924 and 1928, the Cantacuzino Institute invented and produced eight vaccines and three therapeutic sera.[33] It should be remembered here that the Cantacuzino Institute was one of the first institutes in the world, after the Pasteur Institute, to prepare the BCG vaccine according to Albert Calmette's specifications,[34] and Romania was the second country in the world, after France, to introduce BCG vaccination for newborns (in March1926).[35] By 1940, seven prophylactic vaccines, five therapeutic and immunomodulatory vaccines, seven therapeutic sera, and other injectable products were produced.[36] In an advertisement published by the Romanian Medical Movement magazine in 1940, the following vaccines were mentioned: anti-streptococcal, anti-staphylococcal, anti-gonococcal, anti-pneumococcal, anti-typhoid-paratyphoid, anti-cholera, whooping cough (Bordet-Gengou), anti-*E. coli*, influenza, and polymicrobial vaccine broth (staphylococcus, streptococcus, pyocyanic); as were the following toxoids: diphtheria, tetanus, staphylococcus, and streptococcus (i.e., hemolytic streptococcus).

Regarding the production capacity from 1947 to 1964, we can look to the introductory chapter of Ion Mesrobeanu's volume entitled 'Ion Cantacuzino – "Selected Works"' (1965), in which he reviews some of the major stages in the development of production capacity at the Cantacuzino Institute: 'If in the last pre-war years the products that were prepared amounted to between 13,000 and 18,000 litres per year, and in 1948, it reached 22,500 litres, the achievements for 1962 and the plan for 1963 amounted to 60,000-62,000 litres. This significant increase in the institute's production responds to large-scale plans by the Ministry of Health and Social Welfare, which include the complete elimination of several infectious diseases in the coming years, such as diphtheria, tetanus, malaria and rabies. In connection with the continuous expansion of the fight against epidemics, as well as with the desire to continuously increase and improve, in step with the latest scientific discoveries, the range of biological products for diagnosis and control of communicable diseases, the institute has always aimed to expand and improve its preparations. Thus, their number rose from 73 in 1947 to 117 in 1960 and to 174 in 1962'.[37]

In 1951, the Iaşi branch of the Cantacuzino Institute was created,[38] under the leadership of Professor Petre Condrea (1888–1967), a former disciple and collaborator of Cantacuzino. Therewith began the manufacture of adsorbed tetanus vaccine (VTA), tetanus toxoid, anti-*E. coli* bacteriophage and anti-tularemic sera. Intensive research in 1962–1963 led to the patenting in 1966 by Dr. Sylvia Hoişie of the polymicrobial vaccine Polidin, which was in mass production from 1970 to 2010.

In the 1960s the Cantacuzino Institute began producing vaccines against polio: first the Salk vaccine followed by the Sabin vaccine.[39] About this change in the type of vaccines produced, Strebel et al. (1994) write that the 'Cantacuzino Institute in Bucharest, founded in 1921 as a sister institute to the Pasteur Institute in Paris, France, began producing oral poliovirus vaccine in 1962 using Sabin working seeds received from the Poliomyelitis Research Institute in Moscow, USSR. In 1967, vaccine seed virus was received directly from Dr. Albert Sabin, and in 1974,

Cantacuzino Institute was approved by the World Health Organization as an oral poliovirus vaccine production facility. All oral poliovirus vaccine administered in Romania between 1964 and September 1990 was produced by the Cantacuzino Institute'.[40]

Mesrobeanu (1965) also systematically described the evolution of the institute's vaccine portfolio: 'We must also mention the new combination vaccines, such as diphtheria-tetanus bianatoxin and trivaccine against diphtheria, tetanus and whooping cough, both containing the purified diphtheria component. To improve the quality and effectiveness of the tuberculosis vaccine, a lyophilised BCG vaccine was developed. (...) One of the current concerns of the institute is the preparation of an oral vaccine. To this end, the method of cultivating germs in depth is currently being developed, which will allow obtaining the high yields necessary for the preparation of the important quantities of microbial suspension required by this vaccine'.[41]

In 1961, two researchers from the Cantacuzino Institute, Gheorghe Istrati and Teofil Meitert, together with Lucia Ciudin, discovered and developed the world's first live attenuated vaccine to combat dysentery.[42] Starting in 1962, the vaccine was 'used in a limited manner with good results, being internationally recognised, in outbreaks in children's communities'.[43] Also in 1961, Alice Saragea and Paula Maximescu produced the DTP vaccine for the first time in Romania, and that same year DTP was introduced into the national vaccination programme. Since 1974, WHO has recommended the inclusion of DTP in the EPI.[44] In 1977, an inactivated, trivalent split influenza vaccine with aluminum phosphate adjuvant, prepared on embryonated chicken eggs, was made at the Cantacuzino Institute. As Alexandrescu (2013) recalls, 'Romania was the third country in the world to produce a split vaccine after the USA and Denmark. The procedure was developed by a team of researchers which included Ion Niculescu, Ligia Creţescu, Radu Crainic and Claudia Anghel'.[45] In 1977 the first mass vaccination campaign was carried out with the split and inactivated influenza vaccine. In 1989, another vaccination campaign was carried out with a split trivalent influenza vaccine but without adjuvant.[46] In 1987, Gheorghe Dimache introduced intradermal vaccination, for cholera and typhoid vaccines during outbreaks, both of which were produced at the institute.[47] In 1981, a team headed by Elena Ciufecu developed the first batches of a measles vaccine. It was used in the period of 2000–2001 in a mass prophylactic vaccination campaign for the entire population. Since 2004 this vaccine has been replaced with the triple vaccine MMR vaccine.[48]

Until 1990, the Cantacuzino Institute had within its portfolio a range of vaccines that covered all of the diseases with an impact on public health that were included in the EPI.[49] In 1977, global immunization policies were established with the goal of providing universal immunization for all children by 1990; the Romanian government committed itself as a partner in this WHO-coordinated programme. The years following 1990 witnessed the gradual decline of the Cantacuzino Institute. Slowly it was being transformed into a powerless institution incapable of producing even the old vaccines that it still had in its portfolio in the early 1990s, let alone new vaccines based on advanced technologies.

The evolution of the Cantacuzino Institute in the period of 1990–2021

Since 1990, the Cantacuzino Institute has undergone a number of profound changes in the way it is organized as well as in its economic status. The first change occurred as a result of government decision no. 1247/1990, which led to its being transformed from a state institution into *regie autonomă* (a company with autonomous management). Practically, this new status did not lead to an improvement of the institute's financial situation; it had to obtain 90% of its revenues from its own sources and only 10% came from the state through research contracts. With its rich patrimony – consisting of a branch in Iaşi, its headquarters in central Bucharest, a research base spread over 11 hectares in the current residential district Băneasa (Bucharest) and 15 hectares in the village of Dârvari, Ilfov county – the Cantacuzino Institute had a fairly good position on the domestic drug market. At that time, it still had a near-monopoly on large-scale domestic vaccine production, and investments were already being considered for the rehabilitation and refurbishment of some production units. However, following the decision taken by the first government of democratic Romania, after the revolution of December 1989, to transform the institute into an autonomous company, its economic status became uncertain. Now it was neither a public entity financed entirely by the state, nor a private company fully financed by the sale of its products on a competitive market. In fact, as a *regie autonomă*, while it had financial autonomy by law, the managers were politically appointed by the Ministry of Health. In addition, the state could supplement the institute's budget only if its expenses exceeded the revenues from its own sources. This arrangement proved catastrophic in the medium and long term.

From 1991, amidst a gradual reduction in state subsidies, the institute's expenditures for its national activities to monitor the movement of microorganisms were covered by its own revenues, unlike the situation in other countries which provided significant subsidies from the national budget. Moreover, as a result of a decision considered strategic by the Ministry of Health, against the background of an increase in demand for influenza vaccines on the internal market, it was decided that the production of influenza vaccines should become an area of national interest. In the future, the conditions for prioritizing development of this field would have to be created.[50]

As a consequence, the general manager of the Cantacuzino Institute planned to modernize its packaging section for influenza vaccines. In the absence of investments from the state, a project was drawn up by the institute in 1994 that was to be financed by an external loan. The government then borrowed money from the World Bank and used US$4 million of this to re-equip the institute.

However, the budget allocation was used inappropriately. The money was spread over all sections of the institute, no single production line was completely refurbished, and only one ampoule filling machine was purchased for the vaccine section.[51]

In 2002, government decision no. 352/2002 planned to transform the institute once again. From *regie autonomă* it became a 'national research and development institute'. According to Păun (2019), starting with this change of status, a debate arose over whether the production of vaccines at the institute should be continued or stopped permanently. Not everyone agreed with this binary position. According to official documents, the Ministry of Health continued to consider a third way, namely maintaining the production of only essential vaccines such as the influenza vaccine and BCG. So what was actually decided? As a result of the institute's status change, the subject of its activities, in addition to scientific research, included 'the preparation of prophylactic and therapeutic biological products (…) by its own forces and through national and international cooperation, as well as their sale in the country and abroad'.[52] Thus, the institute became a company that could produce, market and sell, both domestically and abroad, without any protection from the Romanian state, like any other domestic or foreign company. In addition, production had to be carried out with no subsidies from the state budget. After the state monopoly law of 1996, the institute's products had no longer benefited from the status of state monopoly products. The provision of the sanitary law of 1930 which had established that quality control was to be done exclusively in-house, by the institute itself, was also abandoned. After 2000, quality control and the marketing authorization authority for local vaccines were transferred to the National Medicines Agency (NMA), which, by law no. 336/2002, imposes the obligation to meet internationally recognized good manufacturing practices (GMP) quality standards. Thus the Cantacuzino Institute's products became subject to external control, something for which the institute was not prepared. Furthermore, given that the old restrictions on the export of Romanian vaccines had been suspended, virtually all vaccine production was now placed on a global market that operated under different rules than those established domestically decades before.

In 2003, the institute reduced production, under the pretext of increasing performance. Only ten vaccines (and other injectables) remained in its portfolio. The following year, the institute began testing a local triple vaccine, the MMR. Although considered a success, it was never mass-produced.

In 2005, a major blow to the Cantacuzino Institute came from its sponsor: the Ministry of Health announced the need for one million doses of influenza vaccine for the 2005–2006 season, and organized a tender for the entire lot, in which, however, for the first time in history, the institute could not participate. The Minister of Health was accused in the press of favouring the institute's competitors. As Professor Mircea Ifrim, secretary of the Academy of Medical Sciences, explained in an interview at the time: 'One million doses of influenza vaccine were put in the specifications, while the [Cantacuzino] Institute could only make

600,000 and that was enough'.[53] As a reaction to the unfavourable press campaign, the health minister announced that he would look for a solution to save the Cantacuzino Institute, which was already facing serious financial problems. A 2005 statement from the Ministry of Health said that very soon 'a package of restructuring measures would be adopted to help the Cantacuzino Institute find private funding to modernize and develop the production of Romanian vaccines'.[54] This gave an important signal that the state was no longer willing to fully cover, from its own funds, the restoration of production infrastructure and that the institute could only hope for funding from external sources.

In the same year, the vaccine packaging section, for which the modernization project had been carried out in 1994, required rehabilitation. This was to be financed with external funds from the International Bank for Reconstruction and Development (IBRD). The new project was based on a study carried out in 2005. This investment strategy had some positive consequences. On the one hand, it allowed the Cantacuzino Institute, in collaboration with the Centre for Military Scientific Research, to sequence the viral genome of the avian influenza virus and to estimate the risks for the Romanian population during the 2005 bird flu epidemic.[55] On the other hand, the investment allowed the institute to increase the production of influenza vaccines in the period of 2006–2007, to which the Ministry of Health also contributed with a subsidy of RON 140,000. This new investment 'consisted of a redevelopment of the area but also infrastructure works. The expansion and modernization of the space and the acquisition of new generation equipment was done with the help of the loan from IBRD'.[56] Moreover, the project led to the commissioning of very modern influenza vaccine production areas that complied with GMP manufacturing standards. For this project, which ultimately cost over 10 million euros, WHO provided technical support and the allocation of R&D projects to maintain an adequate response capacity to pandemic threats in the region.[57]

In this context, it became possible for Romania to participate in the WHO programme to combat the swine flu pandemic in 2009. Shortly after WHO representatives asked the Cantacuzino Institute to produce a pandemic swine flu vaccine, the institute launched on the market a Romanian product called *Cantgrip*®. Regarding this pandemic vaccine, Păun recalls that: 'In the period following the 2005 bird flu wave, an attempt was made to develop a vaccine for special situations, specifically a pandemic vaccine (2009), with the important involvement of human and material resources. Obtaining this type of vaccine was a scientific success, but the presentation in the media, the desire to use this product to obtain political capital, and especially poor management led to financial disaster. The population was reluctant to accept this vaccine in the existing conditions of the market and among other preparations, but also in the context of poorly conducted marketing'.[58]

In 2007, the government decided to borrow from the World Bank, again to provide the necessary funds for the rehabilitation of the Cantacuzino Institute's production lines and to have several areas authorized by the NMA to meet GMP standards. The government also granted a three-year exemption for the compliance of manufacturing processes with GMP rules. This loan from the World Bank was talked about in the press as 'a climax of disaster' for the institute: 'The institute bought complex machinery and paid for training courses and technical assistance services. The old section of the institute, refurbished, worked, but the results were not as expected. The vaccine lots did not comply with European standards'.[59] A major problem with this project was that the Belgian company that won the tender to carry out the World Bank-financed project was delayed in completing the refurbishment. A new deadline was set for December 2010. In the meantime, the institute did not have a GMP production line but a 'GMP-like' production line. To avoid closure, it could only operate on the basis of an annual authorized exemption given by the NMA. As a result of these delays, on 8 February 2010, the NMA sent a notification to the Cantacuzino Institute withdrawing its authorization to operate as a production unit for sera and vaccines. From that moment, the Romanian state's monopoly over the local production of vaccines was *de jure* suspended.

According to a 2014 document issued by the Ministry of Health, the Cantacuzino Institute's portfolio of biological products, was as follows: 'By 2010, the Institute developed the influenza vaccine, BCG, tetanus, anti-staphylococcal and immuno-modulators (Polidin, Cantastim, Orostim)'.[60] Since the Cantacuzino Institute's license for the production and marketing of vaccines was suspended, on 8 February 2010, the Ministry of Health had to rely on imports to ensure its supply of the influenza vaccine and other vaccines for the implementation of the National Immunization Calendar.[61] Regarding the reasons for the drastic reduction of the Cantacuzino Institute's vaccine portfolio, the Ministry of Health cited: 'underfunding and the impossibility of allocating the necessary financial resources for development and refurbishment in order to meet GMP standards'.[62] It went on to add, however, that: 'It should be remembered that the Cantacuzino Institute is a member of the Pasteur Institutes network and has several reference laboratories certified in the WHO/ECDC network.[63] WHO supports the policy of the Ministry of Health for the rehabilitation, refurbishment, modernisation and resumption of influenza vaccines and BCG vaccine production. For the two mentioned vaccines, the institute is seen by the WHO as an important vaccine manufacturer for the Balkans and Eastern Europe'.[64]

In 2013, the production of influenza vaccines was thus resumed at the Cantacuzino Institute, without a license, for the 2013–2014 season, though the production was considered non-compliant following tests performed by the NMA and a laboratory in France and was suspended. Beyond the losses caused by the unsold vaccine stocks, additional losses occurred at the pure water station. To these were added the fine by the Ministry of Health and the institute's increasing debts to the National Agency for Fiscal Administration, followed by the termination of the contract with the National Health Insurance House. Due to arrears in its debt payments, the Cantacuzino Institute was no longer able to participate in public tenders or European project competitions. In fact, in the period of

2011–2014, the Institute recorded only debts and losses: in 2011, its debts were over 4 million euros and its losses 1 million euros; at the end of 2014, this had increased to 5.7 million euros and 2 million euros respectively. During this time the labour force at the institute was also reduced significantly: in 2011, over 620 people worked at the Cantacuzino Institute; at the end of 2014, there were 430 employees, a number set by the government in terms of the number of jobs that could be supported with money from the state budget.[65]

In 2015, the institute's accumulated debts and financial losses were growing, and its sources of financing seemed exhausted. In this context, an inter-ministerial commission met in 2015 with the aim of providing financial recovery solutions. However, the situation was not at all simple to resolve. Twenty years after the competition law adopted in 1996, and inspired by relevant European legislation,[66] came a new blow to national vaccine production. The inter-ministerial commission found that the institute could not receive a subsidy from the state because this would violate the rules on competition. In the 1990s when this law was enacted, this situation was only a possibility but it became real in 2015 when the institute's manager requested state aid. At that time, the Competition Council of Romania (CCR), which had been set up in 2004, referred the matter to the European Commission, which, since 2007, has had oversight over State aid decisions in all EU countries, to ensure that conditions enable the smooth running of the competitive market. Through the CCR, the European Commission thus prevented the intervention of the Romanian state to cover the Cantacuzino Institute's debts and ensure its continued viability.

This led to the government's decision to reorganize the Institute as a scientific research unit, without the production and commercial components that, for several years, had generated only losses. After this change of status, and through its transfer from the Ministry of Health to the Ministry of Education and Research, bringing it under the direct leadership of the National Agency for Scientific Research and Innovation (ANCSI), the Cantacuzino Institute received RON 45 million from the state budget for 2015 to pay its debts, cover employees' salaries and improve 'responsiveness'. The main object of its activities remained R&D, at least in theory. However, the functioning of the Institute remained difficult even after the reorganization, and the new financial arrangements severely affected influenza vaccine production activity.[67] Despite the fact that the number of specialists was reduced to 27, well below the lower limit of 60 employees needed to start mass production of influenza vaccines, the manager of the institute planned to resume production and sent specialists to be trained at the Pasteur Institute in Paris. Following these transformations, through the loss of qualified human resources, but also through underfunding from the state budget, the institute's reference activity was also severely affected and the ability to react in special situations (i.e., epidemics or pandemics, possible bioterrorist attacks, etc.) was much reduced.[68]

Another reorganization took place in 2016 by emergency ordinance no. 96/2016. The Cantacuzino Institute was transferred back from the Ministry of Education to the Ministry of Health. This return meant that the activities carried out at the institute were financed both from its own revenues and from subsidies from the state, granted through the budget of the Ministry of Health.[69] All these changes in the status of the Cantacuzino Institute from 2015 to 2016 were based on the idea that commercial activities at the institute should be completely abandoned and that its entire activity should focus on scientific research. Thus, after the complete suspension of production licenses in 2010, due to the lack of production areas conforming to GMP standards, and after the failure to produce seasonal influenza vaccines in 2013, it was finally no longer possible to produce any vaccines at the Cantacuzino Institute.

A significant change of perspective appeared, however, with the most recent reorganization of the institute carried out by emergency ordinance no. 66/2017. Through it, the National Research & Development Institute 'Cantacuzino' was transformed into a public military institution, of strategic interest, under the Ministry of National Defence, 'in order to revive it and resume the production of vaccines and other products for which it was famous'.[70] Since then, the institute's communication strategy has focused on describing the modernization and refurbishment process and the promise of the institution's military leadership that vaccines will once again be produced at the Cantacuzino Institute. A number of efforts have been made to restore the institute's R&D capacity and to fill vacancies in research laboratories. As a result, in 2017, a group of Romanian research institutes, which included the Cantacuzino Institute and the 'Victor Babeş' Institute, applied for funding and won a grant of RON 165,299 for the research project entitled 'Development of translational research capacity: development of vaccines from concept to preclinical evaluation - ConVAC'.[71] An official document of the Cantacuzino Institute provides more details: 'The objectives of the consortium are to provide the necessary framework for the development of a vaccine through: 1) studies that will ensure the development of the antigen; 2) studies on the optimisation of the formulation of this antigen; 3) development of characterisation of antigen-adjuvant complexes; 4) evaluation of the protection given by antigen-adjuvant complexes; 5) elaboration of the documentation of the modalities of non-clinical studies according to pharmaceutical regulations'.[72] The project duration was set at two years, until the end of 2020.

Regarding the possibility of local production of the anti-Covid-19 vaccine, the Cantacuzino Institute has neither sufficient R&D capacities nor large-scale production capacities. Like other European countries Romania is dependent on the global vaccine market, and the centralized mechanism established by the European Commission for procuring and distributing Covid-19 vaccines. The vaccines were purchased by the European Commission through an advance purchase agreements procedure with vaccine manufacturers.[73] This mechanism is a public–private partnership, though mediated by the European Commission. It is true that 'Member States send orders directly to vaccine suppliers, indicating, for example, the timing and place of deliveries and specifying logistical aspects', but this is a technical aspect of the relationship with producers. To make the collective purchase, 'Funding for the up-front payments will come from the Emergency Support Instrument (ESI)'.[74]

Where do the funds allocated by member countries come from? The payment for Romania's share of vaccines is provided by the government through a new external loan, probably from the European Investment Bank (EIB), as recommended by the European Commission. This new loan is in addition to the loans taken out from the World Bank to cover the costs of the national anti-Covid-19 strategy. As a recent World Bank paper states: 'In response to COVID-19, the Government of Romania activated € 400 million of pre-arranged financial support from the World Bank through the *Catastrophe Deferred Drawdown Option* (CATDDO) facility that the Government negotiated with the World Bank in June 2018. The financing covers a range of interventions to strengthen health services, minimize losses to both the public and private sectors, and safeguard lives and livelihoods overall'.[75] In this context, a task that the Cantacuzino Institute undertook, starting in December 2020, was to purchase the special refrigeration systems needed to keep and preserve the imported vaccines in the country, and thus it became the 'National Vaccine Storage Centre for Covid-19'. Additionally, in the period of 2020–2021, the institute provided the Romanian population with diagnostic services for Covid-19 using specific testing methods based on the RT-PCR technique, with diagnostic kits imported from multinational suppliers.[76]

Conclusions

This chapter has focused primarily on the role played by Ion Cantacuzino and the public institute that bears his name in terms of national vaccine capacity in Romania. Special attention was paid to the continuity of the institutional project conceived by Cantacuzino, starting with the first experimental medicine laboratory that he led, immediately after his return to Romania from his training in France. With Cantacuzino's takeover of the Laboratory of Experimental Medicine at the Faculty of Medicine in Bucharest, in 1901, Romania entered a new stage in the development of its research and production capacity in the field of vaccines. The period of 1904–1911 was dominated by experimental, small-scale production. But starting in 1912, a method of scaling up vaccine production was developed that would later allow Romania to achieve autonomy in its national manufacturing capacity. The health law of 1910 established the state's monopoly on the production of vaccines, and the laws of 1930 and 1943 established the monopoly of a single institution at the national level, namely the Institute of Sera and Vaccines 'Dr. I. Cantacuzino'. The state held a *de jure* monopoly on domestic vaccine production from 1910 until 2010. The Cantacuzino Institute lost its *de facto* monopoly position in the 1950s when other institutes produced, on a small scale, new types of vaccines. The production of vaccines by the Cantacuzino Institute continued to diversify between 1948 and 1989. Thus, a level of national self-sufficiency was reached, which made Romania independent of other states or international companies when it came to ensuring the necessary vaccines for the domestic market.

The strategy used by Cantacuzino to position the institute on the Romanian domestic market on the one hand, and to position Romania internationally in the active fight against infectious diseases on the other, had two major components. The first was related to the establishment of a key national position for the Cantacuzino Institute. The second was related to the establishment of close international collaborations with the main institutions in the world involved in the study of microbiology and that produced vaccines, as well as with the main international organizations of hygiene and public health. If, in terms of vaccine production, Cantacuzino's core aim was to provide the state with an institution capable of meeting the needs of the national population, in terms of strategies to fight and eradicate communicable diseases, the fundamental idea was to develop international cooperation between states in order to prevent and combat diseases that do not recognize historical or political-administrative boundaries. It is therefore not surprising that, after leading a research and production laboratory for two decades, Cantacuzino set up a national institute for sera and vaccines. It is also not surprising that he became involved in Romanian foreign policy and actively supported the League of Nations and the international health programmes run by its Health Commission and its various specialized sub-commissions. Like his contemporaries, Cantacuzino shared a somewhat idealistic view, that the prevention of wars and epidemics could only be achieved through the combined efforts of the community of nations. It is true that in the new international order drawn by the League of Nations, a joint action for the 'actual abolition of war'[77] seemed possible. Additionally, with the establishment of the League of Nations Health Commission, the joint action of member states to eradicate communicable diseases through common policies and internationally standardized methods of prevention and control also came to seem possible.

As shown in this chapter, inspired by the organizational model of the Pasteur Institute in Paris, the Cantacuzino Institute was conceived from the beginning as a public institution with the mission of advancing fundamental biomedical knowledge in the field of microbiology, training local specialists, and combating communicable diseases through the manufacture of biological products and the launching of mass vaccination campaigns. In its first decades, the institute spearheaded the fight against the great epidemics in Europe, making valuable contributions to the eradication of smallpox and reductions in the number of cases of other diseases through the production of vaccines and sera. But starting in the last decades of the communist period, the situation began to change dramatically. After a partial revival in the early 1990s, a new period of decline followed. In the first two decades of the twenty-first century, the situation of the venerable institute became extremely precarious, bringing it to the brink of bankruptcy. Despite much pressures that the institution be either totally closed or privatized, it nevertheless still exists. Its recent takeover by the army has meant that it has remained a public institution with the objectives of providing health services to the Romanian population as a whole, and not just to certain market segments according to a neoliberal logic.

Although the Cantacuzino Institute was not the first institution in Romania to produce vaccines, nor was it the country's first bacteriological research institute, from 1921 to 1990, it did significantly contribute to Romania's position among countries with expertise in vaccine R&D and a rapid response capability in the event of epidemics or pandemics. In this sense, an important role was played by Cantacuzino and his collaborators, as well as some of their successors. However, as we have shown, after the change of the political regime in 1989 and the transition to a market economy, the strategic position of the Cantacuzino Institute was systematically weakened by a combination of factors, but especially by the progressive weakening of the state as a result of its neoliberal transformation and the withdrawal of funding for research, infrastructure development, and the production of domestic sera and vaccines. To this was added a progressive increase in the influence of transnational mechanisms developed by the European Commission and WHO, but also the burden of successive loans from the World Bank, which were used for indiscriminate investments that did not achieve their goals but rather created major long-term debts.

In the case of the Cantacuzino Institute, although the state has made efforts to keep it in the public sphere, calling it 'an institution of strategic interest', and recently investing a large amount of money in infrastructure, research and production, it is also true that state institutions have significantly contributed to its weakening and elimination from the market. Thus unintentionally or otherwise, the state has played the role of intermediary for certain international bodies and some global pharmaceutical companies. Lack of infrastructure, and investment as well as political corruption were some of the factors that caused the institute to decline in the years after 2000. Under pressure from the EU to adopt GMP quality standards, which involved huge investments that the Romanian government could not afford, the Cantacuzino Institute was removed from the market of major European domestic vaccine producers following the 2010 decision to stop local production and after the unsuccessful attempt to produce a seasonal flu vaccine in 2013. Thus it came to be that following the complete suspension of domestic production of sera and vaccines, Romania became totally dependent on vaccines produced by multinational companies.

Notes

1 According to the World Bank website: 'For the current 2021 fiscal year, low-income economies are defined as those with a GNI per capita, calculated using the World Bank Atlas method, of US$1,035 or less in 2019; lower middle-income economies are those with a GNI per capita between US$1,036 and $4,045; upper middle-income economies are those with a GNI per capita between US$4,046 and US$12,535; high-income economies are those with a GNI per capita of US$12,536 or more', https://datahelpdesk.worldbank.org/knowledgebase/articles/906519-world-bank-country-and-lending-groups (Accessed 15/04/2021).

2 https://datahelpdesk.worldbank.org/knowledgebase/articles/906519-world-bank-country-and-lending-groups (Accessed 15/04/2021).

3 The Romanian Senate: HOTĂRÂRE nr. 111 din 21 octombrie 2020 referitoare la Comunicarea Comisiei către Parlamentul European, Consiliul European, Consiliu şi Banca Europeană de Investiţii – Strategia UE privind vaccinurile împotriva COVID-19 – COM (2020) 245 final. Published in MONITORUL OFICIAL No. 1014, 2 November 2020.

4 These studies were carried out by Professor Victor Babeş (1854–1926), who founded the first medical research institute in Romania, in 1887. Within this institute, called the Institute of Pathology and Bacteriology (later called the Institute 'Victor Babeş'), there was a section called the Anti-Rabies Institute which, starting on 6 March 1888, produced the first rabies vaccine in Romania according to an original method, developed by Babeş and his collaborators, based on the methods of Pasteur.

5 M. Damian and A. M. Năşcuţiu, 'Institutul Cantacuzino, opera monumentală a Profesorului Ion Cantacuzino', in C. Ciufecu and M. Neguţ, eds, *Profesorul Cantacuzino. Personalitate de excepţie în conştiinţa poporului român* (Bucureşti: Editura Total Publishing, 2013), 133–143, 134.

6 A. Cerbu, 'Documente mai puţin cunoscute privind înfiinţarea Institutului Cantacuzino', *Bacteriologia, Virusologia, Parazitologia, Epidemiologia*, 1991, 36, 74–93, 75.

7 I. Mesrobeanu, 'Viaţa şi opera profesorului Ion Cantacuzino', in I. Mesrobeanu, ed, *Ion Cantacuzino. Opere Alese [Oeuvres Choisies]* (Bucureşti: Editura Academiei Republicii Populare Române, 1965), 11–42, 20.

8 M. Neguţ, 'Un spirit pasteurian', in C. Ciufecu and M. Neguţ, eds, *Profesorul Cantacuzino. Personalitate de excepţie în conştiinţa poporului român* (Bucureşti: Editura Total Publishing, 2013), 29–40, 33.

9 Mesrobeanu, 'Viaţa şi opera lui Ion Cantacuzino', 19; Cerbu, 'Documente mai puţin cunoscute', 76.

10 L. Pasteur, *Cinquantenaire de la fondation (14.XI.1888 – 14.XI.1938)* (Paris: Institut Pasteur, 1888/1939), 3.

11 Gh. Magheru, 'Profesorul Ion Cantacuzino', in G. Brătescu, ed, *Momente din trecutul medicinii* (Bucureşti: Editura Medicală, 1983), 711–720, 716; Cerbu, 'Documente mai puţin cunoscute', 79.

12 ****Institut de Serologie de Bucarest: 1902 – 1932* (Bucarest: Institut Arts Graphiques 'E. Marvan', 1932), 6.

13 *Ibid.*, 6.

14 *Ibid.*, 6.

15 Cerbu, 'Documente mai puţin cunoscute', 84.

16 *Ibid.*, 78.

17 *Ibid.*, 83.

18 *Ibid.*, 83.

19 *Ibid.*, 84.

20 V. Alexandrescu, 'Vaccinurile Cantacuzino: tradiţie, continuitate, viitor', in C. Ciufecu and M. Neguţ, eds, *Profesorul Cantacuzino. Personalitate de excepţie în conştiinţa poporului român* (Bucureşti: Editura Total Publishing, 2013), 67–75, 68.

21 *Ibid.*, 68.

22 Damian and Năşcuţiu, 'Institutul Cantacuzino', 134.

23 D. Curcă, 'Contribution of Professor Alexandru Ciucă (1880–1972) in the Diagnosis and Eradication of Animal Diseases', *Revista Romana de Medicina Veterinara*, 2018, 28, 49–60, 52.

24 Mesrobeanu, 'Viaţa şi opera lui Ion Cantacuzino', 30.

25 Mesrobeanu, 'Viaţa şi opera lui Ion Cantacuzino', 27; Cerbu, 'Documente mai puţin cunoscute', 76.

26 The relations established with the Pasteur Institute and the entire global network associated with it were very close during Cantacuzino's lifetime. After the regime change of December 1947, when Romania became a member of the communist bloc, the decision was made in Paris that the Cantacuzino Institute should no longer

be part of the network. Membership was re-assigned to the institute in 1991, only after the political regime changed once again in December 1989. Membership was lost again, however, after 2017 when the institute came under military leadership. Fortunately, on the scientific research side, collaboration between the Romanian and French teams continues to make important contributions to the literature.

27 A. Calmette, *La vaccination préventive de la tuberculose par le B.C.G. (Bacille Calmette-Guérin)* (Paris: Masson et Cie. Éditeurs, 1928), 56; J. Cantacuzène, M. Nasta and T. Veber, 'Vaccination par le B.C.G. en Roumanie', *Annales de l'Institut Pasteur*, 1932, 1, 172; J. Cantacuzène, M. Nasta and T. Veber, 'Vaccination des nouveau-nés par le B.C.G. en Roumanie (Resumé de quelques observations)', *Archives Roumaines de Pathologie Expérimentale et de Microbiologie*, 1933, VI, 135.

28 J. Cantacuzène and V. Panaitescu, 'Essai comparé de vaccination anti-typho-paratyphique par la voie sous-cutanée et la voie buccale (Expérience de Moreni)', *Comptes rendus hebdomadaires des séances et mémoires de la Société de Biologie*, 1925, I, 1138–1140.

29 World Health Organization, *Interim Commission & WHO Expert Committee on Malaria Session. (1st : 1947: Geneva, Switzerland). (1947). Expert Committee on Malaria, report on the first session, Geneva, 22–25 April 1947* (Geneva: World Health Organization, 1947), 1. https://apps.who.int/iris/handle/10665/64024 (Accessed 10/02/2021).

30 N. Cajal and R. Iftimovici, *Din istoria luptei cu microbii şi virusurile* (Bucureşti: Editura Ştiinţifică, 1964), 243.

31 D. P. Fidler, 'Germs, governance, and global public health in the wake of SARS', *The Journal of Clinical Investigation*, 2004, 113, 799–804, 799.

32 I. Felix, *Istoria Igienei în România în secolul al XIX-lea şi starea ei la începutul secolului al XX-lea. Partea I* (Bucuresci: Institutul de Arte Grafice 'Carol Göbl', 1901), 55-61.

33 *** *Institutul Cantacuzino 1921–2011: 90 de ani de excelenţă pentru sănătate* (Bucureşti: Editura Total Pubslishing, 2012), 12.

34 J. Cantacuzène, 'Essais de vaccination des nouveau-nés contre la tuberculose par le BCG en Roumanie', *Annales de l'Institut Pasteur*, 1927, 3, 274–276, 274.

35 Cantacuzène, Nasta and Veber, 'Vaccination par le B.C.G. en Roumanie', 172.

36 Gh. Iancu, *Raport special cu privire la importanţa, producerea şi situaţia vaccinurilor Institutului Naţional de Cercetare-Dezvoltare pentru Microbiologie şi Imunologie 'Cantacuzino'* (Bucureşti: Avocatul Poporului, 15 June, 2012), 5.

37 Mesrobeanu, 'Viaţa şi opera lui Ion Cantacuzino', 30.

38 There were two more branches of the Cantacuzino Institute, in the cities of Timişoara and Cluj-Napoca, though they were both closed in 1990. There is very little data about them.

39 Alexandrescu, 'Vaccinurile Cantacuzino', 73.

40 P. M. Strebel *et al.*, 'Paralytic Poliomyelitis in Romania, 1984-1992. Evidence for a High Risk of Vaccine-associated Disease and Reintroduction of Wild-virus Infection', *American Journal of Epidemiology*, 1994, 140, 1111–1124, 1112.

41 Mesrobeanu, 'Viaţa şi opera lui Ion Cantacuzino', 30.

42 Alexandrescu, 'Vaccinurile Cantacuzino', 75.

43 *Ibid.*, 75.

44 *Ibid.*, 73.

45 *Ibid.*, 75.

46 *Ibid.*, 75.

47 *Ibid.*, 74–75.

48 *Ibid.*, 73.

49 *Ibid.*, 70.

50 D. L. Păun, *Modernizarea legislaţiei naţionale în domeniul sanitar şi implicaţii asupra securităţii naţionale* (Craiova: Editura Sitech, 2019), 146.

51 Journalistic investigation conducted by Digi24 (2015): România furată: Institutul Cantacuzino, lăsat fără niciun rol în producţia de vaccinuri antigripale (08.12.2015), https://www.digi24.ro/special/campanii-digi24/romania-furata/romania-furata-institutul-cantacuzino-lasat-fara-niciun-rol-in-productia-de-vaccinuri-antigripale-465618 (Accessed 19/03/2021).

52 Păun, *Modernizarea legislației naționale*, 152.
53 Digi24.
54 Digi24.
55 Păun, *Modernizarea legislației naționale*, 145.
56 *Ibid.*, 145.
57 *Ibid.*, 146.
58 *Ibid.*, 145.
59 Digi24.
60 Ministerul Sănătății, *Răspunsul Ministerului Sănătății la întrebarea domnului deputat Adăscăliței Constantin (3073A/2013), privind producția de vaccinuri în România* (București: Ministerul Sănătății, Cabinet Ministru. Document EN 13081, No. 561/21.01.2014).
61 *Ibid.*, 2.
62 *Ibid.*, 2.
63 The reference laboratories of the Cantacuzino Institute, as well as other laboratories in the EU, periodically undergo an evaluation by European bodies that supervise the activity of monitoring the circulation of microorganisms in EU countries, as well as the training of microbiology specialists. In 2013, the Cantacuzino Institute was evaluated by the ECDC. On this occasion, it was recognized as a training site for the body of public health experts within the European Public Health Microbiology Training Path (EUPHEM). See: https://www.ecdc.europa.eu/en/national-institute-research-development-microbiology-immunology-cantacuzino-nirdmi-euphem (Accessed 10/03/2021).
64 Document EN 13081, No. 561/21.01.2014.
65 Păun, *Modernizarea legislației naționale*, 156.
66 OECD, *Analysis of competition policy and law in Romania* (Paris: Organisation for Economic Co-operation and Development, 2014), [Online] Available at: http://www.oecd.org/daf/competition/Romania-Competition-Law-Policy-2014-EN.pdf (Accessed 23/02/2021).
67 Păun, *Modernizarea legislației naționale*, 154.
68 *Ibid.*, 155.
69 *Ibid.*, 158.
70 Guvernul României, *Ordonanță de Urgență nr.66 din 21 septembrie 2017* (București: Monitorul Oficial, No. 762, 25 September 2017).
71 *** *Raport anual de activitate al Institutul Național de Cercetare-Dezvoltare în Domeniul Patologiei și Științelor Biomedicale 'Victor Babeș'* (București: INCD 'Victor Babeș', 2018), 84.
72 Job vacancy announcement published on the official website of *Institutul Național de Cercetare-Dezvoltare Medico-Militară 'Cantacuzino'* (INCDMC, 2018).
73 This advance purchase agreement is based on the 'Commission Decision of 18.6.2020 approving the agreement with Member States on procuring Covid-19 vaccines on behalf of the Member States and related procedures'.
74 European Commission, *C(2020) 4192 final COMMISSION DECISION of 18.6.2020 approving the agreement with Member States on procuring Covid-19 vaccines on behalf of the Member States and related procedures* (Brussels: European Commission, 2020).
75 World Bank Group, *The World Bank in Romania. Country Snapshot* (Bucharest: World Bank in Romania, April 2020), [Online] Available at: www.worldbank.org/romania (Accessed 20/01/2021).
76 https://cantacuzino.mapn.ro/press_releases/view/20; https://cantacuzino.mapn.ro/press_releases/view/21 (Accessed 20/01/2021).
77 F. P. Walters, *A History of the League of Nations* (London: Oxford University Press, 1952), 1.

8

VACCINE PRODUCTION IN SERBIA

Political and socio-cultural determinants in historical perspective

Vesna Trifunović

The general decline in vaccine production in public sector institutions is typically attributed to global trends in the field of vaccines that have led to an environment favouring large, commercially oriented pharmaceutical companies. In a worldwide neoliberal setting, there seems to be no place left for local manufacturers with a primary focus on national public health and without access to broad markets. While this may be true, the role of local context in understanding the development of public sector vaccine production is as important as the aforementioned global aspect. Given that state vaccine institutes are usually under direct government control, they are likely to be affected by the interaction of local socio-political occurrences with global demands in the production of vaccines. Therefore, the aim in this chapter is to demonstrate the role of specific political, social, and cultural factors in shaping the functions, achievements, and weaknesses of vaccine production in the public sector. To that end, the chapter provides a case study of vaccine production in Serbia in different historical periods characterized by distinct socio-political regimes.

The history of public sector vaccine production in Serbia stretches from the very beginning of the twentieth century up until now. Throughout that period, vaccines have been manufactured in radically different socio-political systems, due to the country's very dynamic history. These include the pre–World War II monarchist system, post–World War II socialist system, followed by the process of post-socialist transformation which began in the 1990s. The succession of those systems, with their specific ideological backgrounds, provides an opportunity for exploring the effects of different political, economic and socio-cultural forces on the organization and conceptions of public sector vaccine production. The approach adopted assumes that social organization and conceptualization of vaccine production are related[1] and that they are significantly shaped by the local socio-political context and its transformations.

DOI: 10.4324/9781003130345-9

The chapter is divided into three main sections, each dealing with one of the indicated historical periods. The aim in the first section is to demonstrate how local vaccine production was established in relation to global tendencies in the field, and the local context, in the last decades of the nineteenth century. This section explores the interaction of political, economic and socio-cultural determinants that led to the founding of the first Pasteur Institute in the country. Special focus is placed on the first ideas, initiatives, arguments, and motives for launching local production, all pointing to specific conceptions and meanings in that regard. The two sections following deal with the organization of vaccine production at the Torlak Institute, which developed under the influence of political, economic, and socio-cultural factors characteristic for the socialist and post-socialist periods in the country's history. Both sections also consider the changing motives and discourses about national vaccine production that emerged in relation to specific socio-political circumstances in socialist and post-socialist contexts.

The sources used for this chapter differ according to the historical period in focus. A number of national publications were used for insights into the founding of a local Pasteur Institute and its activities during the pre–World War II period. In that respect, particularly valuable data were published accounts containing personal views and experiences of the initiators and founders of local vaccine production. Additional sources were official documents, records of formal meetings, and discussions on the establishment of a national vaccine institute that appeared in a national medical journal. The main sources on vaccine production during the socialist and post-socialist periods were a comprehensive publication about the history and activities of the Torlak Institute and qualitative interviews with nine former employees of the Institute. The participants in interviews were different generations of experts who were professionally active during the socialist and/or post-socialist period. Also, some were engaged in the production of bacterial vaccines, some in the production of viral vaccines and some held management positions. The participants were recruited using the snow-ball method and the interviews took place in September and October 2020. In order to protect their identities, the names of interview participants are not revealed. Additional sources for the most recent post-socialist period were available reports about vaccine production at the Torlak Institute, as well as texts and interviews about the Institute's activities published in local media.

The establishment of local vaccine production

Verifying and popularizing the prevention of smallpox by way of a comparatively benign cowpox virus, Edward Jenner replaced risky variolation and introduced a new, promising public health measure in the last decade of the eighteenth century. In the years following Jenner's findings there was no need for organized production of calf-lymph vaccines due to a widespread arm-to-arm practice, also known as Jennerian or humanized vaccination.[2] However, humanized vaccination subsequently revealed its deficiencies, one of the most prominent ones being a risk of transferring other diseases, such as syphilis. This added to already complex political and ideological arguments against vaccination in the nineteenth century[3] and prompted officials in some countries to acknowledge the necessity for the supervision of the quality of lymph supply.[4] Establishing continuous, safe, and regulated lymph production was an important step in securing the reputation of vaccination. Therefore, various countries increasingly endorsed animal lymph and gradually introduced prohibition of arm-to-arm practice. This gave special impetus to creating the first institutes for organized lymph production.[5]

Almost 100 years after Jenner's findings another pivotal discovery marked the history of vaccination when Louis Pasteur developed a rabies antitoxin. Just as in the case of calf-lymph vaccine, this discovery was embraced internationally, only this time regular production was established much sooner with the founding of Pasteur institutes, as discussed in the Introduction to this book. The last decades of the nineteenth century were a golden age of bacteriology, as Robert Koch isolated the bacterial pathogens of some of the most devastating human diseases of the time.[6]

Although production of calf-lymph and rabies vaccines became a universal practice owing to active international knowledge sharing, the actual establishment of local production was determined by specific socio-cultural and political contexts in different countries. First ideas about the founding of a manufacturing institute in Serbia appeared during the last two decades of the nineteenth century. The records of the time indicate that, beside some individually launched initiatives, civilian and military institutions, independently, dispatched physicians in 1884 and 1886 to master lymph production at the Institute in Vienna.[7] Furthermore, in 1889 a former military physician was dispatched to Koch's Institute in Berlin in order to acquaint himself with bacteriology. The aim was to set up a national bacteriological station.[8] For reasons unknown neither of these efforts resulted in the start of local production. A military medical official attributed the failure to the administration's poor response and lack of support.[9] On the other hand, a report submitted by a civilian physician upon returning from Vienna offered more precise hints about the possible causes of the unfinished enterprise:

> Maintaining [fresh] lymph on cows is so expensive that in my opinion it cannot be conducted here. All that could be done would be to procure a recent lymph, then transfer it to calves and further onto arms. Even this could only be done in larger municipalities due to the expenses and lack of skilled personnel.[10]

It could be assumed that the barriers stated in the report were discouraging for the officials. This was a time of turbulent historical and political events, and unfavourable socio-economic conditions. The years of rapid development of microbiology in Western Europe were in many respects challenging in Serbia.

At the time when the aforementioned initiatives for local production were taken, a monarchist system had just been introduced, but the country was still largely underdeveloped compared to modern European states. The majority of the Serbian population was more or less illiterate; civilian medical services lacked experts; and the administration, at an early stage of development, could not grasp the true significance of these major medical innovations.[11] Despite all this, a small group of highly educated civilian and military physicians devotedly followed the latest medical achievements and never deviated from their efforts to apply them in the country. Therefore, the issue of local production was postponed, only to be raised again some years later, but now with two concrete questions addressed to officials and the medical community:

> Should Serbia follow in the footsteps of all other countries and establish an institute for lymph production or is it better to import the finished product as so far? If it is better for us to have an institution of that kind, how can we establish it? Should the state take the matter into its own hands or should it be given to private individuals (physicians) in concession – of course, under state control as it is in other countries?[12]

As indicated, the idea of founding a local institute implied primarily the production of calf-lymph vaccine. However, it soon became clear that the country also lacked an organized response to the enduring problem of rabies infections, and therefore the need for the production of rabies vaccine was also recognized. In both instances Serbia depended on neighbouring Hungary – lymph supplies were acquired from a private institute based in Pest[13] and people were also sent there to the Pasteur Institute for treatment against rabies.[14] Another conclusion that could be drawn from the previous quotation is that a local institute was conceived as an institution under some kind of state jurisdiction and not as an entirely private enterprise. Although state control over vaccine production was a distinctive feature in many European countries,[15] as discussed elsewhere in this book, private institutes were engaged in this activity as well, including that established in nearby Zagreb in 1907. However, the quality of lymph acquired from the private institute in Pest was questioned in Serbia. In practice it often produced strong reactions and complications.[16] This was used as one of the arguments in favour of a state-controlled system, which was also chosen in adherence with the practice of other European countries. Apparently, the dominant opinion of some initiators of local production was that private manufacturers were primarily guided by economic interests and that to ensure quality and safety vaccine production required state supervision and regulation:

> Lymph was mainly produced in private institutes where quantity was more important than quality. In some countries there were no institutes at all, so the lymph had to be procured from abroad and transported, during which it could had been changed and spoiled. In order to eliminate these threats,

> states took the production of lymph into their own hands and thus provided a kind of official guarantee which was worth more than a bare word or conscientiousness of the manager of a private institute.[17]

On the basis of these considerations, the decision was taken to establish a national Pasteur Institute in charge of producing both calf-lymph and rabies vaccines, and under military jurisdiction.[18] The Institute was officially opened in 1900. Economic reasons were stated as the main motivators for starting local vaccine production, given that significant resources were spent yearly on acquiring animal lymph from abroad and treatments against rabies in the Hungarian Pasteur Institute.[19] Additionally, it was recognized that local people had to endure a long and distressing trip to Pest to be treated for rabies.[20] Nevertheless, the motives were not only economic and pragmatic. As some authors point out, vaccines were in the beginning sometimes seen as a symbol of national pride and prestige.[21] This was also the case in Serbia, but the pride of having a national vaccine manufacturing institute was framed in a specific political and ideological discourse. At the grand opening of the Pasteur Institute, one of its founders delivered a speech stating the following:

> With this new achievement, our homeland will gain not only materially but also morally. The whole of Europe, even our greatest enemies, will have to admit to us that Serbia does not lag behind the civilized West in anything now that we have, in addition to many scientific associations and humanitarian institutions, our own Pasteur Institute.[22]

This suggests that the establishment of local vaccine production was also motivated by general political aspirations towards creating the reputation of a modern country and escaping the identification with backwardness. In other words, vaccine production, as a legacy and symbol of the modern world, had an important role in demonstrating the progressiveness of Serbian society and in countering negative cultural connotations that western societies broadly ascribed to the emerging nations in the nineteenth century Balkans. Namely, a view of the whole Balkan region as undeveloped in economic, cultural, and political terms was firmly rooted in western thought during the enlightenment period, when the idea of progress became synonymous with European modernity.[23] In that period, living with the legacy of Ottoman colonization, the Balkans were largely cut off from many of the mainstream intellectual and cultural trends. This isolation was of crucial importance in the formation of the region's inferior image.[24] Having gained independence from Ottoman rule during the nineteenth century, Serbia sought opportunities for political, social and cultural recognition which would include its society and culture being brought into the frame of modern Europe. In that respect, the founding of a national vaccine institute seems to have been considered as an important step in improving the country's status in the international symbolic order and as an act of identification with progressive western societies.

The knowledge about vaccine manufacturing procedures and techniques was initially transferred to Serbia from the institute in Vienna and the Pasteur Institute in Pest, where a comprehensive training on the production of calf-lymph and rabies vaccines had been provided. Know-how in bacteriology was passed from the Pasteur Institute in Paris, leading to the founding of the bacteriological department in the Serbian Pasteur Institute and eventually to the production of a combined vaccine against cholera, typhoid fever and paratyphoid A and B, oral dysentery vaccine, and oral typhoid fever vaccine.[25] Although manufacturing methods were initially copied from foreign institutes, some were also subsequently improved in the course of local production. The innovations occurred during the post–World War I period when Serbia became part of the Kingdom of Serbs, Croats, and Slovenes, later renamed the Kingdom of Yugoslavia. The first significant novelty introduced in the Serbian Pasteur Institute concerned the use of ether in attenuating the virulence of fixed virus, which became an internationally recognized method in the production of rabies vaccine.[26] During the interwar period one more Pasteur Institute was established in Serbia. Being exclusively in charge of the production of rabies vaccines, this Institute pioneered another internationally acclaimed and accepted method. The innovation involved the use of phenol and ether in achieving total inactivation, leading to the introduction of a so-called Hempt's phenol–ether vaccine into widespread international usage.[27]

The innovations with regard to rabies vaccine were no coincidence given the growing problem of rabies infections in the post–World War I period. The disease was gaining momentum, as indicated by the increase in the frequency of treatment by up to 300% compared to the pre-war period.[28] Other communicable diseases also posed a significant threat to the already war-ravaged population. These circumstances propelled the founding of more health institutions in the new kingdom. They included the Pasteur Institute in Zagreb, discussed in another chapter, and the Central Hygiene Institute in Belgrade founded in 1924.[29] This institute largely took over the production of vaccines in Serbia after 1930 when the law on control of biological products was enacted.[30] The Institute in Belgrade was established according to the agreements that had been previously made at the sessions of the Permanent Epidemic Committee of the Ministry of Health. The Committee concurred that the institute engaged in vaccine manufacturing should not be a private, but a state institution, which would guarantee better quality and affordability. Furthermore, it was argued that such an institute would secure the country's independence from external political developments in providing vaccines for the local population.[31] Political and ideological motivations underlying these arguments seem to be consistent with those from the pre-war period, only this time instead of demonstrating progressiveness, a national vaccine institute was viewed as a symbol of the country's independence. This discourse probably stemmed from political concerns about the security of vaccine supply and a sense of political responsibility characteristic of other countries at that time as well.[32] It could also be assumed that the local self-sufficiency discourse partly reflected post-war efforts to establish the sovereignty of a newly formed country.

Upon its opening, the Central Hygiene Institute started producing BCG vaccine with a strain brought from the Pasteur Institute in Paris. The Institute also produced vaccines against typhoid fever and paratyphoid A and B, dysentery, cholera, diphtheria and a combined vaccine against scarlet fever and diphtheria.[33] Besides producing vaccines, the Central Hygiene Institute was engaged in other public health activities and, as a result, the need for a dedicated manufacturing department at a separate location soon arose. The facilities were built at a locality near Belgrade called Torlak, and vaccine production was transferred there in 1930. Prior to the outbreak of World War II, the department also introduced Ramon's methods in producing diphtheria and tetanus vaccines.[34] This department of the Central Hygiene Institute subsequently evolved into a separate institution, later named the 'Institute for Sera and Vaccines Torlak',[35] which became the leading vaccine manufacturer in Serbia during the post–World War II period.

Vaccine production in the socialist period

Following the end of World War II, radical social, economic, and political changes based on communist doctrine enveloped the country, leading to the end of the monarchist system. That meant that vaccine production, which had been taking place in a country called the Kingdom of Yugoslavia, was now being conducted in a country named the Federal People's Republic of Yugoslavia, later renamed the Socialist Federal Republic of Yugoslavia. Specific features of this entirely different socio-political context inevitably reflected on further developments in the field of local vaccine production. In that regard, it is first important to note that the Yugoslav socialist system evolved in a distinctive way, and after the political break with the Soviet Union in 1948 as an alternative to the Eastern bloc. Distinctive characteristics of the Yugoslav system were the conversion of state-ownership over the means of production into social-ownership and a specific model of economy called socialist, or workers', self-management. The model was created with the aim of enabling active participation of workers in governing enterprises conceived as social and not state property. Within these frames, the Yugoslav economic system also went through many modifications that generated its distinct subtypes over the course of time. Thus, the period of the 1960s and early 1970s was characterized as 'market socialism' due to reforms that introduced elements of a market mechanism into the economy.[36]

In geo-political terms, the break with the Soviet Union turned Yugoslavia towards Western democracies which brought about foreign loans, reparations and aid, prompting rapid economic expansion, development and modernization. The country was also one of the initiators of the Non-Aligned Movement, an organization with a strong political and economic agenda that brought together numerous developing states, throughout the world, which were opting for independence from the two power blocs. The support of the West and ties now forged with Third World countries intensified Yugoslavia's foreign relations and involvement in world markets, particularly encouraged by the state's policy to give more freedom to enterprises in their foreign trade operations.[37]

Vaccine production in Serbia, at the time a republic within a larger state, was significantly determined by the aforementioned internal and external political and economic factors. The production continued following the end of World War II, leading early on to the extensive use of locally manufactured BCG, diphtheria and tetanus vaccines.[38] One possible internal impetus for this could be the revolutionary goal of the new regime to reduce morbidity and mortality from infectious diseases which were on the rise in the immediate post-war context. In addition to obvious health-related reasons, ideological motives also underpinned efforts to improve the general health of the population. Namely, in the early post-war period it was important for the socialist regime to legitimize itself by demonstrating the superiority of the new system over the previous one.[39] Intensified and improved vaccine production served to demonstrate the rapid social development and modernization taking place in the established socialist order. Throughout the 1950s, new technologies and novelties were being introduced in the Torlak Institute, such as the production of purified and adsorbed diphtheria and tetanus vaccines, as well as of pertussis vaccine from isolated domestic strains.[40] Shortly afterwards, the components of diphtheria, tetanus and pertussis were combined in a single vaccine, resulting in the production of DTP vaccine. Around the same time, the Virology Sector of the Central Hygiene Institute was transferred to the Torlak location and later merged with the Torlak Institute. This sector first started manufacturing Jonas Salk's inactivated polio vaccine in 1959, but soon reoriented to Albert Sabin's live vaccine. Finally, in the early 1960s, the sector began production of inactivated influenza vaccine.[41] The pioneers of these locally manufactured vaccines were mostly experts trained at leading European institutes,[42] which facilitated the transfer of knowledge and technologies, and additionally contributed to the rise of the Torlak Institute.

These trends in local vaccine production were also possible thanks to wider developments in the vaccines field, starting from 1950, which marked the beginning of the modern era of vaccines.[43] Beside the breakthrough technology of cell culture cultivation of viruses, there was almost no patent protection for vaccines at the time, and knowledge on production techniques was usually freely exchanged between institutions or experts.[44] These factors were especially favourable for initiating the local production of live polio vaccine which was manufactured from the strains provided by Albert Sabin himself and according to his instructions.[45] Yugoslav market socialism and extensive political and economic relations fostered with countries throughout the world further stimulated the mass production of this vaccine which was exported to South America, Europe, Africa and Asia.[46] The Institute also supplied UNICEF, the World

Health Organization and the Pan American Health Organization with its polio vaccine,[47] thus contributing to what later became the Global Polio Eradication Initiative. Mass production and exportation of live polio vaccine included the Torlak Institute into the circle of internationally recognized manufacturers and also brought significant revenues, all of which made this vaccine a particularly important product invested with specific meanings and values:

> [Exportation was important] not just for 'the Torlak', but for the whole country. Big money, great reputation, imagine you vaccinate the whole of South America with a vaccine from Serbia, that was something. The eternal contest for prestige in the world.
>
> [Interviewee 1]

The Torlak Institute was not exclusively responding to national public health needs, but also to commercial opportunities provided by favourable social, economic and political conditions at the time. The participants in interviews who had been actively engaged in the production of vaccines during the 1960s and early 1970s, also referred to those social circumstances as stimulating. According to their accounts, that period in the Institute's history was marked by most up-to-date standards, great work enthusiasm, as well as by the high national and international reputation of the Institute:

> We followed world trends and standards, it was not a closed country, but an open one where seminars, lectures, creating standards often took place in Yugoslavia. When I came [to the Torlak Institute], all our vaccines fitted the world standards, not to mention that we sold polio vaccine in almost 120 countries around the world, which we produced only 3 years after Sabin had made it.
>
> [Interviewee 5]

> There were 20 of us who switched to the production of vaccine [from the Hygiene Institute] and Salk's vaccine was made first... We used to work all day until late at night. So, it was an intensive, hard work with a lot of enthusiasm... 'The Torlak' was an extremely strong institution professionally at that time.
>
> [Interviewee 2]

These accounts suggest that competition for international prestige was an important ideological motivator of local vaccine production during the 1960s and early 1970s. The pride associated with the achievements of the Torlak Institute in that period was framed in a discourse which implied equality with the developed world. In other words, a modern and progressive reputation had been finally demonstrated and acknowledged both nationally and internationally. Consequently, it was in that period that the Torlak Institute became an important national symbol of success and authority in the field of public health, partly owing to the production of vaccines and especially polio vaccine. Interestingly, as discussed in the chapter on Croatia, the Institute of Immunology in Zagreb also experienced its golden age at this time. Favourable local and international circumstances overlapped in their shared Yugoslav context.

However, certain aspects of the Yugoslav socialist system seemingly acted as obstacles to further improvements in local vaccine production. In that regard, the participants in interviews almost unanimously pointed to the self-management model of the economy. As already indicated, that model evolved under the influence of continuous experiments with economic reforms introduced throughout the socialist period. After the so-called market socialism in the 1960s and early 1970s, a period of what was known as 'contractual socialism' ensued with the reforms implemented by the 1974 Constitution and the 1976 Associated Labour Act.[48] The 'associated labour' concept insisted that the market mechanism for resource allocation had to be replaced by mechanisms of social contracts, self-management agreements, and social planning.[49] Thus, the period of contractual socialism was characterized by changes in the formal location of decision-making in the economy. New organizational forms were supposed to enable workers in enterprises to directly and on equal terms exercise their economic and self-management rights.[50]

The self-management system was conceived as collective decision making through referendums and workers' councils as elected bodies with significant influence in devising the policy and business plans of enterprises. Although this system was controversial in practice in terms of the full involvement of workers in the management of enterprises, interviews suggest that workers at the Torlak Institute did participate in at least some important decisions. The aforementioned workers' councils consisted of a number of delegates appointed by the workers and operated according to the guidelines received from the workers. As established by the Associated Labour Act,[51] the structure of workers' council had to correspond to the social structure of workers in the enterprise and the number of delegates had to be proportional to the number of workers engaged in different parts of the work process. Therefore, the council consisted of workers with different social backgrounds and levels of education, and those occupying middle and lower positions sometimes outnumbered and outvoted experts. As one interview participant pointed out, that was the case in the Torlak Institute:

> Technicians always outvoted; workers' councils were ruled by the middle cadre.
>
> [Interviewee 7]

That meant that some key decisions affecting the production of vaccines were not made exclusively by scientists or public health officials, as in many other countries at the time,[52] but also by middle cadres lacking full understanding of various aspects important to the manufacturing process. In that respect, most participants in interviews particularly pointed out that the workers' council sometimes influenced decisions about profit distribution without taking into account the need for further investments:

> Those who didn't have the necessary knowledge voted for what was not in the interest of production. Since there was export [of polio vaccine], there were very good salaries, and in addition to that, there was always a surplus every three months, and then there was outvoting [to divide the surplus to workers]. And some things [necessary for the production] that the managers had to acquire were overruled by the workers' council. That was the negative side.
>
> [Interviewee 3]

> They [workers' councils] maybe had a negative impact on production. In order to start a new process, to buy new technology, it had to go through the workers' council and the management had to make additional efforts to convince workers of the new technological process. I don't believe that workers' councils could have contributed to the production because they were looking to increase wages.
>
> [Interviewee 5]

Despite the specificities of its economic system, Yugoslavia was still a socialist country and revenues in enterprises were largely directed to social purposes. Of these, one of the most important was the provision of housing for workers. The determinants that especially shaped the collective decisions of workers with respect to profit distribution could be identified in dominant cultural values that emerged during the 1970s. As suggested by one analysis, these values were created by a mixture of the prevailing ideology, social goals of the time, and influences coming from the West. The synthesis of these factors generated a widespread pragmatic-consumer orientation that favoured primarily material aspects.[53] Furthermore, the majority of the population accepted the paternalistic policy of the state/party and expected the authorities to provide necessary consumer items and good living standards.[54] It seems that such a paternalistic approach specifically manifested in relations between the workers and some directors in the Torlak Institute:

> At that time [in the late 1970s and 1980s], 'the Torlak' was headed by a political figure, a cardiologist, a terrible mistake in cadre policy... We all felt that it was not good, but it was nice for us, so we kept quiet – salaries were high, we shared surpluses, why would you complain if you were doing well? He [the director] made sure the workers were satisfied. He would approve 2-3 surplus salaries, not thinking about anything else. Such was the situation in his time.
>
> [Interviewee 1]

The paternalistic policy aimed at satisfying the consumer and material needs of workers probably figured as one of the factors that led to a change in the ideological motivations for producing vaccines. In place of previous aspirations towards securing international prestige, in this period the production mainly became driven by financial motives:

> For him [the director] profit was important, export of polio vaccine and nothing else, not expertise, not innovations, not rationalizations...
>
> [Interviewee 5]

Another turning point that possibly led to production being motivated more by economic gain could have been the serious economic crisis that ensued in the 1980s, related to the global recession of that time. The excessive foreign loans that had facilitated modernization and development of Yugoslavia had led to a large external debt. When Western countries started tightening their monetary policies by increasing interest rates, the country had difficulties in meeting its financial obligations. Thus, a substantial portion of revenues that the Torlak Institute generated through the export of polio vaccine was now redirected to the state budget:

> During our best years, we were able to use only up to 12% of our export capital [the rest went to the state]. 'The Torlak' was not the only enterprise that was affected by this. In the end, those leftovers were still large because there were millions of doses sold, but self-managers didn't allow that to be invested in anything.
>
> [Interviewee 6]

All this suggests that a commercial orientation did not necessarily guarantee the development and improvements in vaccine production organized under some kind of state control. As the case of the Torlak Institute indicates, successful production was rather conceptualized as economic potential, to be deployed in the interests of broader political, economic and socio-cultural goals. Parallel to these local developments during the 1980s, significant changes in the field of vaccine production began to occur globally. Advanced biotechnological processes were being applied in the production of new and improved vaccines, while the technology had been patented by large pharmaceutical manufacturers, who were no longer willing freely to collaborate or to share knowledge.[55] Some interview participants ascribe the failure of the Torlak Institute to follow those global trends precisely to the local social and cultural determinants characteristic of that time:

> 'The Torlak' was equal with the world in that first line of vaccines: OPV, diphtheria, tetanus, pertussis, some serums and BCG. But the others were already making preparations, new methods were being introduced, new tests were being done, the groundwork for new vaccines was being made,

> and that had not been done in 'the Torlak' ... It was a socialist country at that moment, they didn't have the way of thinking that people had on the other side of the Berlin Wall. They knew a lot at that moment, but they didn't anticipate what was to come.
>
> [Interviewee 8]

However, these new global developments in the field of vaccines were not the primary influences on local production. Certain political and social processes in the upcoming period had a more immediate effect in that respect. Some of those developments marked the end of the socialist system and the beginning of a long process of post-socialist transformation that installed a new political, economic and social order, along with new cultural orientations.

Vaccine production during the two phases of post-socialist transformation

In the early 1990s, shortly after a civil war had broken out, Yugoslavia ceased to exist. The disintegration of the state had serious social and economic consequences in Serbia. The international sanctions imposed on the country led it into extreme isolation, a drastic fall in living standards, and shortages. Just prior to these developments, initial changes in the economic and political system had been introduced, marking the beginning of a post-socialist transformation. In this process, the self-management system was abolished and basic preconditions were created for the conversion of social property into other forms of ownership, which was supposed to transform the economic basis of the society. However, in contrast to some other eastern European countries which entered the same process after the fall of the Berlin Wall, the first phase of post-socialist transformation in Serbia did not lead to mass privatization of socially owned enterprises, but mostly to their conversion into state ownership. Thus, the 1990s were characterized by the growth of the public sector and by direct state control over a large portion of capital in the economy.[56]

In the first half of the 1990s, developments in local vaccine production were primarily influenced by the devastating effects of international sanctions. Now isolated, the country had lost its Yugoslav and global markets. The measures imposed by the United Nations included an almost complete trade embargo, coupled with a prohibition of fund transfers to and from the country, the disruption of air traffic, and the suspension of all officially sponsored scientific and technical cooperation and cultural exchanges.[57] As previously indicated, the Torlak Institute had already started to lose pace with the emerging technologies in the field of vaccines, mostly due to political and socio-cultural determinants during the late socialist period that affected the way vaccine production was organized and conceptualized. In the early 1990s, specific political events, which led the country into almost complete isolation, created new structural barriers to following the global trends which were in full swing at the time:

> The problem for us was that we were under sanctions, without technological and material possibilities to achieve what was technologically improved. The country was closed for four years. We [the Torlak Institute] had no access to information, and in the meantime, everything changed [in the global field of vaccines].
>
> [Interviewee 4]

> The 1980s were, in my opinion, the last chance to catch up [with the new trends], because in the 1990s they were already releasing the second generation of vaccines, recombinant vaccines, molecular technology. We didn't have that prepared at that moment, but in the 1990s we had an even bigger handicap, and those were sanctions. So not only you could no longer share knowledge, you couldn't go anywhere, you couldn't import anything, you didn't even have a source of income or it was significantly reduced because you could no longer export. Then the disintegration of Yugoslavia, your market suddenly shrank...
>
> [Interviewee 8]

Despite these hardships, the production of vaccines continued by adapting to the unfavourable new circumstances. The organization of influenza vaccine production in particular shows how adjustments to adverse conditions were made through applying social practices that typically emerge in times of crisis. Namely, the period of international sanctions and economic blockade was marked by a rapid development of an informal or 'grey' economy in which virtually all social strata began to participate in the struggle for survival. Judging by the statements of some participants in the interviews, a similar social strategy was used to maintain the production of influenza vaccine in different periods of crisis that emerged during the 1990s:

> Because we were under sanctions, we were removed from WHO membership. The WHO didn't give us a strain for the production of the flu vaccine, so we smuggled it in various ways. We had friends at UNICEF, ***** went to the airport to get a strain for vaccine from a pilot and take it to 'the Torlak'. Under the sanctions, we received a strain from Zagreb for the first year, and then from Vienna, Budapest... And finally, during the bombing, ***** had no choice but to get into a car and go to Bucharest one night to get a strain from a long-time colleague there and smuggle it across the border. We got it [strain] where we had connections, personal acquaintances. 'The Torlak' produced the flu vaccine in that period.
>
> [Interviewee 7]

This recollection also suggests that international cooperation in the field of vaccines, based on strong relations between experts and institutions, were not abruptly interrupted by the new global emphasis on competitiveness and the ending of free sharing. The conditions of extreme social crisis and autarchy in the early 1990s also affected the way local vaccine production was conceptualized and motivated. In that respect, the discourse of self-sufficiency became dominant, attributing a special value to national vaccine production. Furthermore, two main motives for producing vaccines surfaced – to meet the local needs for vaccines in an isolated Serbian society, and to return to the international market once the sanctions had been lifted.

> During the time when there were sanctions, when we had nothing, we survived as a society because we had our own production of vaccines, we had our own vaccines, we didn't depend on anyone. The country that has that has a great advantage because it does not depend on the will of the big manufacturers and on their production. It does not depend on them sending you how much they think they can give you.
>
> [Interviewee 4]

> Because we were under sanctions, we had to produce for ourselves, it was not allowed to import.... We had considerable supplies because we had big plans with India. The director at the time instructed us to make stocks, to have maximum capacities and maximum production.
>
> [Interviewee 5]

Returning to the international market became especially important after comprehensive sanctions were lifted in 1996 following political settlement of the conflicts in former Yugoslavia. However, with the gradual opening of the country, the Torlak Institute soon faced the changing world of vaccines and increasingly became exposed to the influences of global trends. The exportation of polio vaccine was renewed, but primarily to a limited number of countries that acquired vaccines directly through international tenders. Re-establishing cooperation with the UN procuring agencies required the implementation of the WHO's vaccines prequalification programme that had been developed in the meantime with the aim of establishing global standards of quality, safety and efficacy.[58] The programme introduced a new concept of quality by giving increasing importance to good manufacturing practice (GMP). In other words, vaccines were no longer considered of high quality if the end products passed certain tests, but only if the quality was built into every stage of the production process through maintaining and monitoring consistency of production.[59] This further implied the need for adequate control environments, validation of equipment and procedures, and supporting documentation, all of which involved significant costs and efforts for local manufacturers faced with these demands. In Serbia, these requirements were soon implemented through domestic legislation. Thus, the Torlak Institute began a process of adapting to the new set of standards. Due to financial difficulties this proved to be very difficult. The decision was also made to mainly focus on improvements in the production of polio and influenza vaccines, since these were assessed as the most cost-effective.[60] However, the demands of the WHO's prequalification programme proved to be a significant barrier in that respect.

> The then management opted for polio vaccine because it was the vaccine that brought in the most money. They started the reconstruction, doing the most they could at that moment, aiming to obtain prequalification from the WHO, but they didn't get it.
>
> [Interviewee 8]

Consequently, the stringent regulatory requirements seem to have also provoked negative reactions and specific views at the local level on what those requirements were actually about.

> The original strain [Sabin's polio strain] needed to be certified, handed over to them [the WHO] to get a certificate, because without that we were not able to sell in the market that they [the WHO] provided. 'The Torlak' refused that. When you give it to them, then it is theirs, and the only trump card for us was to have the original strain that we could trade with. If you give it to them for certification, that's one of the mechanisms to oppress you and remove you... We are the only ones in the world who have the original strain. The WHO and the Americans were after that, but normally it's not something that you just give away.
>
> [Interviewee 6]

This quote illustrates how international regulatory demands clashed with local views of those demands and values built around a polio vaccine produced by the Torlak Institute. Namely, the Institute has always taken great pride in having Sabin's original strain, which was also perceived as a valuable asset, one of the few remaining resources in re-establishing competitiveness in the global market. Therefore, an internationally required technical procedure was negatively interpreted within the frames of local cultural meanings and economic interests. Similar interpretation was applied to other prequalification demands with respect to equipment, documentation and production facilities. This shows how the field of vaccine production is a sphere of negotiations between local and global concepts and values.

> What is now called GMP existed before, though called differently. It was not at the same level in terms of the numbers of people involved or the volume of paperwork, but the basic principles were known. The risks of pollution were known. It was known where one should or shouldn't enter. Now a whole department deals with some aspects, and there is a hyperproduction of documentation, but the essence is the same... Now all is just about the form – lots of managers and documentation... So, you have big companies that dictate the rules and they trample on everyone. No one

> will shut you down, but they'll make demands that you cannot fulfil. They will make their requests through a control agency in your country.
>
> [Interviewee 8]

The Serbian government failed to provide sufficient financial support for the reconstruction of the polio vaccine production facilities, leading ultimately to its suspension in the Torlak institute.[61] The events with respect to influenza vaccine followed a different path. The production was interrupted when the national control agency did not issue a quality assurance certificate in 2005.[62] From that period efforts have been made to reconstruct the facilities and restore production. To that end, the Torlak Institute eventually joined the WHO's programme Global Action Plan for Influenza Vaccines – a project made possible through joint investments of the Serbian government and a number of international agencies.[63] The accelerated progress in that direction in recent years suggests that cooperation between international agencies and national governments can facilitate maintenance of vaccine production in public sector institutions.

The exposure to global trends additionally provoked confronting perspectives over the implementation of new production processes in the Torlak Institute. Such was the case with an initiative for manufacturing a DTP vaccine with an acellular pertussis component. The main obstacle to further progress in that direction seems to have been the lack of consensus on the issue between the experts involved in the production of that vaccine:

> The idea was to start with the production of an acellular DTP vaccine. We were in the Netherlands in 1999, a team of experts visited the Applikon to see and buy fermenters... We saw the technological process at the Dutch institute, we knew in which direction the world was going. Unfortunately, we never made it. There were others who thought that it would not pass, that the whole bacterial vaccine would still win, because it was more immunogenic, which they were right, but it also gave greater post-vaccination reactions. The minority of us claimed that immunogenicity would not be so important anymore, that the post-vaccination reaction would become more important.
>
> [Interviewee 5]

The decision to continue with the old process of DTP vaccine production was probably also influenced by social determinants and strategies that the Torlak Institute devised in the face of new circumstances. First, there were no wider social pressures to introduce the new technology, as there had never been the controversy over allegedly serious side-effects of the whole cell pertussis component as in some other countries. The aforementioned decision to focus on improvements in the production of polio and influenza vaccines which were assessed as the most cost-effective might also have played a role.[64]

A second phase of post-socialist transformation began in 2000 and led to greater exposure to global trends and regulatory demands, but also to neoliberal influences. Namely, starting from 2000, Serbia took a course in foreign policy that involved returning to international financial and political institutions, and candidacy for EU membership. Therefore, the pressure to comply with international trends and standards in vaccine production became greater. Internal policy was aimed at catching up with global neoliberal developments, which implied the promotion of market economy, competition, economic efficiency and promotion of the private sector.

In line with such a political and ideological turn, the state's policy with respect to vaccine production was mainly oriented towards implementing global requirements and leaving the national manufacturer entirely exposed to external influences. Thus, legislative and executive grounds were provided to meet the international directives and recommendations by introducing a new Law on Medicines and Medical Devices and establishing an independent national control agency (the Agency for Drugs and Medical Devices). On the other hand, there seemed to be no ideological grounds for a long-term government commitment to providing sufficient financial support for the national manufacturer. The newly-promoted neoliberal agenda implied that state-owned enterprises were generally viewed as tokens of an obsolete socialist system which needed to be privatized or closed as unproductive, and not worthy of investment. In other words, there was a commitment to breaking both ideologically and practically with the previous system and its symbols.

> Liberal capitalism... we didn't have to produce anything anymore; everything could be imported. The idea was to shut down everything because it didn't pay off.
>
> [Interviewee 5]

However, the Torlak Institute was generally still recognized as an important symbol of authority in public health, so that privatizing or closing it was probably not considered a politically wise act. Instead, there were certain initiatives for establishing strategic partnerships, which, however, were never realized for undetermined reasons. This placed the Torlak Institute in a peculiar situation – the Institute remained in state ownership, thus depending on government support and directives with regard to the prices of its products,[65] but it was also forced to participate in the market and be a self-financing institution.[66] Moreover, the new political and economic regime encouraged the import of foreign vaccines by newly emerging private firms. This in turn suppressed the self-sufficiency discourse and motivations that had arisen in the 1990s. Some media texts from this period reveal the spread of new public discourse about locally produced vaccines as being of lower quality than imported foreign ones.[67] Such discourse was significantly backed-up by the then-dominant view that the country was generally falling behind global developments due to the previous isolation and various socio-political crises that had marked the period of 1990s.

> Around 2005 there was a stampede of foreign manufacturers. They went to health centres and convinced doctors that they should not give DTP, but Pentaxim, that our vaccine was not good. That is something that companies usually do. 'The Torlak' operated according to the old principles, it never had good marketing or post-marketing monitoring, nor the teams for lobbying. And then we were faced with our vaccines going to waste, parents wouldn't accept them.
>
> [Interviewee 8]

This further suggests that the Torlak Institute was not adjusting efficiently either to global trends in vaccine production, or to the new business rules and practices. However, public discourse about local vaccines changed after the media extensively targeted an affair with the acquisition of vaccines during the swine flu pandemic in 2009/2010. In that process, negative messages about the pharmaceutical industry had a major influence on public trust in foreign vaccines, building further on the emerging anti-vaccine sentiment in the country.[68] The change of discourse was clearly demonstrated by some parents' statements on having no doubts about vaccines produced by the Torlak Institute as opposed to foreign vaccines.[69] Advocating for the domestic production of vaccines also became a self-promoting strategy for some political figures. Apart from placing the issue of national manufacturer into the spotlight, those occurrences did not lead to significant changes in local vaccine production.

The Covid-19 pandemic has proven a much more significant turning point in rethinking the importance of domestic vaccine production. The global race to procure approved vaccines against this disease and their shortages have provided new ideological and political grounds for the current Serbian government to engage in establishing local production. Thus, the first months of 2021 were marked by enthusiastic official statements about initiating the production of Russian vaccine (Sputnik V)[70] at the Torlak Institute and the construction of a completely new factory for manufacturing Chinese (Sinopharm Covid-19) vaccine.[71] (Careful reading of media texts indicates that these vaccines would initially be filled and packaged in Serbia, with the possibility of full production in the future.) The dominant discourse in official announcements refers to the speed of these developments thanks to dedicated state support and cooperation with foreign governments. The first production phase of Sputnik V will allegedly start in late May 2021, that of Sinopharm vaccine in mid-October 2021. Compared to previous extremely slow progress in re-establishing the production of influenza vaccine, this attests to the importance of political commitment in implementing such projects. As expected, the discourse of vaccine self-sufficiency has re-emerged in official statements given the global context of crisis and vaccine shortages. Finally, the motives of economic gain and prestige have also reappeared, reflected in the announcements that Serbia would be the first European country to produce these vaccines and supply the region with them. The developments in this respect will indicate further possible effects of political, economic and socio-cultural determinants on the organization and conceptions of state organized production of Covid-19 vaccines.

Concluding remarks

Besides meeting public health needs, an important feature of vaccine production in the public sector seems to be that it can be an instrument for fulfilling certain ideological functions and broader socio-political goals. As suggested in this chapter, that could be the source of both achievements and weaknesses of state organized vaccine production. Thus, the first section demonstrated how ideological views led to the establishment of a national manufacturing institute primarily under state jurisdiction and opposed the possibility of private ownership. Similarly, organizing vaccine production was not only motivated by pragmatic and economic reasons, but also by broader political ideas, aiming to demonstrate the country's progressiveness and independence. National vaccine production was established despite many structural difficulties at that time, and the groundwork was laid for the first achievements.

The dependence on local context dynamics was further demonstrated in the next two sections, where changing discourses and motivations for vaccine production reflected changing ideological functions and changing socio-political circumstances. Thus, the interaction of favourable political, economic and socio-cultural factors laid a foundation for remarkable achievements in local vaccine production. These achievements were also catalyzed by the ideological motives of the then regime and competition for international prestige. Weaknesses that subsequently emerged were related to the lack of incentives for improvements, coming from transformations in the socialist system and purely financial motives for vaccine production associated with cultural orientations and new economic developments. The pervasive social crisis of the 1990s further impeded possible improvements or innovations. However, maintaining vaccine production in extremely unfavourable circumstances was in itself an achievement: motivated by local public health needs and a self-sufficiency discourse. The weaknesses in the post-socialist period were partly based on cultural resistance and challenges in adapting to global requirements and to the new system advanced by the government with a predominantly neoliberal agenda. All this points to the need to consider specific political and socio-cultural aspects in assessing the fate, the desirability and the feasibility of public sector vaccine manufacturers, and in devising policies for securing their viability. With this in mind, we can now follow how the new circumstances of the Covid-19 pandemic will affect the possibilities of vaccine production in the public sector.[72]

Notes

1 Stuart Blume, 'Towards a History of "The Vaccine Innovation System" 1950–2000', in C. Hannaway, ed, *Biomedicine in the Twentieth Century: Practices, Policies and Politics* (Amsterdam: IOS Press, 2008), 255–286.
2 José Esparza *et al.*, 'Early Smallpox Vaccine Manufacturing in the United States: Introduction of the "Animal Vaccine" in 1870, Establishment of "Vaccine Farms", and the Beginnings of the Vaccine Industry', *Vaccine*, 2020, 38, 4773–4779.
3 Nadja Durbach, "They Might as Well Brand Us': Working-Class Resistance to Compulsory Vaccination in Victorian England', *Social History of Medicine*, 2000, 13, 45–62.
4 Dorothy Porter and Roy Porter, 'The Politics of Prevention: Anti-Vaccinationism and Public Health in Nineteenth-Century England', *Medical History*, 1988, 32, 231–252.
5 Esparza *et al.*, 'Early Smallpox Vaccine Manufacturing in the United States', 4773–4779.
6 Steve M. Blevins and Michael S. Bronze, 'Robert Koch and the 'Golden Age' of Bacteriology', *International Journal of Infectious Diseases*, 2010, 14, 744–751.
7 Ljubomir Stojanović, 'Vakcinalni zavod' [Vaccination Institute], *Serbian Archives of Medicine*, 1903, 3, 112–114; Milan Jovanović Batut, 'Institut za spravljanje animalne limfe' [Institute for the Production of Animal Lymph], *Serbian Archives of Medicine*, 1895, 15/16, 154.
8 Mihajlo Marković, 'Odgovor na "Istinu o Pasterovom zavodu"' [The Answer to "The Truth About the Pasteur Institute"], *Serbian Archives of Medicine*, 1902, 9, 385–403.
9 Mihajlo Marković, *Moje uspomene* [My Memories] (Beograd, 1906).
10 Laza K. Lazarević, 'Izveštaj izaslanika za študiranje kako se proizvodi i neguje animalna limfa na teladima' [An Envoy's Report on Studying How Animal Lymph is Produced and Nurtured on Calves], *Narodno zdravlje*, 1884, 20, 154–156.
11 Vojislav Milojević, *Pasterov zavod u Nišu 1900–1985* [The Pasteur's Institute in Niš 1900–1985] (Niš: Zavod za zaštitu zdravlja u Nišu, 1990).
12 Batut, 'Institut za spravljanje animalne limfe' [Institute for the Production of Animal Lymph], 154.
13 Marković, 'Odgovor na "Istinu o Pasterovom zavodu"' [The Answer to "The truth About Pasteur Institute"], 385–403.
14 Mihajlo Marković, 'Kako je postao Pasterov zavod u Nišu' [How the Pasteur Institute in Nis was Created], *Zdravlje*, 1911, 4, 117–120.
15 Clarissa R. Damaso, 'Revisiting Jenner's Mysteries, the Role of the Beaugency Lymph in the Evolutionary Path of Ancient Smallpox Vaccines', *The Lancet Infectious Diseases*, 2018, 18, 55–63.
16 Ljubomir Stojanović, 'Istina o Pasterovom zavodu' [The Truth About the Pasteur Institute], *Serbian Archives of Medicine*, 1902, 4, 165–166.
17 Ljubomir Stojanović, 'Maja za kalemljenje iz Srpskog Vakcinalnog Zavoda u Nišu' [Lymph for Engraftment from Serbian Vaccine Institute in Niš], *Serbian Archives of Medicine*, 1902, 4, 125–135.
18 Official document about the opening of the Pasteur Institute published in Milojević, *Pasterov zavod u Nišu 1900–1985* [The Pasteur's Institute in Niš 1900–1985].
19 Stojanović, 'Istina o Pasterovom zavodu' [The Truth About the Pasteur Institute], 165–166.
20 Marković, 'Kako je postao Pasterov zavod u Nišu' [How the Pasteur Institute in Nis was Created], 117–120.
21 Alexandra Minna Stern and Howard Markel, 'The History of Vaccines and Immunization: Familiar Patterns', *New Challenges Health Affairs*, 2005, 24, 611–621.
22 'Govor dr Mihajla Markovića' [The Speech of Doctor Mihajlo Marković], *Serbian Archives of Medicine*, 1902, 1, 8.

23 David A. Norris, *In the Wake of the Balkan Myth: Questions of Identity and Modernity* (Basingstoke: Palgrave Macmillan, 1999).
24 *Ibid.*
25 *Torlak: 1930–1995* (Belgrade: Institute for Immunology and Virology "Torlak", 1995), 31.
26 G. P. Alivisatos, 'Die Schutzimpfung gegen Lyssa durch das mit Aether behandelte Virus fixe', *Deutsche Medizinische Wochenschrift*, 1922, 48, 295–296; Milojević, *Pasterov zavod u Nišu 1900–1985* [The Pasteur's Institute in Niš 1900–1985], 126–127.
27 Dušan Lalošević, *Dr Adolf Hempt i osnivanje Pasterovog zavoda u Novom Sadu* [Dr Adolf Hempt and the Establishing of the Pasteur Institute in Novi Sad] (Novi Sad: Medicinski fakultet, 2008).
28 Milojević, *Pasterov zavod u Nišu 1900–1985* [The Pasteur's Institute in Niš 1900–1985], 115.
29 'Rulebook on the Establishment and Organization of the Central Hygiene Institute in Belgrade', *Bulletin of the Ministry of Public Health*, 1924, Belgrade.
30 *Torlak: 1930–1995.*
31 *Ibid.*
32 Stuart Blume, 'The Erosion of Public Sector Vaccine Production: The Case of the Netherlands', in Christine Holmberg, Stuart Blume and Paul Greenough, eds, *The Politics of Vaccination: A Global History* (Manchester: Manchester University Press, 2017), 148–173.
33 *Torlak: 1930–1995.*
34 *Ibid.*
35 The official name of the Institute has changed over time. For the sake of simplicity, "the Torlak Institute" will be used in this paper.
36 Jože Mencinger, 'Uneasy Symbiosis of a Market Economy and Democratic Centralism: Emergence and Disappearance of Market Socialism in Yugoslavia', in Vojmir Franičević and Milica Uvalić, eds, *Equality, Participation, Transition – Essays in Honour of Branko Horvat* (Basingstoke: Palgrave Macmillan, 2000), 118–144.
37 Milica Uvalić, 'The Rise and Fall of Market Socialism in Yugoslavia', Special Report, Dialogue of Civilizations Research Institute, 2018, https://doc-research.org/2018/03/rise-fall-market-socialism-yugoslavia/ (Accessed 18/05/2021).
38 *Torlak: 1930–1995.*
39 Sanja Petrović-Todosijević, '(Dis)kontinuitet bez presedana: zdravstvena politika Jugoslovenske države u prvoj polovini 20. veka' [The (Dis)continuity Without a Precedent. Healthcare Policy of the Yugoslav State in the First Half of the 20th Century], *Tokovi istorije*, 2007, 3, 96–119.
40 *Torlak: 1930–1995.*
41 *Ibid.*
42 *Ibid.*
43 Maurice R. Hilleman, 'Vaccines and the Vaccine Enterprise: Historic and Contemporary View of a Scientific Initiative of Complex Dimensions', The Jordan Report, 20th Anniversary, Accelerated Development of Vaccines 2002, US Department of Health and Human Services.
44 Blume, 'The Vaccine Innovation System', 258.
45 *Torlak: 1930–1995.*
46 *Ibid.*
47 *Ibid.*
48 Mencinger, 'Uneasy Symbiosis of a Market Economy and Democratic Centralism', 118–144.
49 *Ibid.*
50 *Ibid.*
51 'Zakon o udruženom radu' [The Associated Labour Act], *Official Journal*, 1976, XXXII, 53.

52 Blume, 'The Vaccine Innovation System'.
53 Zagorka Golubović, *Savremeno jugoslovensko društvo* [Contemporary Yugoslavian Society] (Beograd: Službeni glasnik, 2007).
54 *Ibid.*
55 Blume, 'The Erosion of Public Sector Vaccine Production', 148–173.
56 Božidar Cerović, *Tranzicija: zamisli i ostvarenja* [Transition: Ideas and Realizations] (Beograd: Centar za izdavačku delatnost Ekonomskog fakulteta, 2012).
57 Vojin Dimitrijevic and Jelena Pejic, 'UN Sanctions Against Yugoslavia: Two Years Later', in Dimitris Bourantonis and Jarrod Wiener, eds, *The United Nations in the New World Order. The World Organization at Fifty* (Basingstoke: Palgrave Macmillan 1995), 124–153.
58 Nora Dellepiane and David Wood, 'Twenty-Five Years of the WHO Vaccines Prequalification Programme (1987–2012): Lessons learned and future perspectives', *Vaccine*, 2015, 33, 52–61.
59 J. Milstien, A. Batson and W. Meaney, 'A Systematic Method for Evaluating the Potential Viability of Local Vaccine Producers', *Vaccine*, 1997, 15, 1358–1363.
60 Report on the Current Situation and Activities at the Institute of Virology, Vaccines and serum "Torlak", http://www.zdravstvenisavetsrbije.gov.rs/index.php?page=4 (Accessed 18/05/2021).
61 *Ibid.*
62 *Ibid.*
63 https://www.euro.who.int/en/health-topics/communicable-diseases/influenza/news/news/2018/5/serbia-reaches-a-milestone-for-influenza-vaccines-production (Accessed 18/05/2021).
64 Report on the Current Situation and Activities at the Institute of Virology, Vaccines and serum "Torlak".
65 http://www.novosti.rs/vesti/naslovna/drustvo/aktuelno.290.html:223430-Vakcine-traze-kredit (Accessed 18/05/2021).
66 *Ibid.*
67 https://www.vreme.com/cms/view.php?id=437761; http://www.politika.rs/sr/clanak/65324/Uvozne-vakcine-ubijaju-Torlak (Accessed 18/05/2021).
68 Vesna Trifunović, 'Framing Vaccination in Post-Socialist Serbia: An Anthropological Perspective', *Issues in Ethnology and Anthropology*, 2019, 14, 507–529.
69 Vesna Trifunović *et al.*, 'Understanding vaccination communication between health workers and parents: A Tailoring Immunization Programmes (TIP) qualitative study in Serbia', *Article in production*, in the future available at: https://doi.org/10.1080/21645515.2021.1913962.
70 https://www.reuters.com/article/health-coronavirus-serbia-vaccine-presid-idUSL1N2KB161 (Accessed 18/05/ 2021).
71 https://balkaninsight.com/2021/03/12/serbia-unveils-plan-to-produce-chinese-vaccine-jointly-with-uae/ (Accessed 18/05/2021).
72 This paper is the result of work in the Ethnographic Institute, financed by the RS Ministry of Education, Science and Technological Development, on the basis of the Contract on realization and financing of scientific research in 2021 number: 451-03-9 / 2021-14 / 200173. from 05.02.2021.

EPILOGUE

States and vaccines in the age of Covid-19

Stuart Blume and Maurizia Mezza

Introduction

In many countries of the world state involvement with vaccinology changed in the 1980s. It did so partly in response to the global forces which came into play at the time: the fall of Communism in east and central Europe and the rise of neoliberalism. Advances in the technology underlying vaccine production also played a role. So too did the demands of increasingly stringent standards of 'good manufacturing practice'. Although these forces expressed themselves differently in different countries, state after state divested itself of the ability to produce the vaccines its public health system needed. In an ideological climate dominated by faith in market forces and in reduced state expenditures, there was little interest in upgrading old institutes to meet new standards. Cost-benefit considerations came to outweigh more expansive notions of state responsibility. Insiders noted a growing divergence between public health needs and the priorities of commercial vaccine producers. A handful of global pharmaceutical companies oriented to global markets was coming to dominate production. At the same time new biotechnology companies began to play an important role in developing new vaccines. Lacking established connections to public health institutions, their focus was typically on achieving maximum commercial gain from their new, rigorously patented technologies.

Around the turn of the millennium the vaccine market was growing far more rapidly than that for pharmaceuticals. Vaccines became a major source of growth for the industry. That vaccines were being reconfigured as 'profitable commodities' attracted little critique. It appeared inevitable.

This was the situation in 2019 when, at the very end of the year, the world's attention turned to China. There were reports of a pneumonia-like disease outbreak apparently linked to a seafood and live animal market in the city

DOI: 10.4324/9781003130345-10

of Wuhan. At the very end of December, a specialist team from the Chinese Center for Disease Control and Prevention was sent to investigate the outbreak, which was already spreading far afield. In January 2020 it was established that the epidemic was caused by a coronavirus. Analysis of genome sequences from infected patients showed that the virus was similar to the one responsible for the 2003 SARS outbreak. The new virus was named SARS-CoV-2, and the disease Covid-19. By the end of January human-to-human transmission had been established. On 11 March 2020, the WHO Director General announced that Covid-19 'can be characterized as a pandemic'. More than 118,000 cases had already been reported in 114 countries, and 4,291 people had died. The situation was expected to deteriorate much further.

Publication of the genetic sequence of the virus pointed the way to development of a vaccine. Within just one month 21 potential vaccines were already under development, in large pharmaceutical companies, university laboratories, and small biotech companies around the globe.[1] Their approaches (or 'platforms') differed. Some were trying established ways of producing vaccines, such as inactivation. A few biotechnology companies which were already working on novel techniques of genetic manipulation now turned their attention to the SARS-CoV-2 virus. Prominent among these techniques was one using messenger RNA (mRNA). This is a novel approach, previously applied mainly to development of novel cancer drugs, though in late 2020 none had yet been licensed. The mRNA molecule enters the body's cells and 'instructs' them to produce the required proteins (in this case the spike proteins of the SARS-CoV-2 virus). Although no licensed human vaccine had been produced like this mRNA vaccines against other infectious diseases, including Ebola and Zika, were already under development. A few laboratories had a head start in applying the technique to a Covid-19 vaccine.

All hopes of return to a normal life were immediately pinned on development of a vaccine. Until that time, countries were forced to rely on largely forgotten ways of controlling infectious diseases: enforced hygiene, quarantine and social distancing, and mask-wearing. The social and economic dislocation was vast. Resistance from libertarians, unaccustomed to any restriction on their right to move when and where they chose, sometimes took violent forms. The build-up of social demand, the expectations (as reflected in media) of a vaccine was unlike anything seen since ringing church bells greeted the licensing of the first polio vaccine in 1955.

The start of 2020 saw the world facing a threat to the lives of its 7.8 billion inhabitants comparable only with the 1918 influenza pandemic. The closures and privatizations of public sector vaccine institutes discussed in earlier chapters meant that by this time, with just a few exceptions, public health systems were wholly dependent on private industry. A variety of constructions and initiatives (such as Public–Private Partnerships and Advance Market Commitments) had previously been designed to 'sensitize' the industry to public health priorities. Where would a vaccine come from?

There was little interest in thinking through the many issues which would have to be faced once a vaccine had been developed. We pointed some of them out in May 2020.[2] How could sufficient vaccine for the world's population be produced? How could rich countries be prevented from monopolizing initially limited supplies? Furthermore, 'There will be pressure to fast-track a coronavirus vaccine. Since there will not have been time to test it in all population groups, side-effects might [...] emerge. An acceptable division of responsibility between states and manufacturers in the event of this happening needs to be established'. Through the first nine months of 2020 these issues were largely avoided. Development of a vaccine was the light at the end of the tunnel! Thereafter normal life could be resumed. Today, more than a year later, we know that our concerns were justified and the hyper-optimism was not.

In this Epilogue we look at the impact of the Covid-19 pandemic on vaccine development and production, and in particular at its consequences for state involvement. At this time of writing (May 2021) the situation continues to evolve. Almost every day brings new disclosures of disruptions to production chains, breaches of contract, warnings of rare and potentially fatal adverse events, desperate shortages in one place, vaccines discarded for want of takers in another. Demands for patent waivers, spearheaded by NGOs from the global south, have until recently been blocked by representatives of the United States, the United Kingdom, and the European Union. But plans for starting or restarting local or regional production are gradually taking shape, a development to which we return at the end of this chapter. It is too soon for a definitive stocktaking. Of necessity our objective here is more modest. On the one hand we highlight some of the most significant developments through 18 months of the pandemic. On the other we try to understand how the consolidations and divergences disclosed in previous chapters may play out in the near future.

The race to produce a vaccine

In May 2020 the *Financial Times* carried an article headlined 'Why vaccine "nationalism" could slow coronavirus fight'. Much of the article was devoted to an emerging rivalry between the United States and China...to the extent that these countries, it was claimed, were throwing everything, including their military might, into the race to be first to produce a vaccine. The article speaks of 'a tussle for national bragging rights'! Was something beyond saving lives, and beyond the commercial interests of individual firms, coming into play?

In China, Russia, and the United States, in particular, the political and diplomatic stakes were soon recognized. Each state was determined to be first to produce an effective vaccine. Consequently, each was deeply invested in vaccine development, though in ways that reflected their differing political economies.

In Russia the leading institution was the Gamaleya Research Institute, founded in 1891 as a private laboratory. Its history is similar to that of many of the institutes described in earlier chapters. In 1919 it was nationalized and later given the name of Nikolai Gamaleya. Gamaleya had studied in Pasteur's laboratory in Paris, had fought epidemics of cholera, diphtheria and typhus, and had organized mass vaccination campaigns in the Soviet Union. The Institute operates under the auspices of the Ministry of Health of the Russian Federation, making it a true PSVI. In 2015 it had developed an Ebola vaccine based on use of an adenovirus vector. Its development of a Covid-19 vaccine, using the same approach, was funded by the State Sovereign Wealth Fund, and involved collaboration with the Russian military. An August 2020 report in the *Financial Times* suggested, however, that Russia had too little production capacity.[3]

In China at least three institutions had key roles. The China National Pharmaceutical Group Co., Ltd. (or Sinopharm) falls directly under the State-owned Assets Supervision and Administration Commission (SASAC) of the State Council. It is very large, with 128,000 employees and a full chain in the industry running from R&D, through manufacturing, to retail sales. Sinovac Biotech Ltd. is a China-based biopharmaceutical company which focuses on the research, development, manufacturing and commercialization of vaccines against human infectious diseases, including hepatitis A and B vaccines and vaccines against various strains of influenza. CanSino Biologics is a private stock exchange-listed company founded in 2009. This company has collaborated with the National Research Council of Canada on development of an Ebola vaccine. All the Chinese initiatives involve collaborations between various institutions, including the military. For example, 'Medical researcher Major General Chen Wei at the Beijing Institute of Biotechnology – part of the Academy of Military Medical Sciences – led the team that developed the vaccine, which included collaborators from government agencies, universities and the Tianjin-based pharmaceutical company CanSino Biologics. In July, the team became one of the first in the world to publish results in a peer-reviewed journal that showed a coronavirus vaccine to be safe and capable of eliciting an immune response'.[4]

In the United States, the Federal government also played a major role, but a more indirect one. Direct government involvement in actually conducting R&D was small. Support was largely directed at vaccine development in private industry. A key funding mechanism was Operation Warp Speed, a partnership involving the Centers for Disease Control and Prevention (CDC), the National Institutes of Health (NIH), the Biomedical Advanced Research and Development Authority (BARDA), and the Department of Defense (DoD). Its goal was to produce and deliver 300 million doses of safe and effective vaccines, with the initial doses available by January 2021.[5] Substantial investments were made in companies with leading candidate vaccines, including Johnson & Johnson (Janssen) and AstraZeneca, and small biotech companies including Novovax and Moderna (founded in 2010).

A few other countries tried to join in the race. The British health secretary was quoted as saying that 'The upside of being the first country in the world to develop a successful vaccine is so huge that I am throwing everything at it'.[6] In April the UK government invested 42.5 million pounds in two UK-based vaccine development programmes. One involved the British-Swedish drug maker AstraZeneca. This company signed a deal with the University of Oxford. By the end of 2020 it would produce up to 100 million doses of a vaccine developed by Oxford scientists. It was said early on that supply to the United Kingdom would be prioritized. However AstraZeneca's contractual commitments would later involve the company in a legal battle with the European Union.

For much of 2020 media reporting suggested that the sole indicator of success was winning this race. Gradually signs that there would not be so clear-cut an outcome emerged. Because the stakes were so high announcements and reactions to them were highly politicized. In Western news media this involved ignoring, or trying to discredit, the prior claims notably of Russia and China. Since little had been published regarding the efficacy of their vaccines, there were justifiable grounds for scepticism. However more was involved than lack of Phase III clinical trial data alone.

The first vaccines to be submitted for regulatory approval in Western Europe (including the United Kingdom) and North America were two mRNA vaccines: one developed by Pfizer together with a young German-based company, BioNTech, the other by Moderna. In the United States, then-Vice President Pence claimed that Operation Warp Speed was partly responsible for the success. In this he was contradicted by the head of Pfizer's R&D, who pointed out that the company had not taken any money from Warp Speed.

A number of vaccines, like that of BioNTech-Pfizer, were developed and produced in cross-national consortia. Many more were developed with funding from multiple sources, both national and international. For example, Novavax, a US-based biotechnology company, has developed a protein subunit vaccine which it calls NVX-CoV2373. Its development received funding not only from the US Department of Defense and Operation Warp Speed, but also from the Oslo-based Coalition for Epidemic Preparedness Innovations (CEPI). Interestingly the Novavax vaccine is 'adjuvated' with a patented substance called Matrix-M. Matrix-M is composed of nanoparticles based on saponin, extracted from the bark of a tree, *Quillaja saponaria Molina*, which grows in Chile. When the US company extracting the component had to close because of the lockdown, Novavax requested an exemption from Chilean President Sebastián Piñera![7]

The complexity of structures and underlying infrastructures proved no barrier to politicians attempting to extract political and diplomatic benefit from humanity's struggles with the SARS-CoV-2 virus.

Vaccine nationalism: the domestic context

Vaccine nationalism is not a precise concept. The claims, counter claims, and accusations that can be (and have been) so labeled are various, ranging from political boasting to the hoarding of vaccines by rich countries. It is convenient to distinguish the forms it takes in domestic as against international contexts. In domestic contexts political credibility and popularity are at stake. But how tackling the pandemic was turned into political capital depended on the nature of a country's political system.

An ideology may be at stake. In some places vaccine nationalism expressed itself in rejection of the products of global capitalism. A domestically developed and produced vaccine promises self-reliance and may bolster both national pride and ideological conformity.

Cuba's Finlay Vaccine Institute developed a vaccine which it named 'Soberana-02'. The virus antigen is chemically bound to tetanus toxoid: a well-established technology with the benefits of thermal stability and relatively low production costs. Phase 3 clinical trials took place in Iran.[8] As discussed in an earlier chapter, the Iranian Supreme Leader Ayatollah Ali Khamenei blocked the importation of vaccine from United States and United Kingdom, despite Iran's having the worst Coronavirus outbreak in the Middle East. He declared that AstraZeneca, Moderna and Pfizer BioNtech vaccines are 'untrustworthy'.[9] The cooperation between Cuba and Iran, which are both under US sanctions, reflects a shared search for self-sufficiency, and less reliance on imports from the West.

India also provides an interesting example. The Serum Institute of India (SII), the largest vaccine producer in the world, rapidly signed an agreement to produce the Oxford/AstraZeneca vaccine. Known as Covishield, the Indian regulator gave this SII vaccine approval for emergency use in early January 2021. Meanwhile an Indian company, Bharat Biotech, was developing its own vaccine (Covaxin). Within hours of emergency authorization being granted to Covishield, there is reputed to have been political pressure from the government to have Covaxin get the benefit of emergency authorization as well, in the name of self-reliance and national pride in an indigenously developed vaccine, even though no results were in yet from the Phase 3 trials.

As of February 2021, more than 70 candidate vaccines in addition to the ones mentioned hitherto had reached the stage of clinical trials. Some were being developed by other Chinese institutes, some by European or American companies. In addition, institutes in a number of other countries were also conducting trials of candidate vaccines.

Thus in Iran a number of vaccines are being developed, as noted in an earlier chapter. In February 2021, the Barekat Foundation claimed success in the first round of human trials, and promised that an Iranian vaccine would soon be available. The Ministry of Defence is also supporting production of the Fakhra vaccine,[10] using an inactivated virus approach.

In Mexico a vaccine called 'Patria' ('Homeland') is being developed under a framework agreement between the Ministry of Health, the National Council for Science and Technology (Conacyt) and the largely state-owned producer, Birmex. 'Patria' has passed the preclinical safety and efficacy tests, and if trials are successful it will be produced by the end of 2021.[11]

Once the first vaccines were approaching licensure, the fact that supplies would be limited for many months had to be confronted. A rapid start to mass vaccination would depend on success in securing supplies: in effect, pushing to the front of the queue. A foretaste of what was to come had been seen at the start of the pandemic as countries competed for limited supplies of protective equipment (gowns, gloves, masks). In the United States the idea of 'America first' led the Trump administration to purchase almost the total available supply of remdesivir, one of the few drugs thought to be an effective treatment for Covid-19.[12] Peter Marks, a senior Trump administration official, compared the global allocation of vaccines to oxygen masks dropping inside a depressurizing airplane: 'You put on your own first, and then we want to help others as quickly as possible'.

Whatever the dubious morality underlying these remarks, they express a logic which appealed to many politicians. In wealthy countries, which claimed limited initial supplies through Advance Market Commitments signed with manufacturers, it was speedy and efficient organization of a vaccination campaign, not vaccine development, which mattered politically. In pursuit of popular support and votes, politicians wanted to boast of successfully vaccinating large swathes of the population. Thus in the United States, where 2020 was overshadowed by a forthcoming presidential election, domestic political gains were very much at stake. The Trump White House was happy to claim that hundreds of millions of Covid-19 vaccine doses would be 'ready to go' by Election Day.[13] They were not. Before vaccination can begin the appropriate regulator must approve a new vaccine on the basis of data from large scale (Phase III) clinical trials. If people are to have confidence in the vaccines offered to them then clearly they must be confident that this approval process is free from commercial biases or political interference.

In the United States the regulator is the Food and Drug Administration (FDA). EU countries rely on the European Medicines Agency (EMA), now based in Amsterdam, whilst the post-Brexit UK is advised by its Medicines and Healthcare products Regulatory Agency (MHRA). The EMA started its rolling review of preliminary data from Pfizer/BioNTech trials on 6 October 2020. The British regulator began some weeks later but by analyzing less data concluded its assessment more rapidly, enabling British politicians to claim a different 'first':

> The UK has become the first western country to license a vaccine against Covid, opening the way for mass immunisation with the Pfizer/BioNTech vaccine to begin next week for those most at risk. The vaccine has been authorised for emergency use by the Medicines and Healthcare products Regulatory Authority (MHRA), before decisions by the US and Europe. .... The MHRA has moved with unprecedented speed to grant emergency use authorisation, having received the final data from the companies on 23 November. It has been carrying out a rolling approval process, scrutinising data from early trials as they came in.[14]

European politicians and regulators were unimpressed. The EMA accused the British of prioritizing speed over public confidence, mainly in order to be able to say 'we were first'. Given the high degree of scepticism which surveys in many countries disclosed, there was an obvious need to balance speed against reassurance. The German health minister stated that his country had explicitly rejected following the route the British had taken, preferring that all of Europe move forwards together in combatting the disease.[15]

The start of 2021 saw a series of acrimonious disputes breaking out. To the anger of many European politicians, vaccination in the European Union was advancing far less rapidly than in Britain, Israel, or the United States (after installation of the Biden administration). Disputes broke out within Europe too, as Member States began to criticize what some saw as the incompetence of the European Commission, which had negotiated on their behalf with manufacturers. Some countries began to negotiate their own side deals, and some of those to the east (Hungary, Slovakia) began importing the Russian Sputnik-V vaccine though this had not been approved by the EMA. An additional complication, and an additional source of friction, followed reports of very rare but serious adverse events following vaccination with the AstraZeneca vaccine. Weighing these risks against the need to bring the pandemic under control led some governments to pause use of these vaccines, even when regulators made different risk assessments.

The achievements that gather support for a government at home do not necessarily attract admiration and prestige internationally. The very opposite may occur. As suggested by the comments of the German minister quoted earlier 'nationalism' can be seen as in opposition to wider solidarity. A government's appeal to its electorate differs from a State's attempts to present itself globally, whether as a hive of innovation or as a global benefactor.

Vaccine nationalism: the international context

In the course of 2020–2021, the global vaccine innovation system was coming increasingly to resemble a complex game: a game in which 'players' competed for political and strategic gains as well as markets and profits. Whatever the economic interests involved, as in the 'Space Race' of the Cold War years national prestige and the rival claims of competing ideologies were at stake. Some commentators were anxious to conclude that the US's 'free market' model, involving several businesses competing with each other, would prove superior to Russia and China's 'public conglomerates' model.[16] Others, of course, thought differently.

In addition to demonstrating the efficacy of one's own vaccine(s), success involved challenging the claims advanced by competitors. The claim that the UK's rapid vaccine approval had entailed regulatory corner-cutting was one instance of this. There were many more.

In the view of western scientists, (as refracted through western media) both China and Russia 'cheated' by announcing the regulatory approval of their locally developed vaccines before the results of Phase III trials had been published and internationally verified. The Chinese government approved the CanSino vaccine, called Ad5-nCoV, for limited use in military personnel in summer 2020, before Phase III trials had been completed. If accepted more widely this could be a major 'propaganda victory' for Beijing.[17] Similarly the first Russian vaccine, named Sputnik V, was registered by the Russian Ministry of Health and approved for distribution in Russia in August 2020. At the time no Phase III trial data had been published. Granting regulatory approval before Phase III results have been internationally verified conflicts with WHO guidelines. The claims made for Sputnik-V attracted widespread scorn in the west: a reflection on the lack of published data but also of the high political stakes. The Russian riposte came months later, following reports of blood-clotting apparently caused by the AstraZeneca vaccine. These reports and responses to them enabled Russian authorities to dismiss Western critique of their Sputnik-V vaccine and to insist on its superiority.

Results of Phase III trials of the Moderna and Pfizer-BioNTech vaccines were announced in November 2020. Both reported efficacy of over 90%: far higher than anyone had expected. A few days later AstraZeneca announced that its vaccine was effective up to 90%, but only when the first dose had been (mistakenly) cut in half.[18] While UK media, echoing head of AstraZeneca R&D Mene Pangalos, spoke about 'serendipity'.[19] *The New York Times* reported 'irregularities' and 'omissions' that have eroded confidence in the vaccine.[20] Moncef Slaoui, the head of the U.S. government's Operation Warp Speed highlighted an additional limitation, which received little attention in the United Kingdom though a great deal elsewhere. The 90% efficacy had only been demonstrated in younger patients, whereas it was elderly people who were most at risk. Other critics went further, suggesting that this vaccine had no value for the elderly. Despite British and European regulators reaching a different conclusion, this slur nourished vaccine hesitancy, leading many to reject the vaccine. Whilst applications for regulatory approval of the Pfizer/BioNTech and Moderna vaccines moved ahead in the United Kingdom, the United States, and the European Union, that for the Oxford-AstraZeneca vaccine was delayed.

A few days after these companies' results were announced, a comparable announcement came from Moscow. Presented with data from 19,000 trial participants, who had received 2 doses of Sputnik-V, western scientists now began to take the vaccine seriously. The Sputnik-V vaccine and the Oxford-AstraZeneca are similar: both use a harmless adenovirus to deliver a gene that codes for the SARS-CoV-2 virus spike proteins. But the Russian vaccine uses two different adenoviruses for the primary and booster shots. This, they claim, makes it more effective. Announcements indicate what is at stake for the Russians: commercially, politically, and diplomatically. According to *The Guardian* newspaper the Russians offered to share their adenoviral vectors with the AstraZeneca scientists, and a trial using both vaccines jointly (one dose of each) has been set up in Moscow.

Claim-making and claim-denying were not the only ways in which countries sought diplomatic benefit. By the second half of 2020, as some candidate vaccines appeared to be effective, collaborating in clinical trials with foreign institutions, and offering future vaccine supplies under favourable terms, were assuming greater importance. Holding out the prospect of technology transfer and future local production could be a major inducement, especially to countries with some remaining competence in vaccine production. In its recognition of how Covid-19 vaccines can best be deployed for diplomatic gain, China has led the way. The fallout from the spread of Covid-19 fuelled mistrust of China internationally, and damaged the global appetite for the exports which had helped drive its growth. A successful vaccine, provided at an affordable price, offered a potential route to address resentment and criticism of China's early handling of the virus, as well as a financial boost for the country's biotech firms.

In early December results of a trial of the Sinopharm vaccine in the United Arab Emirates (UAE) suggested that this vaccine has an efficacy of 86%. Before the year's end Turkey, the UAE, Mexico, Chile, and the state of São Paolo in Brazil were planning to start mass vaccination with this or one of the other Chinese-made vaccines. Though official Chinese media rejected the argument, reports soon suggested that China was using its vaccines to further state interests, in what was termed 'vaccine diplomacy'.

For example, China was said to have promised that 6 million doses of CoronaVac, made by the biotech firm Sinovac, would reach Brazil by January 2021. São Paulo's respected and experienced Butantan Institute, which tested the vaccine, would get raw materials to make millions more. The Sinopharm and Sinovac vaccines are made by classic inactivation processes, an approach which offers far more opportunity for technology transfer than the complex mRNA technology. The fact that Chinese institutions appeared to be offering the possibility of technology transfer and local production will have been a major incentive for a country such as Brazil, which still has public sector vaccine production.

The shipments to São Paolo were said to be part of China's global vaccine diplomacy. According to some western commentators, countries in East and South East Asia were 'wary' of the conditions Beijing might attach to its offers of cheap vaccine.

> ...by virtue of its proximity and the aforementioned advantages, China has loomed prominently in states' strategies for gaining access to a vaccine...A good example is Indonesia, where the state-owned pharmaceutical firm Bio Farma is currently testing a new vaccine made by the Chinese company Sinovac Biotech. If successful, the vaccine will then be produced locally in large quantities. A similar arrangement is currently under negotiation in the Philippines. China has also promised Malaysia, Vietnam, Laos, Cambodia, Thailand and Myanmar priority access to Chinese-made vaccines.[21]

Similarly, the Russian Direct Investment Fund, which markets the Sputnik V vaccine, negotiated contracts to provide it at an affordable price to a number of developing countries. Here too discussions appear to have held out the possibility of future local production. By mid-2021 arrangements had been made for production of the Sputnik V vaccine in Serbia (as noted in an earlier chapter) and in Italy.

Early in the pandemic China, Russia, and the United States were competing in a race to produce the first effective vaccine. By the end of 2020 it was clear that the strategic (non-economic) benefit flowing from having been first – first to produce an approved vaccine or first to begin mass vaccination – would be short-lived. Just as the emergence of mutations in the virus pushed end points further into the future, so the rules of the vaccine game were evolving. From a global perspective, having successfully outmuscled competitors in accumulating scarce vaccine was coming to be seen not as praiseworthy but as selfish and problematic. The UK's speedy rollout was critiqued on the grounds both that it represented a sacrifice of inter-national solidarity and that it meant accepting all conditions imposed by manufacturers. These conditions were not necessarily in people's interests. Perhaps unsurprisingly in the aftermath of Brexit comparisons were drawn between British and European procedures.

> When it came to vaccines, the 27 agreed very early on, under the leadership of Berlin and Paris, to pool procurement. All agreed to guarantee that each would have equal access, proportionate to their population size, and above all, that each would apply the same vaccine purchase conditions. Otherwise, how would, say, Luxembourg or Finland have fared against the pharmaceutical giants? [...] The EU together set out the demands it wanted met in exchange for financial aid aimed at speeding up production (€2.7bn). These demands included refusing to exempt laboratories from civil liability, insisting that the companies owned production lines on EU territory – an essential precaution at a time of temporary border closures – and, finally, reasonable prices. Not all these conditions were imposed by the US, the UK, Canada or Israel.[22]

Britain, this article claims, paid for its head start on the EU both by paying a higher price but also by absolving manufacturers of any responsibility in the event of serious adverse effects emerging.

The criticism levelled at the United Kingdom, and other instances of what is interpreted as vaccine nationalism, rests on two arguments. One relates to the need for solidarity between countries if the pandemic is to be vanquished. The second argument, which may be incompatible with the first, appeals to the importance of open, free and global markets as guarantors of continuing innovation.

Market resistance to vaccine nationalism

The commercial pharmaceutical industry prizes open, global and standardized markets. Its resistance to some of the steps taken in response to the pandemic was hardly unexpected. Measures that enable consumers to act in concert, which from one point of view appear as an expression of solidarity, from a commercial perspective appear threatening. The European pharmaceutical industry is said to have lobbied against joint procurement agreements under which the Commission acted on behalf of all Member States in order to secure equitable access and balanced prices throughout the EU. The industry association (EFPIA) preferred to continue supplying these new treatments through established channels rather than by joint procurement.

Nevertheless, the European Commission and the member states agreed on a joint approach to vaccine procurement. By December 2020 contracts guaranteeing a stated number of doses of vaccine once proven safe and effective had been signed. The EU made different agreements with 6 companies: AstraZeneca, Sanofi-GSK, Johnson & Johnson, BioNTech-Pfizer, CureVac, and Moderna.[23] When it became clear there would be no Sanofi-GSK vaccine in the near future, an agreement with Novavax was signed instead. The industry fiercely resisted attempts to open the deals it struck to public scrutiny. Neither the prices to be paid nor the conditions imposed (notably regarding responsibilities in the event of side effects appearing) were to be made public. Companies demanded secrecy on the grounds of commercial confidentiality, but this suited many politicians too. After all, where companies were granted immunity from damage claims (in the event of adverse events occurring) politicians may want to resist disclosure of the fact. An investigation in Latin America found that a number of governments (including those of Colombia, Peru and Uruguay) refused to disclose the contracts they had signed with Pfizer, citing 'confidentiality clauses' in their contracts. Elsewhere details of 'abusive' contracts leaked out.

In late 2020 some information regarding the likely price of competing vaccines did become public, to the fury of manufacturers. It appeared that AstraZeneca would sell its vaccine to the EU for $3–4 a dose. Moderna, previously a loss-making company, initially said that it would sell its vaccine at something like $50 per dose, and defended the reasonableness of setting a commercial price. It subsequently reduced its price to half of that. However different customers paid different prices. In January 2021 the EU received a smaller quantity of the Pfizer/BioNTech vaccine than it had expected. Pfizer was said to have prioritized production for Israel and the United States because they had paid more. Additionally, Israel was able to secure extra doses because it promised to provide Pfizer with data on community responses to vaccination. Many details of the many deals still remain secret.

Beyond prices, patents are another area in which the industry has defended its commercial interests. In late 2020 Moderna announced that it would not enforce its patents for the duration of the pandemic. In other words, organizations could produce mRNA vaccines like Moderna's without running the risk of a legal challenge. Though this appears pure altruism, it is not.

> Moderna's pledge extends through the duration of the COVID-19 pandemic. After that, it has expressed a willingness to negotiate licenses of its technology, presumably on a fee-bearing basis. Thus, if Moderna achieves

> a broad uptake of its vaccine technology during the pandemic and competitors supply the vaccine to meet global demand, then they will need to obtain a paid license from Moderna to continue in this line of business after the pandemic is over (effectively a 'loss leader' strategy).[24]

As a leader in the field of mRNA product development, the company has an interest in establishing this kind of vaccine as the standard. This is simply one move in a complex process.

In late 2020 India and South Africa proposed to the World Trade Organization a temporary waiver of certain TRIPS (Agreement on Trade Related Aspects of Intellectual Property Rights) obligations, such as patents and intellectual property rights, covering treatments and tools related to Covid-19, as well as vaccines. This would facilitate an appropriate response in countries which lacked the muscle to push to the front of the queue. There had been an early precedent in the case of the ventilators in the EU. At the beginning of the pandemic, in many countries there was a severe shortage of ventilators. Thanks to some companies agreeing to share design specifications the automotive sector could start producing them. Patent free medical treatments, vaccines and devices would also allow manufacturers to begin producing Covid-19 essential medical products.[25] Aligning themselves with the interest of their commercial pharmaceutical companies, the governments of the United Kingdom, United States, Canada, Australia, as well as the EU, opposed these initiatives. The UK government backed up its position with the statement that 'existing IP system allowed for pharmaceutical companies to voluntarily share data and technology, and some had already done so'.[26]

In May 2021 it was announced that the United States was dropping its opposition to patent waivers for the duration of the pandemic.[27] In terms of countering the present pandemic patent waivers are unlikely to lead to a substantial increase in the global supply of effective and reliable vaccines. Unlike simpler drugs, new vaccine production lines require expensive clinical trials and inspection of each batch by a competent regulatory authority.[28] Ensuring safety and potency implies that each production unit consistently meet standards of good manufacturing practice. On the other hand, there can be no doubts as to the moral standing of the claim that the profit motive is incompatible with so existential a struggle.

The multilateral response to vaccine nationalisms

Vaccination limited to a few privileged countries could never control the pandemic. Yet because a few countries had reserved far the largest share of vaccines some forecasts suggested that people in the poorest countries would have no access to vaccine until late 2022. Expediency, as well as morality, pointed to the importance of ensuring vaccine accessibility in poor countries. How was this to be achieved?

In April 2020 an event co-hosted by the Director-General of WHO, the Presidents of France and of the European Commission, and the Bill & Melinda Gates Foundation, led to the 'ACT Accelerator' initiative. This would support and coordinate global effort to fight the pandemic, by integrating efforts across academia, private sector and governments.[29] An important element of the plan was the Covid-19 Global Access Facility, COVAX. Co-led by GAVI, the Vaccine Alliance, the Coalition for Epidemic Preparedness Innovations (CEPI) and the WHO, COVAX was established to guarantee rapid, fair and equitable access to Covid-19 vaccines worldwide, and 'regardless of their wealth'.[30] COVAX is supposed to mitigate the impact of bilateral agreements by encouraging rich countries to cooperate and to support low-income countries as well.[31] The facility invested in a broad portfolio of vaccine candidates. Through investment and its own Advance Purchase Agreements with pharmaceutical companies it sought to speed up the development of effective vaccines. The mechanism required that high income countries commit to acquiring part of what they need through the facility and investing to support vaccine development and manufacture. The goal of COVAX was to have 2 billion doses to distribute by the end of 2021: enough to help countries vaccinate all of the highest priority populations. By December 2020 COVAX involved 190 participating and eligible economies. 92 low-income countries would receive their shipments of vaccine without charge. Whilst the European Union has been a major source of support, the United States joined only after the Biden administration had replaced that of Donald Trump. Deals or Memoranda of Understanding were struck with a number of manufacturers.[32] 1.3 billion doses were to be reserved for the 92 eligible middle- and low-income countries, whose participation was funded by means of a special COVAX Advance Market Commitment.[33] While some companies, including AstraZeneca, joined COVAX others (including Pfizer and Moderna) did not. The AstraZeneca-Oxford vaccine will be available on a non-profit basis 'in perpetuity' to low- and middle-income countries in the developing world.

In late February 2021 the first COVAX vaccines were delivered. 600,000 doses of the AstraZeneca vaccine arrived in Accra, the capital of Ghana. Still, the adequacy of the mechanism continues to attract high level critique. Both the UN Secretary General and the Director-General of the WHO have criticized monopolization of vaccine supply by rich countries. At that time 75% of all vaccinations had taken place in just 10 countries and many countries, perhaps as many as 200, had not administered a single dose. Despite their financial contributions to COVAX, rich western countries had ordered more vaccine than their populations needed, thereby depriving the initiative of an adequate supply. Subsequently other multilateral initiatives emerged, including one negotiated by the African Union on behalf of its 55 member states.[34] This too signed agreements with Pfizer, AstraZeneca/Serum Institute of India, and Johnson and Johnson.

Meanwhile China and Russia were transforming their vaccine production into diplomatic capital. As of April 2021, more than a third of all the vaccine produced in Russia had been sent abroad. Given that half or more of the country's population does not want to be vaccinated, limited supply is in equilibrium with limited demand.[35]

A recent report offers a critical assessment of COVAX, though not on the grounds that it cannot deliver according to planning. In a complex assessment its author concludes that COVAX's obscure multi-stakeholder structure weakens the truly multilateral United Nations system, and that lines of responsibility have been made obscure. Moreover, its market-based approach, which dovetails with the interests of the pharmaceutical industry, undermines:

> Public acceptability of health as a global public good. It implies that only those who have access to purchasing power –or who have non-state bodies attempting to have purchasing power on their behalf– are eligible for access to the medical services to mitigate the impact of COVID or other epidemics. COVAX's focus on protecting commercial markets is also reflected in its granting of 'stakeholder' status to Big Pharma but not to those in need of health services or those who might advocate for an alternative public sector response.[36]

Conclusions

The processes of marketization which began in the 1980s led many governments to close, privatize, or dismantle their public sector vaccine institutes. Denied access to the newest technology, and lacking the investments needed to meet rising standards of Good Manufacturing Practice, public sector institutes were unable to provide vaccines of the quality policy makers (and publics) demanded. Moreover, producing vaccines for small national markets made local production far more expensive than purchasing vaccines on the market. Anxious to reduce state expenditures, convinced of the benefits of free trade, confronted by patent restrictions on all sides, politicians in many countries chose for a more limited demarcation of their responsibilities. These are the changes which lie at the root of the institute closures discussed in most previous chapters. Resistance to those ideas, and competing ideological commitments, helps explains resistance to such closures elsewhere.

Among the processes triggered by the pandemic and discussed in this Epilogue vaccine nationalism has a significant place. Sometimes it expressed itself by convincing the population that everything possible was being done to protect it against the virus. Previously this might have entailed supporting a trusted vaccine producer which responded to the country's health care needs rather than to markets and profit. Now, in many countries, it meant securing privileged access to limited vaccine supplies and the rapid roll-out of a vaccination programme.

In the sphere of international diplomacy 'bragging rights' were acquired differently. Queue-jumping or monopolizing supplies could be painted as a rejection of the solidarity needed to end the pandemic – and sometimes was. Various ways emerged by which diplomatic capital was extracted from successful vaccine development and production. Countries could seek to profile themselves as crucibles of innovation, or as munificent donors. We suggested that the prestige associated with 'having been first to develop a vaccine' was short-lived. Longer-term benefit followed from support for a national (but commercial) producer competing in the global market, or from donations to or contractual arrangements with client-countries.

Political or ideological nationalism (or exceptionalism) led some countries, ones with sufficient resources and skills, to set about developing and producing their own vaccine in place of relying on supply from elsewhere. Low- and middle-income countries with more modest financial and technical resources were faced with two countervailing pressures (or inducements). One came from the market, in which the highest bidder wins. The objections to this are not only moral. Whatever their ideological commitments, most politicians in low- and middle-income countries will surely have had few doubts on this score. They would have to wait years to obtain the amount of vaccine they needed in the open market. The second pressure, or inducement, came through diplomatic channels: much needed vaccines could be obtained cheaply in exchange for accepting a form of clientism.

However the Covid-19 pandemic is also leading to some rethinking regarding the role of the state. This is clearly true in countries where memories of earlier vaccine self-sufficiency and domestic vaccine production are strong, or where the fate of an old institute is still in doubt. Is complete dependence on a profit-oriented and globally-focused vaccine industry wise, or politically responsible? The question is (re)emerging…

Previous chapters have shown something of this. In the Netherlands for instance, a report commissioned by the Ministries of Health and of Economic Affairs in 2020 identified infectious diseases control and vaccine development as a strength in the Dutch Life Science and Health ecosystem. The report proposed '*continuous public private partnership*' around pandemic preparedness. As of May 2021, with the political complexion of a new government still unknown, the fate of *Intravacc* (a final residue of the previous vaccine institute scheduled for privatization) has become uncertain. In Iran the pandemic highlighted the need for a more sophisticated and updated vaccine production line, strengthening the need for vaccine self-sufficiency. In this context, partnerships between public and private sectors should facilitate access to new technologies and facilities for vaccine production. India adopted the slogan of self-reliance to combat Covid-19. However, while on the one hand public debates started questioning the closing of the major PSVIs, on the other hand the announcement of privatization of 300 Public sector companies show that the private sector is still regarded as the biggest actor in manufacturing the vaccines against this pandemic. In Croatia memories of the past glory of the Zagreb Institute of Immunology have been combined with unrealistic musings on how it could have contributed to the global vaccine race. In Serbia there appear to be plans to breathe new life into the country's Torlak Institute. Serbia is to be the first country in Europe to produce Sputnik V as well as the Chinese Sinopharm Covid-19 vaccine. A revitalized Torlak Institute, supplying the region with vaccines, would give Serbia considerable international prestige. Finally, in Sweden the question of national vaccine production returned to the political agenda even before Covid-19. The avian 'bird influenza' A/H5N1, in 2005–2006, and the swine flu (H1N1), in 2009–2010, raised the issue of access to pandemic vaccines and the risks related to Advance Purchase Agreements. Without joint EU procurement of pandemic vaccine, Sweden would have stood at the back of the queue for access to Covid-19 vaccines. Independent vaccinologists have once more proposed national or Nordic vaccine production in collaboration with one of the major pharmaceutical manufacturers. In Mexico, as in Sweden, the question of national vaccine production returned to the political agenda even before the Covid-19 pandemic. The government which took office in 2018 began to reconsider national vaccine production in the interests of sovereignty and national security. These concerns have of course acquired greater saliency in course of the Covid-19 pandemic.[37]

What lessons will be drawn from the strengths and weaknesses of COVAX, and by whom? Is pooling resources to create a powerful purchaser, but then relying on the market to negotiate supplies and prices, the best way to go? Or might resources better be pooled in order to create a collective production competence? This was the thinking behind the (ill-fated) Dutch-Nordic Consortium discussed in a previous chapter. At this time of writing, it appears to be an option under consideration in and for Africa. The African continent has hitherto produced a mere 1% of the vaccines it uses. Concerned by Africa's lack of access to Covid-19 vaccines, its political leaders are planning a major investment and upgrade, in which the continent's few producers will have key roles. These are principally Pasteur Institutes in Algeria, Senegal and Tunisia, and Biovac (a South African public-private partnership). In May 2021 the President of the European Commission announced that the EU would support the establishment of vaccine production hubs in Africa with an investment of one billion euros. A regional regulator, along the lines of the EMA, will also have to be established.[38]

The future organization of vaccine supply is far less predictable than anyone could have foreseen as recently as 2019. What is clear is that vaccine production in the public sector, if it is to be sustained or revitalized, in one form or another, will no longer be the renewed expression of a state's long-established responsibility for the health of its citizens. Just as the upheavals of the 1980s brought about radical change in vaccine science, technology, and industry, so the events precipitated by the Covid-19 pandemic are leading to changes the results of which are still unclear but potentially radical.

Notes

1 DRAFT landscape of COVID-19 candidate vaccines – 18 February 2020. Geneva: World Health Organization, https://www.who.int/blueprint/priority-diseases/key-action/list-of-candidate-vaccines-developed-against-ncov.pdf (Accessed 10/04/2021).
2 S. Blume and M. Mezza, https://www.socialeurope.eu/what-when-theres-a-vaccine (Accessed 30/03/2021).
3 H. Foy, https://www.ft.com/content/874059a6-da43-4c23-b29d-21ed59152124 (Accessed 04/05/2021).
4 D. Lewis, https://www.nature.com/articles/d41586-020-02523-x (Accessed 07/05/2021).
5 https://en.wikipedia.org/wiki/Operation_Warp_Speed (Accessed 06/05/2021).
6 Quoted in R. Milne and D. Crow, https://www.ft.com/content/6d542894-6483-446c-87b0-96c65e89bb2c (Accessed 07/05/2021).
7 B. Borrell, https://www.theatlantic.com/science/archive/2020/10/single-tree-species-may-hold-key-coronavirus-vaccine/616792/ (Accessed 04/05/2021).
8 https://www.wsj.com/articles/iran-cuba-under-u-s-sanctions-team-up-for-covid-19-vaccine-trials-11610481712 (Accessed 10/04/2021).
9 https://www.rferl.org/a/cuban-researchers-to-test-covid-19-vaccine-in-iran/31040770.html (Accessed 29/01/2021).
10 Mohsen Fakhrizadeh Mahabadi (1958–2020) was a brigadier general in the Islamic Revolutionary Guard, an academic physicist, and a leading figure in Iran's nuclear programme. Fakhrizadeh was assassinated in 2020.
11 We thank Ana Maria Carrillo for this information.
12 https://www.aljazeera.com/news/2020/7/1/us-buys-nearly-all-stocks-of-coronavirus-drug-remdesivir (Accessed 29/01/2021).
13 https://www.nbcnews.com/politics/white-house/trump-says-without-evidence-vaccine-could-be-ready-election-day-n1236029 (Accessed 01/10/2021).
14 S. Boseley and J. Halliday, https://www.theguardian.com/society/2020/dec/02/pfizer-biontech-covid-vaccine-wins-licence-for-use-in-the-uk (Accessed 06/05/2021).
15 D. Boffey, https://www.theguardian.com/world/2020/dec/02/uk-put-speed-before-public-confidence-in-vaccine-says-eu-agency (Accessed 06/05/2021).
16 M. Molinari, https://rep.repubblica.it/pwa/editoriale/2020/12/27/news/la_risposta_biotech_dell_occidente-279986536/ (Accessed 04/05/2021).
17 D. Lewis, https://www.nature.com/articles/d41586-020-02523-x (Accessed 06/05/2021).
18 https://www.reuters.com/article/uk-health-coronavirus-astrazeneca-oxford/decades-of-work-and-half-a-dose-of-fortune-drove-oxford-vaccine-success-idUKKBN2832NG (Accessed 06/05/2021).
19 J. Murray, https://www.theguardian.com/uk-news/2020/nov/23/oxford-covid-vaccine-hit-90-success-rate-thanks-to-dosing-error (Accessed 07/05/2021).
20 R. Robbins and B. Mueller, https://www.nytimes.com/2020/11/25/business/coronavirus-vaccine-astrazeneca-oxford.html (Accessed 07/05/2021).
21 S. Strangio, https://thediplomat.com/2020/11/chinas-southeast-asian-vaccine-diplomacy-comes-into-relief/ (Accessed 07/05/2021).
22 J. Quatremer, https://www.theguardian.com/world/commentisfree/2021/feb/14/brexit-britain-eu-covid-vaccination-fiasco (Accessed 07/05/2021).
23 https://ec.europa.eu/info/live-work-travel-eu/coronavirus-response/public-health/coronavirus-vaccines-strategy_en (Accessed 07/05/2021).
24 J. L. Contreras, https://blog.petrieflom.law.harvard.edu/2020/10/21/moderna-covid19-patent-pledge/ (Accessed 07/05/2021).
25 World Trade Organisation, https://www.wto.org/english/news_e/news20_e/trip_20oct20_e.htm (Accessed 07/05/2021).
26 M. Safi, https://www.theguardian.com/world/2020/nov/19/uk-faces-calls-drop-opposition-patent-free-covid-vaccines-wto (Accessed 07/05/2021).
27 https://www.bbc.com/news/world-us-canada-57004302 (Accessed 07/05/2021).
28 We are grateful to Marco Krieger, Fiocruz, for clarification of this point.

29 World Health Organization, https://www.who.int/initiatives/act-accelerator (Accessed 07/05/2021).
30 S. Berkley, https://www.gavi.org/vaccineswork/covax-explained (Accessed 07/05/2021).
31 David McAdams *et al.*, 'Incentivising wealthy nations to participate in the COVID-19 Vaccine Global Access Facility (COVAX): a game theory perspective', *BMJ Global Health*, 2020, 5, e003627.
32 World Health Organisation, https://www.who.int/news/item/18-12-2020-covax-announces-additional-deals-to-access-promising-covid-19-vaccine-candidates-plans-global-rollout-starting-q1-2021 (Accessed 07/05/2021).
33 https://www.gavi.org/gavi-covax-amc (Accessed 07/05/2021).
34 P. Adepoju, https://healthpolicy-watch.news/africa-secures-270m-vaccines-but-who-warns-against-ordering-vaccines-inadequately-trialled/ (Accessed 07/05/2021).
35 J. Yaffa, https://www.newyorker.com/news/daily-comment/russia-beat-the-world-to-a-vaccine-so-why-is-it-falling-behind-on-vaccinations (Accessed 28/04/2021).
36 H. Gleckman, 'COVAX. A global multistakeholder group that poses political and health risks to developing countries and multilateralism', *Amsterdam: Friends of the Earth/Transnational Institute*, 2021, 11.
37 We thank Ana Maria Carrillo for this information.
38 A. Irwin, https://www.nature.com/articles/d41586-021-01048-1 (Accessed 04/05/2021).

INDEX

ACT Accelerator, 212
Advance Market Commitment (AMC), 82, 122, 132, 169, 200, 205, 212, 215
Advance Purchase Agreement. *See* Advance Market Commitment
adverse effects following immunization, 71, 119, 132, 201, 206, 209. *See also* encephalitis; narcolepsy
Africa, 7–8, 24, 29, 96, 183, 211–12, 215
AIDS, 27
algorithm, 155
anthrax, 3, 94–95, 141–42
antibiotics, 5. *See also* penicillin
AstraZeneca, 202–4, 206–7, 210, 212
attenuation. *See* vaccine
austerity, 33, 35, 37, 39
Australia, 91, 211; Australian Commonwealth Serum Institute, 12; CSL Ltd., 11
Austria-Hungary, 92–93
avian flu. *See* influenza
Azerbaijan, 138, 140, 142

Babeş, Victor, 156–59, 169, 173n4
Bacillus Calmette–Guérin (*BCG*) vaccine 4, 23, 41n12, 71–72, 77, 94, 113, 115–16, 118–20, 124–26, 131, 141, 160, 162–63, 165, 167, 182–83, 187. *See also* tuberculosis
bacteriology 3–5, 11, 44, 46–47, 49–53, 57, 65–72, 74–75, 77–78, 79–80, 92, 95, 111, 114, 156–158, 172, 173n4, 178, 181
Balkans, 3, 167, 180; war, 89, 159, 188–90
Bharat Biotech International, 131, 133, 204
Bharat Immunologicals and Biologicals Ltd., 112, 115
bankruptcy, 90, 101–2, 105, 171
Barekat Foundation, 148, 204
Barekat Pharmaceutical Group, 148
Batson, Amie, 15
BCG Vaccine Laboratories (BCGVL). *See* India
Beck, Miroslav, 99
Behring, Emil, 3, 12, 47, 67
Behringwerke, 12
Belarus, 94
Berlin, 3, 46, 52, 92, 178, 209
Berlin Wall, 188
Biden, Joe, 206, 211
Bill and Melinda Gates Children's Vaccine Program, 16
Bill & Melinda Gates Foundation, 212
Bilthoven Biologicals (BBio Ltd.), 35, 37, 40, 102
Bilthoven Unit System, 23–24
Biogen, 11
biosecurity, 117, 134, 150
bird flu. *See* influenza
Brexit, 205, 209
Britain. *See* United Kingdom
Butantan Institute, 13, 208

Calmette, Albert, 4, 160, 162; *See also* BCG vaccine
Canada, 5, 28, 202, 209, 211; Canada Development Corporation, 12
Cantacuzino, Ion, 156–61, 171–72
Cantacuzino Institute, 155–57, 159–72, 175n63
CanSino Biologics, 202, 206
Centers for Disease Control and Prevention (CDC); *See* United States
Central Research Institute (CRI), 110, 112, 116, 120, 126, 127, 135n25
Children's Vaccine Initiative (CVI), 10, 15–16, 38
China National Pharmaceutical Group Co., Ltd. *See* Sinopharm
China Center for Disease Control and Prevention, 200
cholera, 4, 21, 51, 92, 111, 138–39, 140, 202; vaccine, 48–49, 51, 66, 81, 94–95, 111–14, 116, 125, 140–42, 158, 162–63, 181–82
Chowdhury, Javid, 114, 122
Coalition for Epidemic Preparedness Innovations (CEPI), 203, 212
Cohen, Hans 9, 23–24, 26, 40
Cold War, 2, 5–9, 83, 206
colonialism 3–4, 8, 22, 39, 44, 47, 96, 111, 143, 180
Congo, 98
conjugation technologies. *See* vaccine
Connaught Laboratories, 5, 12
contracts, 99–101, 133, 164, 167, 201, 203, 208, 210, 214. *See also* Advance Market Commitment
Cormick, John, 138
corporate interests, 10
COVAX, 150, 212–13, 215
Covaxin, 133, 204
Covid-19: pandemic, xiii, 1–2, 17, 29, 36–37, 40, 59, 65–66, 84, 90–91, 105, 110, 133, 148–51, 170, 194–95, 199–203; vaccines, 2, 39, 59, 84, 131, 133, 148, 150, 155, 169, 175n73, 194–95, 201–15; virus, 29, 170, 207
cowpox, 2, 3, 21, 70, 92, 177
Croatia, 17, 89–109, 185, 215; Bacteriological Institute, 92. *See also* Gutschy, Ljudevit;
Edmonston-Zagreb measles vaccine strain. *See* measles; Institute of Hygiene, 92–95; Institute of Immunology Zagreb (IMZ), 89–92, 95–106, 185, 215; Leningrad–Zagreb mumps vaccine strain, 94; *Radovi Imunološkog zavoda Zagreb*, 97; Visia Croatica, 102–4. *See also* self-managerial socialism; Yugoslavia
CSL Ltd. *See* Australia
Cuba, 13, 141, 148, 150, 204
Czechoslovakia, 94

Developing Country Vaccine Manufacturers Network (DCVMN), 39
diagnostics, 55, 65–68, 74, 78, 80, 95, 114, 170
diphtheria 3, 8, 20–22, 27, 31, 41n9, 46–49, 53, 67, 74–75, 94–96, 115, 121, 125, 142, 162–63, 182–83, 187; antitoxin 3, 5, 16, 44, 46–47, 49, 55, 65–70 73, 94, 116, 125, 139, 157; toxin, 27, 67, 94
DNA technology. *See* vaccine
Doha Declaration, 13
dysentery, 51, 74, 94, 114, 163, 181–82

Eli Lilly, 7, 76
Egypt, 9, 141
encephalitis, 31, 72, 76
Enders, John, 6
Epidemic: avian flu, 59, 166; cholera, 51, 92, 138, 140, 158, 202; influenza, 54, 69; malaria, 138; measles, 138; pertussis, 31; plague, 44, 111, 138, 140; polio, 20, 23, 75; smallpox, 45–46, 48, 53, 72, 76, 115, 138; tuberculosis, 138; typhus, 51, 138, 140; typhoid fever, 49, 53, 92, 140, 158, 160
epidemic preparedness, 39, 40, 81, 203, 212, 214
epidemiology, 6, 51–53, 55, 65, 67, 75, 80, 82–83, 92, 95, 116, 132, 140, 159–60; epidemiological surveillance, 8, 78, 80, 83
eradication campaigns: diphtheria, 8; infectious diseases, 91, 93, 171; malaria, 162; measles, 1, 8, 80, 98, 143; pertussis, 8; polio, 8–9, 21, 39, 91, 147, 184; smallpox, 8–9, 21, 41n7, 49, 56, 59, 76–77, 80, 140, 171, 184; tetanus, 8; tuberculosis, 7–8, 160
European Centre for Disease Prevention and Control (ECDC), 84, 156, 167
European Investment Bank (EIB), 170
European Medicines Agency (EMA), 40, 205–6, 215
European Union (EU), 38, 101, 105, 155, 168, 172, 193, 201, 203, 206–7, 211

Evans, Peter, 15
Expanded Programme of Immunisation (EPI). *See* World Health Organisation

Finlay Institute, 13, 148, 204. *See also* Cuba
Fiocruz Institute, 13
FitzGerald, John G., 5
Flexner, Simon, 75
flu. *See* influenza
Food and Drug Administration (FDA). *See* United States
Forum for the Advancement of Immunization Research (FAIR) 24, 39. *See also* polio
Franco, Francisco 44–45, 48, 52–55, 58, 63n73, 64n90
Franco-Prussian War, 5

Galambos, Louis, 11
Gallardo, Eduardo, 52, 54
Gallardo, Florencio Pérez, 52, 54–56
Gamaleya, Nikolai, 202
Gamaleya Research Institute, 13, 201
Gard, Sven, 74–75, 79
GAVI (Global Alliance on Vaccines and Immunization), 16, 28, 39, 130, 132, 212
gender, 49
genetic engineering, 26, 29
Gispen, Rijk, 22
GlaxoSmithKline (GSK), 28–29, 37–38, 43n45, 82, 120–21, 210; SmithKline Beecham, 10
global health, 2, 9–16, 26, 28, 39, 90
Global Polio Eradication Initiative (GPEI), 39, 184. *See also* World Health Organization
global public goods, 39, 213
globalisation, 12, 13–16, 80, 132
good manufacturing practices (GMP). *See* World Health Organization
Gutschy, Ljudevit, 92. *See also* Croatia

Haemophilus influenzae type b (cHib), 25, 27–28, 29, 35, 38, 42n27, 121, 125
Haffkine, Waldemar, 4, 111
Haffkine Bio-Pharmaceutical Corporation Ltd., 120–21, 133
Haffkine Institute, 111, 114
Harvard University, 6
Hayflick, Leonard, 97
Henderson, Donald, 8
hepatitis A, 202
hepatitis B, 10, 26–27, 38, 120–21, 125, 131, 202
HIV, 151. *See also* AIDS
Hong Kong, 5
Hong Kong flu. *See* influenza
human diploid cell strains (HDCS), 97–98
Hungary, 179, 206

Ibáñez, Julián Sanz, 52
Ikić, Drago, 95, 97–99
inactivated polio vaccine (IPV), 6, 20, 23–24, 31, 55, 65, 75–76, 95, 98, 142, 148, 162, 183–84
India, 4, 17, 38, 98, 99, 110–37, 140, 197, 204, 211, 214; BCG Vaccine Laboratories (BCGVL), 110, 113, 115–16, 118–20, 122, 124, 126, 130, 133, 134n10; Central Research Institute (CRI), 110–12, 115–16, 118, 120, 123–24, 126–27, 133; criminal investigation, 123; independence, 17, 115–16, 132; Integrated Vaccine Complex (IVC), 117, 119, 123, 130–31, 133; Universal Immunisation Programme (UPI), 119, 129
Indo-China War, 8
Indonesia, 15, 39, 208
influenza: avian (bird) (A/H5N1), 59, 82, 159, 166, 215; Hong Kong flu (H3N2), 56; Spanish flu (H1N1), 52, 69, 200; swine flu (H1N1), 83, 155 166, 194, 215; vaccination campaign, 163, 165–66; vaccines, 51, 54, 56, 59, 74–75, 82, 97–98, 111, 116, 125, 162–65, 167–69, 183, 189–90, 192, 194, 202innovation, 6, 22–23, 25–26, 32, 34, 40, 52, 111, 116, 118, 139, 147, 179, 181, 187, 195, 206, 209, 214
Institute for Translational Vaccinology (Intravacc). *See* the Netherlands
Institut Mérieux 9, 11–12, 23–24
intellectual property, 13, 36, 110, 132, 147, 211. *See also* patents
International Bank for Reconstruction and Development (IBRD), 166
international cooperation, 14, 54, 80, 84, 95–99, 141–42, 165, 188–90, 192, 194, 204, 212
International Federation of Pharmaceutical Manufacturers' Associations (IFPMA), 16
International Monetary Fund (IMF), 100, 132

International Vaccine Institute (IVI), 11
InterVax, 101
Iran, 17, 138–54, 204, 214; Article 44 of the Constitution, 145–46; Center for Disease Control, 143 National Development and Vaccination Plan (NDVP), 150–51; Razi Vaccine and Serum Research Institute, 139, 141–42; Vaccination Act, 140

Japan, 31
Jenner, Edward, 2, 138, 177–78
Johnson & Johnson, 81, 202, 210

Karolinska Institute (KI), 56, 65–70, 75, 81, 84
Klebs, Albert, 3
Kling, Carl, 68–70, 72–75
Klink, Ab, 20
knowledge exploitation, 33, 39
knowledge transfer, 9–10, 25, 33, 90, 97–98, 178, 181, 183, 187, 189
Koch, Robert, 3–4, 159, 178; Institute for Infectious Diseases, 3, 52, 92, 159, 178
Koprowski, Hillary, 98
Kreeftenberg, Hans, 28

Latin America. *See* South America
League of Nations, 93, 141, 156, 160, 171
liability, 7, 209
licence, 7, 11, 23, 25–27, 37–38, 90, 98, 101, 118, 121, 139, 144, 167, 169, 200, 204–5, 210–11; *See also* patents
Illera, Luis Rodríguez, 52
Lymph: animal, 21, 42n38, 45, 70, 76, 92, 111–113, 115, 161, 177, 178, 179, 180, 181; human, 22, 178

malaria, 4, 10, 111, 138, 160; *See also* eradication campaigns
mandatory vaccination, 2, 45, 53, 57, 70–73, 77, 94
marketing, 7, 12, 38, 41n12, 80–81, 101, 161, 165–67, 194, 208
marketization, 81, 213
Marshall Aid Plan, 7, 22, 94
Mashrouteh Revolution, 139, 144
measles, 1, 80, 138; Edmonston-Zagreb measles vaccine strain, 98–99; measles, mumps, rubella (MMR) vaccine, 25, 31, 56–57, 59, 79, 97–98; vaccine, 6, 25–26, 57, 77, 94, 98, 115–16, 123, 125, 142–43, 163; *See also* eradication campaign
Medical Research Council Laboratories (London), 97
Medicines and Healthcare products Regulatory Agency (MHRA), 205
MedImmune, 11
meningitis, 28–29
Merck, 11, 25–26, 95
Mérieux, Charles, 24. *See also* Institut Mérieux
messenger RNA (mRNA), 148, 200, 203, 210–11
Millennium Development Goals, 143
Mirza, Abbas, 138
mistrust 45, 151, 208
Mexico, 98, 204, 215
Moderna, 202–4, 207, 210–12
Moorhead, Paul, 97
monkeys, 23, 27, 68, 75–76, 97
monopoly 28, 32, 71, 80, 132, 146, 156, 160–61, 164–65, 167, 170, 201, 212, 214
Muraskin, William, 2

narcolepsy, 83
neoliberalism 13–14, 59, 80, 110, 132, 171–72, 176, 193, 195, 199
Netherlands, The, 9, 12, 17, 20–43, 73, 76, 91, 144, 192, 214; Central Laboratory of the Blood Transfusion Service (CLB), 27, 41n19; Dutch National Immunization Programme (NIP), 20, 22–23, 25–34, 38, 40, 41n10, 43n45; Dutch Nordic Consortium 30, 33–34, 39, 215; Institute for Translational Vaccinology (Intravacc), 29, 35–37, 40, 42n33, 43n42, 214; National Institute of Public Health and the Environment (RIVM), 20, 22–35, 37–39, 41n7, 41n12, 41n19, 42n23, 42n33, 42n37, 42n38, 43n45; Netherlands Vaccine Institute (NVI), 34–35, 37–39, 42n38, 42n41
Nobel Prize, 50–51, 67
Non-Aligned Movement, 96, 182
Novovax, 202

Olin, Gunnar, 74–75
Olin, Patrick, 80
Operation Warp Speed, 202–3, 207
Oral Polio Vaccine (OPV), 6, 24, 39, 55, 76, 95, 98, 112–13, 115–16, 120–23, 125, 162–63, 183–84, 187, 191
Ottoman Empire, 3, 139, 180

Pan American Health Organization (PAHO), 1, 184
Pandemrix, 83
parasitic diseases, 10
Pasteur, Louis, 3, 5, 12, 48, 157, 173n4, 178
Pasteur Institute, 3–5, 22, 47–48, 50–52, 67, 75, 92, 110, 112–14, 116, 120, 125, 139, 140–42, 147–48, 150, 156–57, 159–60, 162, 167–68, 171, 173n26, 177–82, 202, 215
Pasteur Mérieux, 9, 11
Pasteur Mérieux Connaught, 12, 28. *See also* Sanofi Pasteur
patents, 6, 10, 11, 13–14, 23, 25, 30, 32, 38, 90, 97, 146–47, 162, 183, 187, 199, 201, 203, 210–11, 213
Patria (vaccine), 204
penicillin, 5–6, 94
Pentaxim, 194
pertussis (whooping cough), 8, 20, 22, 27–28, 31, 35, 37, 41n8, 43n45, 55, 57, 74–75, 80, 94–96, 115, 121, 130, 142, 162–63, 183, 187, 192; acellular vaccine, 27, 31, 35, 41n8, 43n45, 80, 130, 192; whole cell vaccine, 28, 31, 35, 41n8, 130, 192
Perum Bio Farma Ltd., 39
Pfizer, 203–5, 207, 210, 212
pharmaceutical R&D, 7, 15, 26, 33–36, 39, 42n33, 43n52, 66, 90, 92, 94, 99, 111–12, 115, 122, 147, 148, 151, 156, 165–66, 168–69, 172, 202–3, 207
Philips-Roxane Laboratory, 98
plague, 5, 44, 47, 111, 138, 140–41; vaccine, 48, 111–12, 114
pneumococcal vaccine, 7, 28, 30, 48–49, 125, 129, 162
Poland, 94, 98
Polidin, 162, 167
polio (poliomyelitis), 1, 6–9, 12, 20, 23–24, 31, 38–39, 55, 59, 65–66, 74–77, 91, 904, 97–98, 111, 141–43, 147, 162–63, 183–87, 190–92, 200; *See also* eradication campaigns; inactivated polio vaccine; Oral Polio Vaccine
Poolman, Jan, 27–29, 37, 43n45
post-marketing monitoring, 194
post-socialist transformation, 89, 91, 172, 176–77, 188–93
Praxis Biologicals, 27
privatisation, 10, 12–15, 17, 20–21, 23, 35–37, 39–40, 42n37, 43n42, 81–82, 91, 99–104, 132–33, 143, 145–48, 151, 171, 188, 193, 200, 213–14
public health, 1–16, 20–21, 33, 36, 39, 44, 46–47, 53–59, 85, 89, 91–96, 99, 101, 104–6, 118, 130, 132–33, 138–40, 143, 151, 157, 159, 169, 171, 176–77, 182, 184–85, 193, 195, 199–200; needs, 10, 184, 195
public-private partnership, 10, 130–31, 133, 145, 169, 200, 215

quality control, 8, 13, 15, 21, 25, 27–28, 34–35, 41n7, 51, 55, 71, 116–17, 119, 165, 172, 178–79, 190, 192, 213
quarantine, 1, 3, 56, 66, 139, 200

rabbit: brain, 73; serum, 52; vaccine (naurovaccine), 73
rabies vaccine, 3, 9, 23, 48–51, 55–56, 92, 112–14, 116, 125, 141, 155, 178–81
Rajchman, Ludwik, 93
Reinders, Geert, 21, 40
Remdesivir, 205
rinderpest, 21, 142
risk assessment, 84, 206
Rockefeller Foundation, 16, 44, 52–53, 93
Rockefeller Institute for Medical Research, 52, 75
Romania, 17, 155–75; Cantacuzino-Sion law, 161; Laboratory of Experimental Medicine, 156–59, 161, 170; National Institute of Sera and Vaccines 'Dr. Cantacuzino.' *See* Cantacuzino Institute
Roosevelt, Franklin D., 6
Roux, Emilie, 3–4, 46–48, 67, 140
rubella (German measles), 6, 25–26, 31, 41n9, 56–57, 59, 79–80, 94, 97–98, 107n26, 125, 142–43
Ruitenberg, Joost, 26, 41n19
Russia, 3–4, 13, 51, 121, 194, 201–3, 206–9, 213

Sabin, Albert, 6, 55, 116, 162, 183–84. *See also* Oral Polio Vaccine
Salk, Jonas, 6, 24, 75. *See also* inactivated polio vaccine
sanctions, 143, 145, 149–51, 188–90, 204
sanitary measures, 3, 93
Sanofi Pasteur, 12, 28, 76, 123, 124. *See also* Pasteur Mérieux Connaught
SARS, 14, 59, 200
SARS-CoV-2. *See* Covid-19

Selander, Edvard, 67, 69
self-managerial socialism, 89–99, 182, 185, 187–88
self-sufficiency, 9, 15, 32, 72, 115–16, 130, 155, 170, 182, 190, 193–95, 204, 214
Serbia, 17, 98, 159, 176–98, 209, 215; Agency for Drugs and Medical Devices, 193; Associated Labour Act, 185; Central Hygiene Institute (Belgrade), 93, 181–83; Torlak Institute, 98, 177, 182–94, 215.*See also* self-managerial socialism; Yugoslavia
Serum Institute of India, 20, 28, 35, 37, 40, 99, 120–21, 133, 204, 212
September 11, 2001, 34, 39
Shibasaburō, Kitasato, 3
Shin, Seung-il, 11, 12
Silobrčić, Vlatko, 90, 100
Sinopharm, 194, 202, 208, 215
Sinovac Biotech, Ltd., 202, 208
Slaoui, Moncef, 207
Smallpox: epidemic, 2, 21, 34, 45–46, 111, 115, 138; eradication campaign;
vaccination campaign, 4, 16, 44, 48–49, 53, 70, 72–74, 76–77, 91, 138–39, 177. *See also* Jenner, Edward; vaccine, 2, 8, 21–22, 45, 48–49, 51–52, 55–56, 58, 65–66, 70–71, 75, 92, 94–95, 111–12, 115, 140–41, 158, 161
SmithKline. *See* GlaxoSmithKlineSoberana (vaccine), 148, 204. *See also* Cuba
social determinants of health, 149
South America, 96, 183–84
Soviet Union, 7–9, 94, 162, 182, 202
sovereignty, 91, 105, 118, 150, 182, 215
Spain, 2, 17, 44–64, 73, 82; Alfonso XIII Institute, 44–45, 47–48, 50–53, 58; civil war, 44–45, 47, 52–54, 58–59; conflicts of interests, 57–58; Institute of Military Hygiene (IHM), 44–45, 47, 49; National Institute of Bacteriology and Hygiene, 46; National School of Health (ENS) 50, 52–55; National Vaccination Institute (INV), 44–46
Spanish flu. *See* Influenza
Sputnik V vaccine, 194, 206–9, 215
staphylococcal infections, 75
Štampar, Andrija, 93
sulphonamide, 6
Sweden, 17, 31, 65–88, 91, 215; Drug Side Effect Board, 79; Infectious Disease Control Institute (*Smittskyddsinstitutet*, SMI), 81; Medical Products Agency, 79, 83; National Board of Health and Welfare (NBHW), 65, 79, 81–83; SBL Vaccin AB, 66, 81; Statens bakteriologiska laboratorium (SBL), 65–66, 68–85; Swedish Serum Institute, 69; Valneva, 81, 84
swine flu. *See* influenza

technology transfer, 4, 12, 16, 25, 28, 30, 33, 37, 39, 97–98, 123, 181, 183, 208
tetanus, 8, 49, 57, 68–69, 143, 162; anti-tetanus serum, 49, 69, 94, 113, 125, 157; tetanus vaccine, 20, 22, 29, 31, 50, 53, 55, 74–75, 94–95, 111, 115–6, 121, 142, 162–63, 167, 182–83, 187, 204
Trade-Related Aspects of Intellectual Property Rights (TRIPS), 13, 147
Trump, Donald, 205, 212
trust, 45, 68, 98, 151, 194, 204, 208
tuberculosis, 3–4, 7–9, 21, 23, 48, 51–53, 68, 70–71, 80, 111, 138, 141, 160, 163. *See also* Bacillus Calmette–Guérin (*BCG*) vaccine; eradication campaign
typhoid, 5, 21, 48–51, 53, 75, 92, 94–96, 111–15, 125, 140–41, 158, 160, 162–63, 181–82
typhus, 5, 48, 51, 75, 138, 140–41, 202

Ukraine, 94
United Kingdom (UK), 3–5; 13, 29, 80, 111, 132, 138, 144, 151, 201–9, 211
United Nations (UN), 188, 213; UNICEF-WHO Joint Committee on Health Policy, 9; United Nations Children's Fund (UNICEF), 1, 9, 16, 28, 39, 96, 121, 130, 181, 189; United Nations Development Programme (UNDP), 9; United Nations Relief and Rehabilitation Administration (UNRRA), 94
United States, 6–8, 11, 13, 25, 27, 30, 34, 47, 57, 67, 71, 75–76, 78–80, 94, 97–99, 121, 144, 149, 201–7, 209–12; Bayh-Dole Act, 11; Centers for Disease Control and Prevention (CDC), 121, 159, 202; Food and Drug Administration (FDA), 78, 79, 121, 205; National Foundation for Infantile Paralysis (NFIP), 6; Office of Technology Assessment (OTA), 7
Universal Immunisation Programme. *See* India
USSR. *See* Soviet Union

Vaccine: adjuvants, 163, 169; attenuated, 3, 6, 10, 24–25, 55, 76, 94, 98, 107n26, 163, 181; combined, 22, 26, 55, 57, 95, 98, 115, 181–83; conjugation technologies, 26, 29–30, 38; diplomacy, 201, 203, 207–8, 213–14; hesitancy, 143, 194, 207; inactivated, 6, 10, 20, 23–24, 26–27, 39, 55–56, 73, 75–76, 79, 116, 142, 148, 163, 181, 183, 200, 204, 208; markets, 1, 10–12, 15–16, 23, 27, 30, 32–34, 45, 78, 89, 91, 95–96, 100–1, 105, 119, 132, 144, 148, 155–56, 159–61, 164, 168–69, 171–72, 176, 188–91, 199, 206, 209–11, 213–15; nationalism, 201, 203–214; price, 8, 11, 28, 56, 69, 80, 82, 96, 119–120, 122, 124, 127, 131, 133, 193, 208–10, 215; recombinant, 10, 11, 26, 27, 30, 38, 84, 100; shortage, 110, 118–19, 131, 133, 150, 194–95, 201
van Hemert, Paul, 23, 40, 41n12
van Wezel, Anton, 23, 40
van Wezel process, 25, 39
veterinary medicine, 46, 48, 50, 57–58, 65, 67–69, 72, 74, 77–78, 142, 156, 161
virology, 6, 8, 11, 22, 44, 47, 52–56, 74, 77, 99, 183

Wistar Institute, 76, 97–98
whooping cough. *See* pertussis
World Bank, 14, 16, 100, 132, 155, 164, 166–67, 170, 172
World Health Organization (WHO), 7, 10, 14–16, 90, 163, 166–67, 172, 189–92, 200, 207, 212; Expanded programme of immunization (EPI), 8, 24, 39, 57, 91, 98, 115, 139, 155; good manufacturing practices (GMP), 13, 35, 37, 40, 91, 99, 116–19, 121–24, 131, 133, 147, 165–67, 169, 172, 190, 191; prequalification programme, 39, 142n27, 121, 190–91; Primary Health Care (PHC), 139, 142–43; UNICEF-WHO Joint Committee on Health Policy, 9; World Health Assembly (WHA), 7, 14. *See also* eradication campaign
World Intellectual Property Organisation (WIPO), 147
World Trade Organization (WTO), 13, 146–47, 151, 211
World War I, 4–5, 51–52, 58, 92–93, 140, 160, 181
World War II, 5, 7, 22, 94, 111, 141, 144, 176–77, 182–83
Wyeth Lederle, 30

yellow fever, 13, 113, 116
Yersine, Alexandre, 5
Yugoslavia, 9, 17, 89–100, 181–90. *See also* Croatia; Serbia

Zhdanov, Victor, 8